Research in Criminology

Series Editors
Alfred Blumstein
David P. Farrington

Research in Criminology

Delbert S. Elliott
David Huizinga
Scott Menard

Multiple Problem Youth

Delinquency, Substance
Use, and Mental Health
Problems

Springer-Verlag
New York Berlin Heidelberg
London Paris Tokyo

Delbert S. Elliott
David Huizinga
Scott Menard
Institute of Behavioral Science
University of Colorado at Boulder
Boulder, CO 80309, USA

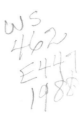

Library of Congress Cataloging-in-Publication Data

Elliott, Delbert S.
  Multiple problem youth: delinquency, substance use, and mental
  health problems/Delbert S. Elliott, David Huizinga, Scott Menard.
  p. cm.—(Research in criminology)
  Bibliography: p.
  ISBN 0-387-96925-X (alk. paper)
  1. Juvenile delinquency—United States. 2. Youth—United States—Drug
  use. 3. Youth—United States—Mental health. I. Huizinga, David. II. Menard,
  Scott. III. Title. IV. Series.
  HV9104.E447   1988
  362.7′4′0973—dc19   88-38132

Printed on acid-free paper

© 1989 by Springer-Verlag New York Inc.

Typeset by TCSystems, Inc.
Printed and bound by Edwards Brothers Inc., Ann Arbor, Michigan.
Printed in the United States of America.

9 8 7 6 5 4 3 2 1

ISBN 0-387-96925-X Springer-Verlag New York Berlin Heidelberg
ISBN 3-540-96925-X Springer-Verlag Berlin Heidelberg New York

Contents

Preface

In April 1984 the Alcohol, Drug Abuse, Mental Health Administration (ADAMHA) and the Office of Juvenile Justice and Delinquency Prevention (OJJDP) held a State-of-the-Art Research Conference on juvenile offenders with serious drug, alcohol, and mental health problems. This conference reflected the growing concern over multiple-problem youth, the possibility of a common set of underlying causes linked to these different forms of problem behavior, and questions about how to identify multiple-problem youth and develop treatment strategies that address this more complex pattern of problem behavior and its precipitating causes. This book attemps to address the major epidemiological and etiological issues raised at this conference and is an extended version of a paper presented there by the first two authors (Elliott & Huizinga, 1984).

It seems particularly appropriate that the data and analyses presented here rely heavily on the National Youth Survey, a ten-year longitudinal study involving a national sample of adolescents, which has been jointly funded by the National Institute of Mental Health, the National Institute of Drug Abuse, the Office of Juvenile Justice and Delinquency Prevention, and The National Institute of Justice. This funding pattern reflects the common interest in the relationship between these forms of problem behavior and the complex set of issues that confront us in our efforts to deal with multiple-problem youth.

We would like to acknowledge the contributions of the many persons associated with the National Youth Survey (NYS) and those who contributed directly and indirectly to the preparation of this volume. Linda Kuhn and Judy Armstrong-Laurie (NYS Field Supervisors) are largely responsible for our success in obtaining high quality interviews and maintaining a high participation rate over the ten years of the NYS. Bertha Thomas (the NYS Librarian), more than any other person, is responsible for the quality and documentation of the NYS data set. Her standards for accuracy and completeness are unexcelled in survey research. Although too numerous to mention by name, we also wish to thank our field staff, trackers and interviewers, and the research assistants who were responsible for the collection, editing, and coding of our interviews.

Other members of the NYS research team contributed to the analyses and interpretations offered here. In particular, we acknowledge the contributions of Frank Dunford, Barbara Morse, and Finn Esbensen. Phyllis O'Meara and Dorothy Watson assisted in the preparation of the manuscript and stuck with us through the many revisions of text and tables. We are also grateful for the encouragement and assistance of Dr. Jim Breiling, our Project Monitor at the Antisocial and Violent Behavior Branch of the National Institute of Mental Health.

Finally, we wish to thank the members of the NYS youth panel, who have been willing to share their experiences, perceptions, and beliefs, their failures and successes, and their hopes for the future. In the final analysis, it was their willingness to stick with us over ten years of their lives and endure multiple, repeated interviews that made this volume possible.

Del Elliott, David Huizinga, Scott Menard

1

Introduction

Study Objectives

Historically, the study of adolescent problems and disorders has involved independent inquiry into specific problems such as delinquent and antisocial behavior, substance (tobacco, alcohol, and illicit drug) use and abuse, suicide, teenage pregnancy, runaway, and mental illness. This division emerged out of the traditional interests and specializations of the various academic disciplines and has been perpetuated by the present organization of federal and state agencies supporting research and program development in these areas and by the current organization of federal, state and community treatment and support services for adolescents with these problems. Yet there is reason to question the usefulness of this division in the light of recent research (Bachman, 1987; Donovan & Jessor, 1985; Elliott, Huizinga, & Ageton, 1985; Huba & Bentler, 1984; Jessor & Jessor, 1977, Osgood et al, 1988) in which it is suggested that these adolescent problems may have a common etiology and frequently involve concomitant forms of behavior. Should this be the case, there would be a compelling reason to question the appropriateness of the present organization of social control and treatment agencies that tend to focus rather narrowly on a particular problem form with little coordination between agencies and little attention to the more general nexus of problems that characterize clients.

Although there is a fairly extensive body of knowledge about each of these problem behaviors, relatively little is known about their joint distributions in the adolescent population, their temporal ordering or developmental progression into multiproblem patterns, and whether these problems are causally related to one another, have independent causal antecedents, or are different manifestations of a common causal syndrome.[1] Baseline epidemiological and etiological data are critical to

[1] Several recent studies involving national samples have focused on one or more of these issues (see Bachman, 1987; Donovan & Jessor, 1985; Osgood et al.,

the development of new prevention and intervention strategies and to a more effective integration and coordination of existing services and strategies to deal with youth who exhibit multiple forms of problem behavior

Our objective in this book is to present national baseline epidemiological and etiological data on the joint occurrence of delinquent behavior and alcohol, drug, and mental health (ADM) problems. Specifically, we propose to address each of the following questions.

1. What patterns of joint delinquent-ADM problems are found within the adolescent population?
2. What proportion of youth exhibit each multiple problem pattern, and how are youth exhibiting these patterns distributed in the general population by age, sex, race, class, and place of residence?
3. How do these patterns differ with regard to the frequency of each type of behavior?
4. Is there a particular temporal order or developmental sequence in the onset of these behaviors or disorders that is more likely than others?
5. Can we identify a common set of causes for these problems?
6. What is the predictive effect of joint involvement in these behaviors on subsequent long-range "career" or chronic involvement in crime or ADM disorders? (For example, does the presence of heavy drug use with crime during adolescence increase the risk of a long-range criminal career and, if so, is the effect additive or interactive?)

In addressing the epidemiological issues above we have relied upon data from the National Youth Survey (NYS), an ongoing longitudinal study involving a national probability sample of U.S. adolescents. In the discussion of the etiological issues and risk factor models we will review both the results of predictive analyses involving NYS data and the findings from other predictive studies based upon large representative samples. Our general approach can be described as involving general population surveys employing self-reported measures of delinquency and ADM problems. After describing the NYS and the unique suitability of this study for assessing the relationship between delinquent behavior and ADM problems behaviors over the adolescent and early adult years, we will review a number of issues involved in the measurement of delinquency and ADM problems and then present the specific measures employed in the NYS.

1988). These studies and several others involving local samples (Huba & Bentler, 1984; Nurco, Shaffer, Ball and Kinlock, 1984; Zabin et al., 1986) will be reviewed in later chapters, where their findings are relevant to particular issues being addressed.

The National Youth Survey

The National Youth Survey, funded primarily by the U.S. Department of Health and Human Services through the National Institute of Mental Health (NIMH) with supplemental funding from the U.S. Department of Justice through the Office of Juvenile Justice and Delinquency Prevention (OJJDP) and the National Institute of Justice (NIJ), is a projected longitudinal study of delinquent behavior, alcohol and drug use, and problem-related substance use in the American youth population.[2] To date, seven waves of data have been collected on this national youth panel covering the period from 1976 to 1986. The data reported here are limited to the first six waves of data and cover the 7-year period from 1976 to 1983.

The NYS employed a probability sample of households in the continental United States based upon a self-weighting, multistage, cluster sampling design. The sample was drawn in late 1976 and contained 2,360 eligible youth aged 11–17 at the time of the initial interview. Of these, 1,725 (73%) agreed to participate in the study, signed informed consents, and completed interviews in the initial (1977) survey. An age, sex, and race comparison between nonparticipating eligible youth and participating youth indicates that the loss rate from any particular age, sex, or racial group appears to be proportional to that group's representation in the population. Further, with respect to these characteristics, participating youth appear to be representative of the total 11- through 17-year-old youth population in the United States as established by the U.S. Census Bureau (Elliott, Ageton, Huizinga, Knowles, & Canter, 1983).

Respondent loss over the six surveys was relatively small (13%). Comparisons of participants across the six waves indicated that loss by age, sex, ethnicity, class, place of residence, and reported delinquency did not substantially influence the underlying distributions on these variables. It was thus concluded that the representativeness of the sample with respect to these variables was not affected in any serious way by the losses over the six surveys. For a more detailed analysis of attrition see Elliott et al. (1983).

Annual involvement in delinquent behavior and specific ADM problem

[2] The work reported here was supported by a series of grants (MH27552) from the Center for Studies of Crime and Delinquency, NIMH, for the period June 1975 through May 1986. Supplemental funding (78-JN-AX-0003) for the second and third years of the study was received from OJJDP and supplemental funding (83-IJ-CX-0063) for the collection of arrest data was received from the NIJ. The points of view or opinions expressed here are those of the authors and do not necessarily represent the official position or policies of the Department of Health and Human Services or the Department of Justice.

behaviors was self-reported by members of the youth panel in confidential, personal (face-to-face) interviews. In most instances these interviews occurred in the respondent's home. If the situation at home was such that privacy could not be guaranteed, arrangements were made to conduct the interview in some other setting where privacy was assured. Respondents were guaranteed that any information they provided in the interview was confidential and could not be released to any person or agency without their written consent. All data collected were protected by a Privacy Certification from the U.S. Department of Justice or a Certificate of Confidentiality from the U.S. Department of Health and Human Services.

The NYS is well suited to address both the epidemiological and etiological questions posed. The study was specifically designed to obtain baseline epidemiological data and to test an integrated theoretical model explaining delinquency and drug use (Elliott, Huizinga, & Ageton, 1985); it involves a representative national sample with adequate representation of all adolescent age groups; comprehensive measures of delinquent behavior as well as substance use and problem use are available, providing both prevalence and frequency estimates of each behavior and their joint occurrence annually over a 5-year period (1976–1980) and comparable data for 1983; and the longitudinal design affords the opportunity to examine the temporal ordering of the onset of specific behaviors or problems over the adolescent years. Although adolescent mental disorders were not a primary focus in the early years of this study, measures of several mental health problems were obtained as predictors of delinquency and problem use of alcohol and drugs and are available for the first 5 years of the study. More attention was given to mental disorders on the sixth wave of the study, which incorporated parts of the NIMH Diagnostic Interview Schedule (Hesselbrock, Stabenau, Hesslebrock, Mirkin & Mey 1982; Robins, 1981; Robins, Helzer, Croughan, Williams, & Spitzer, 1981a,b) and a major set of questions on the use of mental health services.

The Measurement of Delinquent Behavior and ADM Problem Behaviors.

Although self-reported survey measures of delinquency, substance use, and mental illness have come to dominate epidemiological research in these areas, some important limitations of self-reported measures need to be addressed. Self-reported survey measures were initially developed as an alternative to measures obtained from clinical records or from police or court records. Both conceptual and methodological problems were associated with the use of clinical and law enforcement records to identify persons involved or not involved in these problems or to estimate the frequency and distribution of these forms of deviant behavior in any specific population. Conceptually, theories of deviance made an important distinction between deviant behavior and official responses to deviant behavior, and between persons involved in deviant acts and persons apprehended for these behaviors or treated for these disorders (Becker, 1963; Cicourel, 1968; Gibbs, 1966, 1972; Kitsuse, 1962, 1972; Kitsuse & Cicourel, 1963; Lemert, 1951, 1972, 1974; Schur, 1969). With the emergence of these theoretical distinctions in the 1960s, law enforcement and clinical records came to be viewed as direct measures of official response or treatment, but as indirect and in some instances inadequate measures of delinquent behavior or ADM problems.

The assertion that clinical and justice system records were still useful as indirect measures of these behaviors raised serious methodological questions about the representativeness of these records. Are offenders processed in the juvenile justice system a representative subset of all offenders? Are their recorded offenses a representative subset of their actual offenses? Are youth in drug treatment programs or under psychiatric care for mental disorders representative of all drug abusers and all mentally ill adolescents? Although there is still some debate over the representativeness of official delinquency records (Elliott & Ageton, 1980; Hindelang, Hirschi, & Weis, 1979, 1981), most researchers consider it too questionable to rely upon clinical and law enforcement data for measures of delinquent behavior and ADM problems, particularly for studies of the distribution of these behaviors and disorders in the general population. For research on the causes of delinquency or ADM problems the difficulty is not so much that persons with a clinical or law enforcement record are incorrectly assigned to the problem (experimental) group, but that those without such a record are incorrectly assigned to the non–problem (control) group.

Out of a concern over "hidden" delinquency and "hidden" ADM problems (i.e., delinquency and ADM problems that were not captured by or represented in official records) researchers developed self-reported measures of these behaviors and disorders. Self-reported measures were designed to be more direct measures of problem behaviors or disorders that could be used with large representative samples to assess the prevalence and frequency of these problems in the general population and to provide an accurate classification of persons having or not having these problems. The findings from early self-report studies in each of these problem areas appeared to confirm the unrepresentativeness of clinical and law enforcement records and the inaccuracy of classifications based upon these data (Erickson & Empey, 1963; Gold, 1966, 1970; Gold & Reimer, 1975; Porterfield, 1946; Robins, 1975; Short & Nye, 1957; Srole, Langner, Michael, Opler & Rennie, 1962; Williams & Gold, 1972). Self-reported measures clearly provided a new and different picture of the magnitude and distribution of these problems in the general population. The popularity of self-reported survey measures of delinquency and ADM problems has grown tremendously over the past two decades, and for many today it is the preferred measure, particularly for epidemiological studies.

Self-reported measures of adolescent problems do appear to be more direct measures that avoid the selective biases and other apparent shortcomings of clinical and law enforcement record measures. However, as employed in current research, these measures also have a number of limitations. Several critics of the self-report method have questioned the reliability and validity of these measures (Bentler & Eichberg, 1975; Nettler, 1974; Reiss, 1975; West, 1973). However, the weight of the available evidence indicates that these measures have good to excellent levels of reliability and acceptable levels of validity as compared with other social science measures. This conclusion holds for self-reported measures of delinquency, alcohol and illicit drug use, and mental disorders (Akers, Massey, Clarke, & Laver, 1983; Ansel, Mandel, Mathias, Mason, & Hocherman, 1976; Bachman, O'Malley, & Johnston, 1978; Bale, 1979; Ball, 1967; Blackmore, 1974; Bonito, Nurco, & Shaffer, 1976; Chaiken & Chaiken, 1982; Clark & Tifft, 1966; Cox & Longwell, 1974; Dentler & Monroe, 1961; Eckerman, Bates, Rachal, & Poole, 1971; Elliott & Voss, 1974; Erickson & Empey, 1963; Farrington, 1973; Gandossy, Williams, Cohen, & Harwood, 1980; Gibson, Morrison, & West, 1970; Gold, 1970, 1977; Groves, 1974; Hackler & Lautt, 1969; Hardt & Peterson-Hardt, 1977; Hesselbrock, Stabinau, Hesselbrock, Mirkin, & Mey, 1982; Hindelang, Hirschi, & Weis, 1981; Hirschi, 1969; Jessor, Graves, Hanson, & Jessor, 1968; Jessor & Jessor, 1977; Johnston, Bachman, & O'Malley, 1979; Kulik, Stein, & Sarbin, 1968; Marquis & Abner, 1981; Megargee, 1972; Parry, Balter, & Cisin, 1971; Petersilia, 1978; Petzel, Johnson, & McKillip, 1973; Short & Nye, 1958; Single, Kandel, & Johnson, 1975).

The fairly extensive body of research on self-report measures indicates that deliberate falsification is a relatively rare event. There are, however, some problems related to the accuracy of recall, chiefly having to do with forgetting particular events or forgetting the temporal location of events recalled. Nevertheless, the use of shorter reporting periods, aided recall, and various bounding techniques substantially reduces this source of error (Garofalo & Hindelang, 1977; Loftus & Marburger, 1983; Sudman & Bradburn, 1983).

In self-reported delinquency (SRD) research there is also evidence that respondents sometimes report relatively trivial events that would not be considered delinquent acts if observed by law enforcement agents (Elliott & Huizinga, 1983, 1988; Gold & Reimer, 1975; Huizinga & Elliott, 1986). This latter problem is limited primarily to minor offenses; there is little evidence that trivial events are reported in response to most questions about serious criminal acts (Elliott & Huizinga, 1983, 1988). However, given that most earlier SRD measures were heavily weighted with nonserious offenses and that the proportion of trivial responses to nonserious items is sometimes substantial, there is evidence that these measures significantly inflated earlier estimates of the prevalence and frequency of delinquent behavior. This source of error can also be reduced or corrected through the use of detailed follow-up questions about reported events (Elliott & Huizinga, 1983), although this technique has seldom been used. This same potential source of error may be present in self-reported measures of mental disorders such as the NIMH Diagnostic Interview Schedule (Robins et al., 1981a). Another potential source of inflation in earlier self-report studies is classification error, such as the use of overlapping categories that could result in counting the same event more than once (Elliott & Ageton, 1980; Elliott & Huizinga, 1988).

In sum, deliberate falsification, recall error, classification errors, and the reporting of trivial events are all potential sources of invalidity present in self-reported measures (Elliott & Huizinga, 1988). We believe that the evidence suggests that the reporting of trivial events may be the greatest of these potential sources of error in self-reported measures. In general, however, self-reported measures appear to be reasonably valid measures. Further, good survey procedures can substantially reduce many of the potential sources of inaccuracy.

More serious limitations are associated with self-reported instrument construction problems and with the use of particular sampling strategies. There are two major criticisms of the construction of most of the self-reported measures.[3] First, the items included in these measures are not representative of the behavioral domain being measured. This problem is particularly serious in the case of SRD measures, in which trivial and nonserious forms of delinquent behavior are greatly overrepresented but serious violations of the criminal code are either underrepresented or omitted altogether. The focus of most earlier SRD measures was thus upon relatively trivial, nonserious forms of delinquent behaviors. Second, many self-report measures use normative response categories (e.g., often, sometimes, occasionally) or truncated frequency categories (e.g., never, once or twice, three or more times). Neither response set is adequate for very precise frequency estimation. There is also evidence that numerical estimates based upon these response categories severely truncate the true distribution of responses (Elliott & Ageton, 1980). With the above set, for example, any number of behaviors in excess of two is collapsed into a

---

[3] There are other less serious construction problems that are not discussed here (e.g., item overlap, leading to double counting of offenses; ambiguous item wording, resulting in an inappropriate classification of offenses; and problems related to the generality or specificity of item wording) that have implications for the number of offenses reported. There are also a number of problems associated with the construction of scales using subsets of items. For a detailed discussion of these problems see Elliott and Ageton (1980), Elliott, et al., (1983), Elliott and Huizinga (1988), and Hindelang et al. (1981).

single "high" category. Although this procedure may allow for some discrimination between youth at the low end of the frequency distribution, it clearly precludes any discrimination at the high end. A youth involved in three shoplifting offenses during the reporting period receives the same "delinquency score" as a youth involved in 50 to 100 shoplifting events during the period. These response sets are particularly problematic when the reporting period is a year or longer and when high-frequency items such as petty theft, truancy, marijuana use, beer use, or carrying a concealed weapon are included in the measure.

Given the truncated frequency distributions and the restricted behavioral range of many earlier self-reported measures, the only distinctions possible were very fine gradations between relatively nondelinquent youth or youth with relatively low levels of drug use. Earlier self-reported measures simply have not captured differences that have any real program or theory relevance. This limitation calls into question many of the earlier self-reported findings regarding delinquent behavior. Several recent self-report studies have shown that—with proper representation of offenses, controls for offense seriousness, and response sets that afford better offending rate estimates—the differences between self-reported research findings and those based upon official record data are far less than suggested by the earlier SRD studies (Elliott & Ageton, 1980; Elliott & Huizinga, 1983; Hindelang, 1978; Hindelang, Hirschi, & Weis, 1979, 1981).

There has also been some confusion over the use of prevalence and frequency rates in the earlier comparisons of self-reported and official record measures (Biderman, 1972; Elliott, 1982; Elliott & Huizinga, 1988; Reiss, 1975; Tracy, 1978). The prevalence rate refers to the proportion of youth in the population who are active offenders during a given period; frequency rates refer to the average number of offenses per person in the population (or per active offender) during a given period. Given the above-noted problem with response sets, it is not surprising that the vast majority of SRD studies (and many early substance use studies) were limited to estimates of prevalence that were inappropriate for use in comparison with official arrest data (e.g., Uniform Crime Reports) since the latter provide frequency estimates (e.g., see Hindelang et al., 1981). Unfortunately, very few SRD studies have obtained reasonable estimates of the frequency of offending.

A second major limitation concerns the use of probability samples. Whereas the use of self-reported measures in probability samples of the general population provided a solution to the limited generalizability of clinical samples and official records measures, this method frequently fails to capture enough high-frequency, serious cases (e.g., chronic index offenders, heroin addicts, or schizophrenics) for any meaningful analysis of these groups. Yet these groups are often the most visible and problematic within the community. Simply stated, relatively rare events or patterns of events are problematic for general survey designs and, unless the samples are quite large, it is difficult to focus upon very serious problem groups.

There are several possible solutions to this sampling problem. Increasing the sample size is an obvious solution, but this approach is often difficult to justify on cost grounds. A more cost-efficient strategy would be to stratify the sample in such a way as to overrepresent specific high-risk groups while retaining the ability to generalize back to the general population. Robins (1975) has also suggested that we accumulate the relatively few serious cases obtained from separate general population samples for a study of more serious crime, drug, or mental health problems. There are special problems associated with each of these solutions, and in practice the limited number of serious cases obtained in general population surveys continues to be a significant limitation on self-reported studies using general population surveys. In part, this problem is a function of the use of cross-sectional data. Unless one uses lifetime recall measures, the prevalence of low-base-rate behavior will be low in any given year or on any given survey. With longitudinal prospective data, the numbers accumulate over time and are more substantial and recall periods can be relatively short. Also, measures of antecedent variables are available over reasonable recall periods with longitudinal prospective data.

NYS Measures of Delinquency and ADM Problems

DELINQUENT BEHAVIOR

Special attention was given to the above criticisms of self-reported measures in developing the delinquency and ADM problem measures for the NYS. Delinquent behavior was conceptualized as a parallel measure to official arrest (i.e., as behavior proscribed by criminal statutes and carrying some risk of official action if observed or reported to the police). The SRD measure included 40 offenses that were representative of the full range of offenses reported in the Uniform Crime Reports (UCR). Any specific act that involved more than 1% of the UCR-reported juvenile arrests during the study period was included in this measure. With the exception of homicide, all UCR Part I (Index) offenses were included. These crimes are those included in the FBI's measure of serious crime. All but one of the UCR Part II offenses were included, together with a number of status offenses. Nearly all items involved a violation of criminal statutes. The response set involved an open-ended frequency estimate for each offense. For those reporting frequencies of ten or more on a particular offense, a set of categorical responses which ranged from "monthly" to "two to three times a day" was also used. The two sets of responses are highly correlated. In this report the open-ended frequency responses are utilized for more precise epidemiological estimates, and the categorical scores are used in analyses involving theory testing (Elliott et al., 1985; Elliott, 1985). This decision was based upon the fact that the frequency responses are most readily interpreted, and are more comparable with official record measures. The categorical scores are better suited to the theory testing work because they have slightly better psychometric properties and because the interpretation requirements are less demanding.

The recall period is slightly over 12 months, inasmuch as each respondent was interviewed between January and March of each year and reported on his or her delinquency involvement over the preceding calendar year. Anchoring techniques were employed to facilitate accurate recall of events in the reporting period, and detailed follow-up questions were asked on the fourth and subsequent surveys to evaluate the reporting of trivial events.

ALCOHOL AND DRUG USE MEASURES

Although a number of drug-related offenses were included in the SRD measure (e.g., selling marijuana, being drunk, buying liquor for a minor), questions involving the personal use of alcohol and illicit drugs were included in a separate measure of drug use. This measure included seven drug substances: alcohol (beer, wine, and hard liquor; see Appendix A), marijuana, hallucinogens, amphetamines, heroin, cocaine, and barbiturates. Questions about the personal use of these seven substances were asked of all panel members on each of the annual surveys. Questions about the use of a more extensive set of drug substances were included in the second and third surveys for a subsample of youth in the national youth panel (see Elliott & Knowles, 1981; Elliott, Ageton, Huizinga, Knowles, & Canter, 1983; Huizinga & Elliott, 1981). This subsample was also asked a much more detailed set of questions about first use, quantity used, reasons for using, drug sources and reasons for terminating use of drugs. However, it was not possible to obtain national estimates of the incidence or prevalence of use for this extended set of drugs for any but the 12, 14 and 16 year old cohorts. The estimates of drug use reported in this volume are thus limited to the seven drug substances mentioned above.

The general format of drug use questions was similar to that employed with the SRD measure. The general question for the set of drug use items was "In the past year how often have you used . . . ?" The reference period for drug use, like delinquent offenses, was the last calendar year. The response set for the first and second surveys was a categorical set involving nine frequency categories ranging from "never" to "two to three times a day." Starting with the third survey and for all subsequent surveys, the dual open-ended and categorical response set utilized with the SRD measure (described previously) was employed for the drug use measure.

Delinquency and Drug Use Scales

Three sets of delinquency–drug use scales were constructed. These sets vary by the level of offense homogeneity and seriousness. The first set is called offense-specific scales and involves a very tight, homogeneous grouping of offense items, both with respect to the nature of the acts involved and their degree of seriousness. The items in these scales also have very similar prevalence and general offending (frequency) rates, so that no one offense can dominate the scale. The second set, offense-category scales, involves more general classes of behaviors and more internal variability with respect to seriousness and relative frequency of occurrence. The final set, the summary scales, is the most general and heterogeneous classification of offenses. The specific scales included in each of these sets are identified in Table 1.1, together with the specific offense items included in each scale.

Data presented in this report are limited to the offense-specific scales, two offense category scales (Illegal Services and Public Disorder) and two summary scales (General Delinquency C and Index offenses). We have deliberately excluded all status offenses and focused on more serious forms of delinquency, and, except for General Delinquency C and Index scales, there are no overlapping items among the remaining scales; that is, they are all independent. We prefer to rely primarily upon the offense-specific scales since they are the most homogeneous and least subject to the kinds of distortions that result from combining offenses of different seriousness and relative frequency of occurrence. The use of these scales should provide a more complete and accurate picture of delinquency involvement than would the use of the more general scales. No data on specific individual offenses are presented here, but they are available elsewhere (Elliott et al., 1983; Flanagan & McGarrell, 1986).

The Drug Use scale includes use of hallucinogens, amphetamines, barbiturates, heroin, and cocaine. Independent estimates are made for alcohol use and marijuana use; that is, use of these substances is treated separately and neither is included in the Drug Use scale.

Prevalence Rates, General Offending Rates and Individual Offending Rates

Prior self-report studies of delinquency and drug use have often confused prevalence rates and offending (frequency) rates. Prevalence refers to the number of persons in a population who report one or more offenses of a

TABLE 1.1. Delinquency scales—National Youth Survey.

Offense-specific scales	Offense-category scales	Summary scales
Felony Assault	*Illegal Services*	*School Delinquency*
(1) Aggravated assault	(1) Prostitution	(1) Damaged school property
(2) Sexual assault	(2) Sold marijuana	(2) Cheated on school tests
(3) Gang fights	(3) Sold hard drugs	(3) Hit teacher
		(4) Hit students
Minor Assault	a *Public Disorder*	(5) Strong-armed students
(1) Hit teacher	(1) Hitchhiked illegally	(6) Strong-armed teachers
(2) Hit parent	(2) Disorderly conduct	(7) Stole at school
(3) Hit students	(3) Public drunkenness	(8) Skipped classes
	(4) Panhandled	
Robbery	(5) Obscene calls	a *Home Delinquency*
(1) Strong-armed students		(1) Damaged family property
(2) Strong-armed teachers	a *Status offenses*	(2) Runaway
(3) Strong-armed others	(1) Runaway	(3) Stole from family
	(2) Skipped classes	(4) Hit parent
Felony Theft	(3) Lied about age	
(1) Stole motor vehicle	(4) Sexual intercourse	*Index offenses*
(2) Stole something > $50		(1) Aggravated assault
(3) Broke into bldg/vehicle	*Crimes Against Persons*	(2) Sexual assault
(4) Bought stolen goods	(1) Aggravated assault	(3) Gang fights
	(2) Gang fights	(4) Stole motor vehicle

Summary scales (continued)
a *General Delinquency A*
*(1) Damaged family property
*(2) Damaged school property
*(3) Damaged other property
(4) Stole motor vehicle
(5) Stole something > $50
(6) Bought stolen goods
*(7) Runaway
*(8) Lied about age
(9) Carried hidden weapon
(10) Stole something < $5
(11) Aggravated assault
(12) Prostitution
*(13) Sexual intercourse
(14) Gang fights
(15) Sold marijuana
*(16) Hitchhiked
(17) Hit teacher
(18) Hit parent
(19) Hit students
(20) Disorderly conduct

Minor Theft
(1) Stole something < $5
(2) Stole something $5–$50
(3) Joyriding

[a] Vandalism
(1) Damaged family property
(2) Damaged school property
(3) Damaged other property

Drug Use
(1) Hallucinogens
(2) Amphetamines
(3) Barbiturates
(4) Heroin
(5) Cocaine

(3) Hit teacher
(4) Hit parent
(5) Hit students
(6) Sexual assault
(7) Strong-armed students
(8) Strong-armed teachers
(9) Strong-armed others

General Theft
(1) Stole motor vehicle
(2) Stole something > $50
(3) Bought stolen goods
(4) Stole something < $5
(5) Stole something $5–$50
(6) Broke into bldg/vehicle
(7) Joyriding

(5) Stole something > $50
(6) Broke into bldg/vehicle
(7) Strong-armed students
(8) Strong-armed teachers
(8) Strong-armed others

(21) Sold hard drugs
(22) Joyriding
*(23) Bought liquor for minor
(24) Sexual assault
(25) Strong-armed students
(26) Strong-armed teachers
(27) Strong-armed others
*(28) Evaded payment
*(29) Public drunkenness○
(30) Stole something $5–$50
(31) Broke into bldg/vehicle
(32) Panhandled
*(33) Skipped classes
*(34) Didn't return change
*(35) Obscene calls

General Delinquency C
Same as General Delinquency
A except that items with
asterisk (*) are omitted.

---

[a] Not available for 1977 and 1983.

given type or who report using a specified drug within a designated period of time. The unit of analysis (i.e., what is counted) is persons. The prevalence rate is typically expressed as the percentage of persons in the population who have reported some involvement in a particular type of offense or use of a particular drug. The time interval involved is usually designated, as in an annual prevalence rate, a 3-year prevalence rate or a lifetime (ever) prevalence rate.

General offending rates refer to the number of offenses or drug use occasions that occur in a given population during a specified time interval, expressed as a rate per some population base. In this case, it is offenses or drug use occasions, not persons, that are being counted. General offending rates may be expressed as an average number of offenses per person in the population, or as the number of offenses per some population base (e.g., per 100, 1,000, or 100,000 persons). For example, the Federal Bureau of Investigation's annual report of arrests (UCR) involves an arrest rate per 100,000; the National Crime Survey (NCS) reports the general victimization rate as a rate per 1,000 persons or households (Sparks, 1981). As in the case of prevalence, the period of time involved is usually designated (e.g., monthly offending rate, annual offending rate, lifetime offending rate).

In this report all rates are annual rates; prevalence rates are expressed as percentages and general offending rates as rates per 1,000 (i.e., as the mean number of offenses or drug use occasions per 1,000 persons in the general sample or subsample or type, the same method of reporting used by the NCS). The prevalence rate for a scale is thus the percentage of persons in the population or some subgroup who report some involvement in at least one of the offenses included in the scale. General offending rates for scales are the average number of offenses reported for all offenses in the scale combined, multiplied by 1,000, for persons in the specified population.

Occasionally we will make reference to individual offending rates. In this case we are referring to the average number of offenses of a given type per *active offender* (for that type of offense) during the specified time interval. By definition, the minimum individual offending rate is 1.00. The individual offending rate can be derived directly from the prevalence rate and the general offending rate; that is, the general offending rate divided by the prevalence rate equals the individual offending rate. Given this relationship we will systematically present prevalence and general offending rates in the tables and will not present individual offending rates. The reader can easily calculate them from the data given. When it will help the interpretation of particular patterns of prevalence and general offending rates we will refer to individual offending rates; however, there will be no systematic presentation or discussion of this frequency rate. Whenever we use the more generic term offending rate, we will be referring to the general offending rate as defined above.

Reliability and Validity of SRD and Drug Use Scales

Reliability analyses for the NYS scales included the calculation of an internal consistency measure (Cronbach's alpha) for each scale each year; a 4-week interval test-retest correlation; and a measure of absolute accuracy in test-retest scores. These three measures of reliability were obtained for the total sample and for each of the major demographic subgroups (see Huizinga & Elliott, 1986). With one exception, reliabilities were adequate to excellent for the total sample and all demographic subgroups (e.g., test-retest reliabilities ranged from .7 to .9 in the total sample). The exception involved the minor assault prevalence scale, which had marginal (.50 to .67) reliabilities in some demographic subgroups.

Validity analyses included (1) an analysis of detailed follow-up questions to determine whether the self-report items in the SRD inventory were eliciting appropriate responses, (2) an analysis of the proportion of reported behaviors that were too trivial to be considered delinquent offenses, (3) a comparison of arrest records and self-reported offenses in the year of arrest, and (4) an analysis of the pattern of relationships between the SRD scales and a set of independent predictor measures. In general, all of these analyses confirmed the validity of these self-reported scales: 96% of responses were judged appropriate to the specific question asked; two-thirds of responses were judged to be delinquent acts (i.e., nontrivial behaviors); approximately 80% of arrests were matched with self-reported offenses in the same year (the higher the frequency and seriousness of reported offending, the greater the probability of an arrest); and the pattern of relationships between SRD and predictor measures was as expected for the total sample and specific demographic subgroups.

As an additional validity check we compared the NYS national prevalence rates for alcohol and marijuana use with those reported by Johnston, Bachman, and O'Malley in the Monitoring the Future (MTF) study. These data are presented in Table 1.2. For both alcohol and marijuana use, the prevalence estimates are quite similar. The largest difference between these two national probability samples involves the prevalence of marijuana use in 1977 (3.8%), alcohol use in 1980 (4.0%) and marijuana use in 1983 (4.3%). However, all of these differences are within the confidence intervals of the NYS estimates; that is, none of the differences in Table 1.2 is statistically significant.

There were two important qualifications to the general conclusion regarding the validity of these scales. First, there were generally higher rates of trivial events reported for nonserious than for serious offense items. There was an unusually high proportion of trivial events reported for offense items in the minor assault scale (over 75% for all demographic subgroups). Unless corrected, prevalence and offending estimates based upon responses to this scale are seriously inflated estimates of minor

TABLE 1.2. Annual prevalence rates for alcohol and marijuana use: The
National Youth Survey and Monitoring the Future studies 1977–1983.

	Prevalence of alcohol use		Prevalence of marijuana use	
	NYS[a]	MTF[b]	NYS[a]	MTF[6]
1977	48.6	47.6	83.2	87.0
1978	51.8	50.2	88.9	87.7
1979	49.8	50.8	85.8	88.1
1980	52.8	48.8	85.4	87.9
1981		46.1		87.0
1982		44.3		86.8
1983	41.0	42.3	83.0	87.3

[a] National Youth Survey, youths aged 18.

[b] L.D. Johnston, P.M. O'Malley, and J.G. Bachman, *Use of Licit and Illicit Drugs by American High School Students 1975–1984*. Data refer to prevalence of use during the last 12 months by high school seniors.

assault offenses. The tendency to report trivial events was not related to age, sex, race, class, or place of residence (rural or urban). As a result, this problem does not affect comparisons by these variables, since the error is a constant. However, it does affect the magnitude of prevalence and offending rates as generalized to any population.

The second concern is that the comparison of arrest and self-reported offenses revealed a lower rate of matching for blacks than for whites. Hindelang et al. (1981) reported a similar finding. Whether this phenomenon reflects a race-related error in the official records or in the self-reported measure (or both) is unclear, but it does suggest some caution when comparing delinquency rates for blacks and whites. With these two qualifications, we conclude that the NYS measures have acceptable reliability and validity. Detailed analyses of the reliability and validity of the NYS measures are available (Elliott & Huizinga, 1988; Huizinga & Elliott, 1986).

Mental Health Problem Measures

SOCIAL ISOLATION/LONELINESS AND EMOTIONAL PROBLEMS

Two mental health problem scales are included in the analysis of ADM problems, a Social Isolation/Loneliness scale and an Emotional Problems scale. Conceptually, the first measure was designed to capture what Weiss (1973) refers to as social and emotional isolation, loneliness stemming from the frustration of needs for belongingness and social connectedness to primary groups, the absence of close relationships, or psychological deficits in these relationships. Prior research has linked isolation and loneliness to a number of adolescent problems such as drug addiction (Holzner & Ding, 1973; Konopka, 1966; Pittel, Calef, Gryler, Hilles, Hofer, & Kempner, 1971), suicide (Horton, 1973), prostitution (Konopka, 1966), alcoholism (Rosenberg, 1969), sexual exhibitionism (Basquin & Trystram, 1966), and delinquency (Brennan & Auslander, 1979; Russel, 1973; Tanner, 1973). The Social Isolation/Loneliness scale used in this report is a ten-item scale with items reflecting perceived isolation from one's family and peers, and general feelings of loneliness in each of these social contexts. Sample items are: "I feel like an outsider with my family," "I don't feel that I fit in very well with my friends," "I feel close to my friends," "Sometimes I feel lonely when I'm with my family." In addition to a general Social Isolation/Loneliness scale, three five-item subscales are available, each reflecting social isolation/ loneliness in a particular social context (i.e., the family, school, and peer group). All of these scales have acceptable psychometric properties with reliabilities (alpha) ranging from .65 to .82 (see Elliott, Huizinga, & Ageton, 1985).

The Emotional Problems scale is an eight-item subscale from a modified version of the Klein et al. (1978) Negative-Labeling scale. The items in the general scale are descriptive phrases (e.g., are well liked, have a lot of personal problems, do things that are against the law, are often upset) and respondents are asked how much they think parents and peers would agree or disagree with each of these descriptions of them. Klein factored the original set of 24 items and found three general factors, which he labeled sick (emotional problems), bad (delinquent, unruly), and good (conforming). For the NYS, additional scale analyses reduced the items in each set to four. The Emotional Problems scale is composed of the four emotional problems items repeated for perceived agreement by parents and peers (i.e., eight items). Perceived agreement to these same items by teachers was also obtained on the first three surveys but these items were not included in the general scale since they were not available for all five surveys.

The Emotional Problems scale reflects the degree to which respondents perceive that parents and peers view them as having emotional problems. It is a measure of *perceived* labeling by parents and peers as a person with emotional problems. It is not a direct measure of self-reported emotional problems. Both the general eight-item scale and the two-item subscales have acceptable levels of reliability and homogeneity (alpha coefficients ranging from .7 to .8).

The Social Isolation/Loneliness and Emotional Problems scales are highly correlated (.85 in 1980) and may be reasonably approximated by a single four-item subscale of the Emotional Problems scale. The four items involve emotional problem labeling by one's family, and the scale formed by combining them is correlated highly with both Social Isolation/

Loneliness (.83 in 1980) and Emotional Problems (.98 in 1980). After the fifth wave of data collection only the emotional problem labeling by family items were retained in the NYS interview schedule. The other items involving Social Isolation/Loneliness and Emotional Problems were replaced in later years by measures of depression and utilization of mental health services. The relationship among the earlier and later mental health problem measures is detailed in Appendix B. For 1976–1980, the measure of mental health problems is a combination of the Social Isolation/Loneliness scale and the Emotional Problems scale. For subsequent years, only the family subscale of the Emotional Problems scale is used, and Depression and Utilization of Mental Health Services are considered separately.

Depression

In order to determine the extent of depression and depressive symptoms among youth aged 18–24, the sixth wave of the NYS incorporated elements of the NIMH Diagnostic Interview Schedule (DIS) (Robins et al., 1981a). The DIS was designed to be consistent with current psychiatric diagnostic systems: (1) the American Psychiatric Association, *Diagnostic and Statistical Manual of Mental Disorders* (DSM-III); (2) the Feighner Criteria (Feighner et al., 1972); and (3) the Research Diagnostic Criteria (Spitzer, Endicott, & Robins, 1978). An abridged version of the DIS has recently been used in the NIMH Epidemiological Catchment Area (ECA) Program (Regier et al., 1984). Available reports indicate that both the reliability and validity of the DIS are quite good (Helzer, Robins, Croughan, & Welner, 1981; Hesselbrock et al., 1982; Robins et al., 1981b, 1982).

The NYS measure of depression is essentially identical to that in the NIMH-DIS. Although interview probes are embedded in the NYS instrument to facilitate interviewers' correct use of probes and enhance reliability (the DIS uses a detached interviewer probe flowchart), both measures should yield equivalent information. Generally, both lifetime and 6-month rates for the total NYS sample (8.4% and 5.5%, respectively) approximate those found in the ECA site in New Haven, Connecticut (7.5% and 5.2%). Both samples reveal a fairly large sex differential in the 6-month prevalence rate for depression. The percentage of males and females in the NYS reporting a major depressive episode (3.1% and 8.0%) also compares with those found in New Haven (3.9% and 6.4%). Differences in depression rates between the NYS and ECA project sites may be partly attributable to sample design. Prevalence rates from New Haven, the only ECA site coincident with a standard metropolitan area, may be expected to closely reflect estimates from a national survey (see Regier et al., 1984; see also Robins, Helzer, Weissman, Orvaschol, Gruenberg, Burke, & Regier, 1984, for a fuller description of the ECA study and sample design). In general, preliminary analyses of depression rates among the NYS sample appear consistent with recent rates reported by the ECA program, thus providing some confidence in the validity of the NYS depression measure.

UTILIZATION OF MENTAL HEALTH SERVICES

The use of mental health services within the NYS sample is examined by means of a set of items modeled after those employed in the NIMH ECA program (see Shapiro et al., 1984). These items measure outpatient use of health services for help with emotional, nervous, drug, alcohol and/or general mental health problems, both "ever" and during the year prior to the interview. Services include private practice psychiatrists, psychologists, physicians, spiritualists, herbalists or natural therapists, mental health centers, psychiatric, drug, or alcohol clinics, social service agencies, and self-help or community agencies. Additional items assess the type and extent of inpatient admissions by hospitals or other treatment programs for mental health problems.

When NYS and ECA prevalence rates for ambulatory use of formal mental health services (physicians, psychiatrists, clinics, etc.) and inpatient hospital and treatment center admissions are compared, NYS annual hospital admissions for 18- to 24-year-olds are comparable to ECA annual hospital admissions for 18-year-olds (0.9 for NYS, an average of 1.0 for the ECA sites). Comparing NYS annual prevalence with ECA 6-month prevalence of utilization of general medical providers, the NYS rate is, predictably, about twice the ECA rate. For mental health visits and utilization of mental health specialists, the NYS annual prevalence rate is more than twice the ECA 6-month prevalence rate. As with depression, then, NYS prevalence rates are somewhat higher than ECA prevalence rates, but still similar, and the difference may be attributable to differences in sampling between the NYS and ECA samples.

The full set of mental health utilization measures includes friends, clergy, self-help groups, and other nonprofessional sources of help, as well as physicians, outpatient clinics, and other professional sources of help. In this report we have used a subset of the total list that reflects only professional mental health care (physicians, psychiatrists, mental health clinics, outpatient facilities) in our measure of mental health service utilization. Limiting the scale to professional practitioners and facilities enables us to focus on mental health problems of sufficient severity that individuals sought professional attention.

Problem Use of Alcohol and Drugs

Scales reflecting problem use of alcohol and problem use of drugs were obtained for the third and successive surveys. These measures were patterned after the problem alcohol use measure developed initially by

Cahalan (1970) and modified by Jessor and Jessor (1977). These scales each involve six items, reflecting negative social consequences of alcohol or illicit drug use. The general form of the items was: "How many times in the last year have you had problems with your family because of your use of alcohol?" Different life areas were reflected in each item (friends, spouse/girlfriend/boyfriend, physical fights, physical health, arrests by police). Responses ranged from "never" to "more than six times." Only respondents reporting some alcohol or drug use were asked these questions. Both of these scales had acceptable levels of reliability (.70 to .73).

Delinquency and ADM Problem Typologies

Several typologies are utilized in the following analyses. The NYS delinquency typology was developed and validated earlier in a study of delinquent careers (Dunford & Elliott, 1984). Four delinquent types were identified on the basis of the frequency and seriousness of their offenses.

1. *Nondelinquents.* Youth engaging in fewer than four total offenses and no index offenses.
2. Exploratory delinquents. Excluding those classified as nondelinquents, youth with 11 or fewer total offenses and no more than one index offense.
3. *Nonserious delinquents.* Youth with 12 or more total offenses and no more than two index offenses; or with two index offenses, regardless of the number of total offenses.
4. *Serious delinquents.* Youth with at least three Index offenses.

Using this classification scheme, youth in the NYS were placed into one of these four delinquency types for each of the six study years. This typology was validated using official arrest histories, social psychological predictor measures, self-reported delinquency scales, and demographic variables (Dunford & Elliott, 1984).

A TYPOLOGY OF DRUG USERS

To identify groups or types of drug users, a typology of drug users based on the kind and frequency of drug use was developed. The definition of the types was based on previous analyses of the NYS drug data (Brennan et al., 1981; Huizinga, 1982; Huizinga & Elliott, 1981; Johnson & Huizinga, 1983). The annual type definitions are as follows:

1. *Nonuser.* No use of any drug four or more times.
2. *Alcohol use.* Use of alcohol four or more times but no use of any other drug four or more times.

3. *Marijuana use.* Use of marijuana four or more times, and possibly use of alcohol, but no use of other illicit drugs four or more times.
4. *Polydrug use or multiple illicit drug use.* Use of amphetamines, barbiturates, hallucinogens, cocaine and/or heroin four or more times.

The requirement of drug use four or more times in order to be considered a drug user was based on the notion that it was more appropriate to place people whose drug use was very infrequent or experimental in the nonuse category. The typology is thus designed to measure nonexperimental use of particular drugs.

The above categorization provides a hierarchical unidimensional scale in the sense that a given type meets the requirement for all preceding types. Although the types are not intended as a scale, it should be noted that they form a reasonably good Guttman Scale, achieving a coefficient of reproducibility of more than .99 for the entire NYS sample on the first survey. Johnston, O'Malley, & Eveland (1978) utilized a similar scale and also report that it had Guttman-like properties. This scale also is consistent with research findings regarding the developmental sequence of drug use (Jessor, Donovan, & Widmer, 1980; Kandel, 1975, 1978; Kandel & Faust, 1975). All NYS respondents were classified into one of these four drug user types each year.

A Classification of Problem Substance Users

A simple dichotomy was used to type those experiencing negative social consequences of alcohol and illicit drug use. Users were considered problem users if they reported negative social consequences on four or more occasions for alcohol or on four or more occasions for illicit drugs. Problem Substance Users were those persons classified as Problem Alcohol Users and/or Problem Drug Users. Problem use of either alcohol or illicit drugs was sufficient for classifying a youth as a Problem Substance User in any given year. Those youth classified as non–problem users on both scales were thus classified as Non–Problem Substance Users.

Mental Disorder Classifications

These classifications are based upon simple dichotomies of the Emotional Problems scale and the Social Isolation/Loneliness scale. Youth with scores of 26 or greater on the Emotional Problems scale were classified as having emotional problems; those with scores of 25 or less were classified as not having emotional problems. At a minimum, those classified as having emotional problems reported that some combination of parents or peers agreed with at least two of the four descriptive phrases characteriz-ing them as having emotional problems while neither agreeing nor disagreeing with the remaining descriptive phrases. Those with Social Isolation/Loneliness scale scores of 30 or greater were classified as socially isolated/lonely. A score of this magnitude requires at least some agreement with statements describing the respondent as socially isolated or lonely.

For 1976–1980 those classified as either having emotional problems or (inclusively) being socially isolated or lonely were classified as having a mental health problem. For 1983, those having a score of 13 or higher on the family subscale for emotional problems (corresponding to a score of 26 on the Emotional Problems scale) were classified as having a mental health problem. This classification maintains continuity in the conceptualization of mental health problems between 1976 and 1983. Prevalence and frequency of depressive symptoms and utilization of mental health services are considered separately but not included as part of our delinquency-ADM typologies because the latter two measures are unavailable for 1976–1980.

The typologies used in this chapter are presently unique to this and other studies based on the National Youth Survey. They are empirical typologies that rely specifically on the data from the NYS and are constructed to reflect increasing seriousness. For the offense and drug use typologies, increasing variety of delinquent or alcohol and drug problem behavior occurs as well. Our typologies are thus offense- or behavior-centered, rather than offender- or individual-centered (see Gibbons, 1987, p. 205).

There are two reasons for using the seriousness of problem behavior as the basis for constructing our typologies. First, as studies by the Rand Corporation suggest (Chaiken & Chaiken, 1982; Petersilia, Greenwood, & Lavin, 1977), the most serious criminals in the prison population (violent predators) account for more robberies (per capita) than robbers, more burglary than burglars, and more drug dealing than drug dealers. In other words, among those convicted and sentenced to prison, there are few specialists, but there is a pronounced tendency for increasing seriousness of offending to be accompanied by a wider variety and by increased rates of offending. Second, an extensive review by Gibbons (1987) of proposed typologies and empirical research on them indicates that previous criminal typologies have usually been criminal-centered and have usually failed to receive empirical support. The previous literature on delinquent or criminal typologies most applicable to the present study is that from the Rand Corporation studies (Chaiken & Chaiken, 1982; Petersilia et al., 1977) of incarcerated felons.

Less has been written on typologies of alcohol and drug use. Alcoholism and drug addiction are commonly distinguished from psychological dependency, and both are distinguished from simple use of alcohol and other drugs; moreover, users of different types of substances are often discussed separately. Kandel (1982) indicates that there is a normal progression in alcohol and drug use, from nonuse to (1) beer and wine, then to (2) cigarettes or hard liquor, then to (3) marijuana, and finally to (4) other illicit drugs, with each of the earlier stages being prerequisite to the subsequent stages. The drug user typology allows for this progression, with stages 1 and 2, both of which involve the use of drugs that are legal for adults, combined. Kandel's research suggests that users of illegal drugs (including marijuana) are more likely to be involved in delinquency and other problem behaviors and to experience psychological stress. There is also a fairly substantial literature (Collins, 1981; Donovan & Jessor, 1985; Elliott et al., 1985; Gandossy et al., 1980; Graham, 1987; Gropper, 1985; Hammersley & Morrison, 1987; Inciardi, 1981; Jessor & Jessor, 1977; Johnson, Goldstein, Preble, Schmeidler, Lipton, Spunt & Miller, 1985; Parker & Newcombe, 1987) linking drug and alcohol use with criminal behavior. We would expect, therefore, some overlap among the serious and nonserious offender types, polydrug and marijuana users, and those classified as having mental health problems; and also higher rates for all types of problem behaviors for those classified as serious delinquents, as polydrug users, or as having mental health problems.

As noted earlier, the NYS data do not contain clinical diagnoses of emotional problems or structured interview components to identify diagnostic categories. To identify adolescents with emotional problems, an emotional problems scale and a loneliness scale were used. Using the classification described, the mental health measure provides a reasonable identification of youth evidencing self-perceived emotional problems. When combined with delinquent behavior, those identified as having emotional problems might well be classified as displaying an antisocial conduct or personality disorder.

2
The Demographic Distribution of Delinquency and ADM Problems

There is a substantial literature on the relationship between criminal behavior and age, sex, race or ethnicity, social class or status, and place of residence. The earliest examples of this literature may be found in the work of the French cartographers Guerry and Quetelet (see Vold & Bernard, 1986, pp 131–132), and contemporary examples abound. Although it is not as extensive, a similar literature exists on the relationships of alcohol and drug use with these same demographic variables; most of it (like the popularity of the drugs with which it is concerned) developed since World War II (see, e.g., Kandel, 1980). Only the literature on alcohol use and its associated problems is substantially older. The available literature on demographic correlates of adolescent mental health problems is much less extensive, rarely involves representative national samples, and often focuses on a single mental health problem such as depression (e.g., Kandel & Davies, 1982).

In the discussion that follows, the literature on each of the demographic correlates is selectively reviewed and findings from the National Youth Survey (NYS) regarding the relationships of delinquency and alcohol, drug, and mental health (ADM) problem behaviors to sex, race, social class, age, and place of residence are presented. The conclusions derived from past literature will be compared with those obtained from the NYS data.

In the tables that follow, each of the demographic variables is dichotomized except sex, which is a natural dichotomy. Race is dichotomized into white and black; the results of using white and nonwhite have also been examined and are almost identical to the white-black comparison because blacks in the NYS sample numerically dominate the nonwhite group. For social class, we compare middle and lower class, omitting working class, using the Hollingshead two-factor index of social class.[1]

---

[1] This measure combines the principal wage earner's occupation and education into a single index, from which five social classes may be constructed. Because of low frequencies in some of the categories, we have combined the top two classes to form a middle class, the bottom two to form a lower class, and retained the middle category as the working class.

For age comparisons the youngest and the oldest cohorts are used (ages 11 and 17 in 1976, 15 and 21 in 1980, and 18 and 24 in 1983). The choice of the oldest and the youngest cohorts maximizes the difference in age for a sample whose respondents are generally close in age. For place of residence, we compare urban and rural in 1976, 1980, and 1983.[2]

For each of the dichotomous categories of the demographic variables, prevalence rates and mean general offending rates (or use rates, or scale scores) are presented separately. The correlation between the demographic variables and the prevalence or general offending rates are also presented using Pearson's r. Statistical significance of differences in prevalence is tested using Chi-square (χ^2); for the differences in general offending rates (means) and correlation coefficients, t-tests are employed.[3]

In an effort to summarize briefly six waves of data collection spanning 8 years,[4] data are presented for 1976 when the panel was aged 11–17, for 1980 when the panel was aged 15–21, and again for 1983 when the panel was aged 18–24. This permits three cross-sectional views and an 8-year longitudinal perspective on change in the youth panel. In those cases where findings from these three waves do not accurately reflect the demographic distributions for all six waves, this fact will be noted in the text.

---

[2] The place of residence classification is based on U.S. Census descriptions of the cities, towns, and areas where respondents lived. Urban areas are central cities of a Standard Metropolitan Statistical Area (SMSA) or an urbanized area with a population of 100,000 or more; suburban areas are central cities of an urbanized area with a population of less than 100,000 or any part of an SMSA not previously classified as urban, or any community with a population of 25,000 or more; rural areas are cities or places not included in an SMSA or part of a central city in an urbanized area with a population less than 25,000.

[3] Because the NYS uses a stratified cluster sample, the calculation of variance estimates by standard (SRS) formulas underestimates the true variance. A measure of the relationship between the standard formula variances (S^2) and the estimated variance based on the stratified cluster design (V^2) is the design effect (DEFF), DEFF $= V^2/S^2$. For the NYS, the DEFF for most item estimates is small, e.g., the DEFF for over 80% of the prevalence estimates is ≤ 1.3; for general offending rates over 80% is ≤ 1.4. Because the DEFF is generally quite small, we have not attempted to adjust for the DEFF in the statistical tests presented in Tables 2.1–2.5. In comparison with tests that adjusted for design effects (see Elliott et al., 1983), there are no substantive differences in conclusions. The exact DEFF for each item estimate is presented in Elliott et al., 1983.

[4] In wave 6, data were collected for 1981, 1982, and 1983. However, only the 1983 data are fully comparable with data collected in 1976–1980. For 1981 and 1982, the recall period was for more than 1 year, many variables (particularly attitudinal variables) were not collected, and other variables were measured differently. Specifically, delinquency in 1981 and 1982 was not measured by frequency. Individual offense prevalence was measured, and multiple-item delinquency scales were coded as categorical variety scales (i.e., how many of the different offenses comprising the scale the respondent had committed).

Two preliminary comments about differences in general offending rates by demographic categories are in order. First, even when the correlation coefficients are statistically significant, they are almost always small (less than .30); this result indicates that the relationships between problem behavior (as measured by general offending rates, use rates, or scale scores) and demographic variables are weak. More precisely, demographic group membership appears to be a poor predictor of individual rates of problem behavior. This weak prediction arises in large measure because every demographic group has a large number of persons with no delinquency or ADM problems, and the presence of these persons in *both* groups being compared reduces the predictive value of group membership and the correlation coefficient. This explanation of *why* our ability to predict individual rates of problem behavior is weak in no way changes the fact *that* our ability to predict is weak.

Second, despite the low correlation coefficients, some of the mean differences are not only statistically significant, but are substantial as well (whether one uses absolute differences or ratios of means). For example, the male-female differences in general offending rates for Index offenses in 1976, 1980, and 1983 are 1297, 687, and 504 per thousand, respectively, and the ratios of male to female Index offending rates in those same years are 5.0, 3.7, and 7.0 to 1, respectively, despite weak correlations between −.10 and −.15 (all correlations and differences significant at .001 or better). What this result indicates is that our ability to predict relative *group* levels of delinquency is considerably better than our ability to predict *individual* levels of delinquency, based on group membership.

In contrast, the correlations are generally higher for those cases in which the difference in prevalence is statistically significant. Most correlations, however, are still weak, again reflecting the presence in all categories of substantial numbers of nonoffenders, nonusers, and individuals without mental health problems. With prevalence, as with general offending rates, there are often substantial group differences, but with the exception of alcohol and marijuana use among those aged 11 and those aged 17, membership in a particular demographic category is not a strong predictor of individual delinquency or ADM problems.

Sex, Delinquency, and ADM Problems

PAST RESEARCH

Whether official statistics on arrest or self-report data on behavior are used, males have a higher prevalence of delinquent and criminal behavior than females (Blumstein et al., 1986; Clark & Haurek, 1966; Dentler & Monroe, 1961; Elliott & Voss, 1974; Elliott et al., 1983; Gold, 1970; Gold & Reimer, 1975; Hood & Sparks, 1970; Nye & Short, 1957; Slocum & Stone, 1963). This finding is especially true for more serious offenses

(Gold & Reimer, 1975; Hindelang et al., 1981; Sarri, 1983). Males also tend to have a higher frequency of delinquent behavior, insofar as frequency has been measured in past studies (Clark & Haurek, 1966; Elliott et al., 1983; Gold & Reimer, 1975; Williams & Gold, 1972). Based on prior research, then, we would expect to find that males have significantly higher prevalence and general offending rates than females and that this difference should be most pronounced and consistent for more serious offenses.

Males also have higher prevalence rates of alcohol, marijuana, and other illicit drug use, although the differences between males and females appear to be decreasing over time (Gold & Reimer, 1975; Jessor, 1979; Kandel, 1980, 1982; Penning & Barnes, 1982). Women, however, are more likely than men to use psychoactive drugs under medical super-vision, whereas men are more likely to use psychoactive drugs without medical supervision (Kandel, 1980). There is little in the literature to indicate whether similar differences exist between male and female use rates, as opposed to prevalence, but the most reasonable expectation is that they would parallel prevalence rates. Thus we would expect males to have higher prevalence and use rates for alcohol, marijuana, and other illicit drugs.

Evidence on the prevalence of mental illness by sex suggests that men have a higher prevalence of personality disorders than women, but women have a higher prevalence of affective disorders and neurosis (Dohrenwend & Dohrenwend, 1976; Robins et al., 1984; Murphy, Sobol, Neff, Olivier, & Leighton, 1984). In particular, prevalence rates for depression are higher among women than men, and girls score higher on the average than boys on scales for depression (Kandel & Davies, 1982). According to Kessler, Reuter, and Greenley (1979), and Shapiro et al. (1984), women are more likely to seek out mental health care. We may expect, then, that females will have higher prevalence and scale scores for depression, and higher prevalence of mental health service use. We would also expect mental health service use rates to be as high or higher for females as for males. Considering the construction of our mental health problem measure (emotional problems plus social isolation), it seems more likely that this measure would reflect personality disorders than manic-depressive psychosis or neurosis. If this assumption is in fact true, we would expect males to have higher prevalence of mental health problems on our measure than females, and as high or higher mean scale scores.

NATIONAL YOUTH SURVEY FINDINGS

Delinquency

Sex differences in delinquency and ADM problems are presented in Table 2.1. With one exception (robbery in 1983) all the differences in prevalence and all of the correlations between prevalence of offenses and sex are

TABLE 2.1. Sex differences in delinquency and ADM problems.

Type of problem		Prevalence rates			Mean general offending rates (per 1,000)		
		Male	Female	r	Male mean	Female mean	r
Felony assault	1976	23.6[c]	9.0	−.20[c]	774[c]	217	−.13[c]
	1980	12.9[c]	4.6	−.14[c]	449[c]	124	−.10[c]
	1983	11.2[c]	2.5	−.17[c]	239[c]	58	−.10[c]
Felony theft	1976	16.2[c]	7.6	−.13[c]	968[a]	325	−.05[a]
	1980	12.5[c]	4.1	−.15[c]	679[b]	170	−.07[b]
	1983	12.3[c]	3.7	−.16[c]	757[b]	119	−.07[b]
Robbery	1976	7.7[c]	2.4	−.12[c]	486[b]	67	−.07[a]
	1980	2.8[b]	0.7	−.08[b]	164	38	−.04
	1983	0.5	0.0	−.05[a]	7	0	−.05[a]
Index offenses	1976	29.2[c]	10.8	−.23[c]	1620[c]	323	−.13[c]
	1980	17.8[c]	6.5	−.17[c]	944[c]	257	−.10[c]
	1983	14.4[c]	3.4	−.19[c]	588[c]	84	−.11[c]
Minor assault	1976	63.9[c]	34.9	−.29[c]	11259[b]	3347	−.07[a]
	1980	30.1[c]	10.3	−.24[c]	1925	394	−.05[a]
	1983	10.4[c]	3.0	−.15[c]	356[c]	68	−.09[c]
Minor theft	1976	25.4[c]	14.7	−.13[c]	2447[a]	752	−.04[a]
	1980	20.1[c]	8.6	−.16[c]	1063	1118	.00
	1983	14.6[c]	6.6	−.13[c]	780	675	−.01
Illegal services	1976	6.6[a]	3.9	−.06[b]	1832	336	−.04[a]
	1980	16.4[c]	4.6	−.19[c]	7974[b]	670	−.07[b]
	1983	13.3[c]	3.0	−.19[c]	7258[b]	295	−.08[c]
Public disorder	1976	46.0[c]	37.6	−.09[c]	9374	3306	−.08[c]
	1980	52.2[c]	42.8	−.09[c]	13867[c]	6440	−.09[c]
	1983	58.5[c]	36.5	−.22[c]	10775[c]	3993	−.10[c]
Vandalism	1976	44.2[c]	25.6	−.19[c]	4371[b]	862	−.06[b]
	1980	23.0[c]	7.0	−.22[c]	941[c]	301	−.10[c]
	1983	10.5[c]	2.2	−.17[c]	441[c]	35	−.09[c]
General delinquency	1976	76.2[c]	52.1	−.25[c]	24481[c]	6638	−.10[c]
	1980	59.2[c]	35.1	−.24[c]	22092[c]	6128	−.09[c]
	1983	53.0	27.1	−.26[c]	17339[b]	6294	−.08[c]
Alcohol use	1976	49.3[c]	42.8	−.07[b]	9220[c]	5511	−.08[c]
	1980	81.9	79.7	−.03	55678[c]	32228	−.14[c]
	1983	89.1	87.2	−.03	75040[c]	39406	−.20[c]
Marijuana use	1976	18.5	16.0	−.03	7726	6664	−.02
	1980	46.4[a]	40.9	−.05[a]	43909[c]	17785	−.14[c]
	1983	47.8[c]	38.7	−.09[c]	44783[c]	19970	−.12[c]
Polydrug use	1976	5.2	5.6	.01	1273	900	−.01
	1980	19.4[b]	13.5	−.08[c]	7084[a]	3841	−.05[a]
	1983	24.7[b]	18.0	−.08[c]	9320	7117	−.02
Problem substance use	1976	NA	NA	NA	NA	NA	NA
	1980	14.5[c]	5.6	−.15[c]	8.22[c]	6.93	−.12[c]
	1983	10.5[c]	4.4	−.12[c]	9.98[c]	8.06	−.15[c]

TABLE 2.1. *Continued*

Type of problem		Prevalence rates			Mean general offending rates (per 1,000)		
		Male	Female	r	Male mean	Female mean	r
DUI/DWI	1976	NA	NA	NA	NA	NA	NA
	1980	NA	NA	NA	NA	NA	NA
	1983	54.9ᶜ	32.8	−.22ᶜ	30174ᶜ	7326	.15ᶜ
Mental health	1976	12.0	12.6	.01	39.8	39.3	−.03
problems	1980	5.0	6.2	.03	36.1ᶜ	34.8	−.09ᶜ
	1983	5.9	6.1	.00	16.2	16.0	.02
Depression	1976	NA	NA	NA	NA	NA	NA
(symptoms)	1980	NA	NA	NA	NA	NA	NA
	1983	22.2ᶜ	31.7	.11ᶜ	.52ᶜ	.94	.14ᶜ
Mental health	1976	NA	NA	NA	NA	NA	NA
service use	1980	NA	NA	NA	NA	NA	NA
	1983	4.9ᶜ	10.8	.11ᶜ	760	1178	.03

$p \le .05$.
$p \le .01$.
$p \le .001$.

statistically significant (a negative correlation reflects a higher rate for males). Three differences (robbery in 1980 and 1983, and illegal services in 1976) are not as pronounced, but are in the expected direction and, with the one exception noted above, significant at .05 or better. The differences in general offending rates are not as strong as those for prevalence. Males have higher offending rates for felony assault, felony theft, and Index offenses generally, but the differences for robbery in 1980 and 1983 are small, in part reflecting the small number of cases of robbery in 1983. The pattern remains consistent for these more serious offenses, however, with males consistently having higher general offending rates. For minor offenses (with the exception of minor theft in 1980 for which male and female rates are nearly the same), males again have consistently higher general offending rates than females, and with four exceptions (minor theft in 1980, as noted above; minor theft in 1983; and minor assault in 1980 and illegal services in 1976), both the mean differences and the correlations are statistically significant at the .05 level or better.

These results are consistent with our expectations that males would have consistently and substantially higher rates of general offending and prevalence. The difference is more pronounced for prevalence than for general offending rates, and for general offending rates it is more pronounced and consistent for summary scales (Index offenses and general delinquency) than for offense specific scales. The difference between males and females is weakest for minor theft. Although male prevalence is higher for this offense category, general offending rates for females are close to those for males, especially for 1980 and 1983. This finding suggests that although fewer females are involved in minor theft, those individuals may commit that offense more often than males who are involved in the same crime. Indeed, the mean *individual* offending rate for females in 1980 is 13.0 offenses per active offender compared to 5.3 for males; for 1983, these mean individual offending rates are 10.2 for active female offenders compared to 5.3 for active male offenders. Conklin (1986) also cites evidence from official statistics that suggests that larceny may be the one offense for which female involvement, relative to males, may have increased over time. In general, however, the NYS data are in agreement with past research on male-female differences in prevalence and general offending rates, with males having substantially and consistently higher rates than those for females on both measures.

Drug Use

Although the prevalence of alcohol use among males is higher for 1976, the difference between males and females is not statistically significant for 1980 or 1983, suggesting that the differences in male and female alcohol use prevalence disappear after the age of 15. Use rates, by contrast, are higher for males in all three of the years in Table 2.1. For marijuana use, the differences in both prevalence and use rates are not significant for 1976, but are significant for 1980 and 1983. Once again, males have the highest prevalence and use rates, and the differences in use rates are greater than the differences in prevalence. Polydrug use is similar for males and females in 1976, but males have significantly higher prevalence rates in 1980 and 1983. Unlike marijuana use, however, male-female use rates are significantly different only for 1980, although the direction of the differences (males have higher use rates) is consistent for all three years.

For two other indicators of alcohol or drug problem behavior, problem substance use and driving while under the influence of alcohol or drugs (DUI), males have much higher prevalence and offending rates (for DUI) and scale scores (for problem substance use). Both of these are consistent with the pattern of heavier use among males than among females. Again, the general picture that emerges is one of higher male involvement in alcohol and drug use, and problem behavior connected with alcohol and drug use. Moreover, the differences in problem use measures of alcohol and drugs are much more pronounced than those associated with prevalence and frequency of use.

Mental Health Problems

As expected, females have higher prevalence rates of both depression and mental health service use. Females' scale scores (number of depressive symptoms) are also higher than those for males, again as expected. All of these differences are statistically significant. Although the rate of mental health service use is higher for females than males, this difference is not statistically significant. Calculating individual use rates reveals that those males who do use mental health services do so at a higher rate than females (mean individual use rates of 15.5 for males vs. 10.9 for females using mental health services).

Differences in prevalence of mental health problems are not in the expected direction. Although this finding is not statistically significant, females have a higher prevalence of mental health problems than males, as measured by a combination of emotional problems and social isolation. Mental health problem scale scores, in contrast, are higher for males than for females, but the difference is statistically significant only for 1980. For both prevalence and scale scores, the differences are very small, even when they are statistically significant, and the overall results suggest that there are no substantive mental health problem differences between males and females on this measure. Taken together, these results confirm our expectations with regard to depression and mental health service use, but fail to confirm our expectations with respect to the mental health problem measure. It seems likely, based on these results, that our mental health problem measure is tapping a different dimension of mental health problems than the other two mental health measures.

Race, Delinquency, and ADM Problems

Past Research

When official arrests are the sole criterion for determining the relationship between race and criminal or delinquent behavior, there is no question that blacks have higher rates of arrest (and by implication involvement in delinquency and crime) than whites (Pope & McNeely, 1981). With the advent of self-report measures, however, the question arose whether arrest rates accurately reflected race differences in criminal or delinquent behavior. Several self-report studies (Chambliss & Nagasawa, 1969; Elliott & Voss, 1974; Epps, 1967; Gould, 1968) found no difference between whites and blacks, and Gold (1970) found no difference when social class was controlled. Williams and Gold (1972) found no racial difference in frequency (which was poorly measured in that study), but did find that blacks were more likely to commit more serious offenses than whites. Hirschi (1969) and Slocum and Stone (1963), on the other hand, did find slight differences by race.

More recent research (Elliott & Ageton, 1980. Hindelang et al., 1981) indicates that there are racial differences in self-reported delinquent behavior, at least for more serious types of crime. Using the first wave of the NYS data (1976), Elliott and Ageton found that blacks had higher offending rates for predatory property crimes and for a measure of general delinquency which (unlike the measure used in the present study) included status offenses and other fairly trivial offenses. Hindelang (1978) came to a similar conclusion based on his analysis of personal crimes involving lone offenders from the National Crime Survey (NCS) victimization data. Both studies concluded that the representation of blacks among those arrested exceeded their involvement in crime as indicated by NYS and NCS data, but that the general patterns of race differences were accurately reflected in all three measures. Based primarily on the more recent studies, then, we would expect blacks to have higher prevalence and general offending rates than whites, particularly for more serious offenses. This expectation must be qualified, however, because (1) most self-reported offender studies have not found significant race differentials and the NYS analysis, which did find a significant difference, was limited to the first year's (wave) data; and (2) there is some evidence that blacks are more likely to conceal their involvement in delinquency than whites (Hindelang et al., 1981; Huizinga & Elliott, 1986).

Although some earlier studies found higher prevalence of marijuana use among blacks (see Penning & Barnes, 1982, for a historical review), more recent studies have found, particularly among younger age groups (Jessor, 1979), that marijuana use is higher among whites or else that there is no difference in use between whites and blacks (Penning & Barnes, 1982). According to Kandel's (1980) review, whites use more marijuana, tobacco, alcohol, and pills than blacks, but blacks use more heroin. Given the measures used in the present study, and the relatively low frequency of heroin use compared to cocaine, barbiturates, amphetamines, and hallucinogens, we may expect higher prevalence and use rates of alcohol, as well as marijuana and other illicit drugs, among whites than among blacks.

What little literature exists on the relationship between race and mental illness may be quickly summarized: There is no consistent pattern of racial differences in mental illness (Dohrenwend & Dohrenwend, 1969; Little, 1983; Robins et al., 1984). We therefore have no basis to expect racial differences in prevalence or scale scores on the mental health measures in the NYS data, except insofar as race may be associated with socioeconomic status, to be discussed in the next section.

NATIONAL YOUTH SURVEY FINDINGS

Delinquency

Racial differences in prevalence of offending as presented in Table 2.2 are generally consistent. Blacks have higher prevalence rates for the more serious offenses (felony assault, robbery, and total Index offenses), but whites have higher prevalence rates for the less serious offenses and for general delinquency. The exceptions in Table 2.2 are robbery in 1980, minor assault in 1976 and 1980, and public disorder in 1976, none of which

TABLE 2.2. Race differences in delinquency and ADM problems.

Type of problem		Prevalence rates			Mean general offending rates (per 1,000)		
		White	Black	r	White mean	Black mean	r
Felony assault	1976	15.4[b]	22.5	.07[b]	415[a]	1035	.11[c]
	1980	8.7	9.3	.01	301	204	−.02
	1983	6.1[a]	9.9	.06[a]	107	236	.06[b]
Felony theft	1976	12.2	13.9	.02	747	413	−.02
	1980	8.5	7.5	−.01	393	474	.01
	1983	7.6	9.4	.03	470	176	−.02
Robbery	1976	4.3[b]	8.5	.07[b]	277	282	.00
	1980	1.7	3.1	.04	95	190	.02
	1983	0.2	0.9	.05[a]	3	9	.03
Index offenses	1976	18.8[c]	29.1	.09[c]	911	152	.05[a]
	1980	12.2	13.3	.01	611	606	−.00
	1983	8.2[a]	12.5	.06[a]	314	297	−.00
Minor assault	1976	50.1	52.9	.02	7151	11637	.03
	1980	19.9	22.7	.03	1225	907	−.01
	1983	7.6[a]	3.9	−.05[a]	243[a]	90	−.03
Minor theft	1976	21.5[a]	15.1	−.06[b]	1937[a]	506	−.03
	1980	14.9	12.8	−.02	929	1783	.03
	1983	11.4[a]	6.4	−.06[a]	624	567	−.00
Illegal services	1976	4.9	7.4	.04	1111	1620	.01
	1980	11.7	9.3	−.03	4480	3469	−.01
	1983	8.4	7.7	−.01	1885	11901	.08[c]
Public disorder	1976	44.1[c]	32.0	−.09[c]	6825	6660	−.00
	1980	52.3[c]	25.7	−.20[c]	11992[c]	1664	−.09[c]
	1983	53.0[c]	27.5	−.19[c]	8692[c]	1725	−.08[b]
Vandalism	1976	36.1	32.4	−.03	2037	6880	.06[b]
	1980	16.2	11.5	−.05[a]	664	434	−.03
	1983	6.3	6.1	−.00	216	142	−.02
General delinquency	1976	65.3	64.6	−.01	15983	20342	.02
	1980	49.2[a]	40.9	−.06[a]	14021	12418	−.01
	1983	42.1[b]	32.3	−.07[b]	10532	15767	.03
Alcohol use	1976	49.6[c]	34.0	−.11[c]	7923	6456	−.02
	1980	84.9[c]	61.1	−.22[c]	50736[c]	18310	−.14[c]
	1983	90.6[c]	76.0	−.17[c]	61527[c]	38107	−.10[c]
Marijuana use	1976	18.2	15.1	−.03	7021	9467	.03
	1980	44.7	41.2	−.03	33617	25659	−.03
	1983	44.5	40.8	−.03	32041	40288	.03
Polydrug use	1976	6.0[a]	2.3	−.06[b]	1247[b]	178	−.03
	1980	18.5[c]	7.1	−.11[c]	6151	2708	−.04
	1983	23.1[c]	9.9	−.12[c]	7359	8738	.01
Problem substance use	1976	NA	NA	NA	NA	NA	NA
	1980	11.6[b]	4.5	−.09[c]	7.99[c]	5.86	−.14[c]
	1983	8.1	4.7	−.05[a]	9.38[c]	7.20	−.12[c]

TABLE 2.2. *Continued*

Type of problem		Prevalence rates			Mean general offending rates (per 1,000)		
		White	Black	r	White mean	Black mean	r
DUI/DWI	1976	NA	NA	NA	NA	NA	NA
	1980	A	NA	NA	NA	NA	NA
	1983	50.1[c]	18.8	−.23[c]	21297[c]	5394	−.08[b]
Mental health	1976	10.0[c]	21.2	.13[c]	38.8[c]	42.5	.16[c]
problems	1980	4.8[a]	8.8	.06[b]	34.8[c]	38.0	.15[c]
	1983	5.5	8.6	.05[a]	15.8[c]	17.3	.11[c]
Depression	1976	NA	NA	NA	NA	NA	NA
(symptoms)	1980	NA	NA	NA	NA	NA	NA
	1983	27.2	21.5	−.05[a]	.73[c]	.52	−.05[a]
Mental health	1976	NA	NA	NA	NA	NA	NA
service use	1980	NA	NA	NA	NA	NA	NA
	1983	8.4	6.4	−.03	943	1113	.00

[a] $p \leq .05$.
[b] $p \leq .01$.
[c] $p \leq .001$.

are statistically significant. Only about half of the differences in Table 2.2 (and the associated correlations) are statistically significant.

To some extent, the use of the years 1976, 1980, and 1983 in Table 2.2 is misleading relative to differences in the prevalence of serious offenses by race. Although the prevalence rates for blacks were equal to or greater than those for whites in all 6 years of the study for felony assault, robbery and Index offenses, these differences failed to achieve statistical significance in more years than not. Differences in felony assault and Index offenses were significant only in 1976, 1979, and 1983; differences in robbery were significant only in 1976 and 1978. The findings relative to race differences in the prevalence of serious offenses is thus quite mixed, with significant differences found in less than half of the study years. With regard to the generally higher prevalence rates for whites on nonserious offenses and general delinquency, the conclusion from the data in Table 2.2 holds for all study years. Further, with the exception of public disorder in 1980 and 1983, none of the correlation coefficients involving race is larger than .10 in magnitude, indicating very weak relationships between race and the prevalence of different types of offenses.

Racial differences in offending rates, with few exceptions, are not statistically significant. General offending rates of felony assault are significantly higher for blacks than whites only in 1976 and 1983. For 1976, 1980, and 1983, general offending rates for public disorder are higher for whites than blacks. There is otherwise little consistency to the pattern of racial differences in general offending rates, and no evidence of strong racial differences. Underreporting by blacks may affect these estimates for all the years examined, and the extent of underreporting is difficult to determine. These comparisons, then, should be interpreted cautiously. What does seem clear is that whites are definitely *not* more heavily involved, and may be less involved than blacks, in serious offending. With this exception, the patterns of racial differences are weak or unclear.

Drug Use

Whites are consistently more likely (prevalence) to use alcohol, as well as marijuana and other illicit drugs, and the differences for alcohol and polydrug use prevalence are statistically significant. For marijuana use, however, the differences between whites and blacks are small and not statistically significant, a result consistent with some previous research. For 1976, the differences in use rates and the correlations between use rates for alcohol, marijuana, and polydrug use are not statistically significant, except for the difference (but not the correlation) in polydrug use, which is significantly higher for whites. Differences in rates of marijuana and polydrug use are not statistically significant for 1980 or 1983, but whites have significantly higher rates of alcohol use for both of the later years. Whites also report higher prevalence rates and offending rates or scale scores for DUI and problem substance use. In general, these patterns are consistent with those found in recent, previous studies.

Mental Health Problems

Both prevalence rates and mean scale scores are higher for blacks than for whites, on the mental health problem measures. This result was unanticipated on the basis of previous research. Depression, by contrast, appears to be more concentrated among whites than among blacks, while the mental health service use difference between the two groups is not statistically significant. Overall, these equivocal results reflect what little literature exists on racial differences in mental health problems and service utilization. There is some indication that there may be racial differences in particular types or forms of mental health problems, with neither race having clearly higher rates of mental health service use. It is possible, however, that these differences reflect social class differences between whites and blacks rather than race differences.

Social Class, Delinquency, and ADM Problems[5]

PAST RESEARCH

Most early anonymous self-report studies show no relationship between social class or socioeconomic status and delinquent behavior (Akers, 1964; Allen & Sandhu, 1967; Chambliss & Nagasawa, 1969; Dentler &

---

[5] We use the term "social class," "social status," and "socioeconomic status" interchangeably. Marxian distinctions between bourgeoisie and proletariat, Weberian distinctions among class, status, and party, and other fine distinctions used in the stratification literature are largely ignored.

Monroe, 1961; Elliott & Voss, 1974; Epps, 1967; Farrington, 1973; Gould, 1968; Nye, Short, & Olson, 1958; Pfuhl, 1970; Porterfield, 1943). This evidence, compiled over a span of 30 years, ranges from rural farm areas to large cities, and includes samples in Hawaii, Washington, Kansas, Michigan, and California. It covers a wide variety of juvenile offenses from "incorrigibility" and truancy to robbery and aggravated assault. In a number of interview studies (Erickson & Empey, 1965; Gold, 1966; Reiss & Rhodes, 1961) a weak inverse relationship was found between delinquency and social status. Gold (1970) found a weak relationship between low socioeconomic status and delinquency for males but not for females. One anonymous questionnaire study on English youths (McDonald, 1969) also found such a relationship. By contrast, two interview studies (Arnold, 1965; Voss, 1966) found the opposite association, that is, high-status youth were slightly more prone to delinquency. Based upon a review of these early studies of social class and delinquency, Tittle, Villemez, and Smith (1978) concluded that social class was unrelated to criminal or delinquent involvement.

The findings of the early studies of self-reported delinquency and social class were plagued by methodological problems. They often included only trivial offenses (to the exclusion of more serious offenses) and used truncated frequency categories that made accurate estimation of general offending rates impossible. In more recent studies, however, when serious delinquency is included, it does appear to be linked to social class, with lower-class youth reporting higher prevalence and frequency of delinquency (Elliott & Ageton, 1980; Elliott & Huizinga, 1983; Hindelang et al., 1981).

A related point is that most studies of social status have measured the social status *background* of the respondents, rather than the social status of the respondent himself or herself. Hirschi (1969, p. 82) argues

. . . it is apparent that the child not likely to be going anywhere (but down) is likely to commit delinquent acts. The class of the father may be unimportant, but the "class" of the child most decidedly is not.

Pine (1965) found that downward social mobility was indeed associated with delinquency. Although the present study uses the current social class of the subject's parents, it should be borne in mind that an alternative measure of the respondent's *own* status (as we use the respondent's own race, sex, age, and the place of residence) might well yield a stronger relationship between social status and delinquent behavior. Another possible measure of social class not used here would be the social class status of the area in which the individual lives. This has been shown to be related to delinquency in studies involving both official and self-report data (Clark and Wenninger, 1982; Johnstone, 1978; Lander, 1954; Schuerman & Kobrin, 1986; Shaw & McKay, 1942). Despite questions raised by the earlier literature on self-reported delinquency and social class and despite the distinction among different measures of social class noted above, our expectation is that social class will be inversely related to prevalence and general offending rates for at least the more serious forms of delinquency.

Recent research on alcohol and drug use reveals no clear differences by social class, except that marijuana prevalence may be higher among college students (Jessor, 1979), among upper and middle classes (Penning & Barnes, 1982), or just among high-socioeconomic-status college students (Kandel, 1980). Overall, past research leads us to expect little difference by social status in the prevalence or use rates of alcohol, marijuana, or other illicit drugs.

In contrast with the uncertainty over the relationship between social class and delinquent behavior, and the apparent lack of any relationship between social status and use of alcohol, marijuana, and other illicit drugs, social class has been found to be a consistent and important predictor of mental health problems, with those in the lowest class having consistently higher prevalence rates of mental illness or mental health problems than those in the middle or upper class (Dohrenwend, 1975; Faris & Dunham, 1965; Hollingshead & Redlich, 1958; Srole & Langner, 1979). This may not be true, however, for all types of mental illness. In particular, although the prevalence of schizophrenia and personality disorders are highest in the lowest social classes, there is some tendency for the higher social classes to have higher prevalence rates of neurosis and manic-depressive psychosis (Dohrenwend, 1975). Specific to depression, there may be no difference by social class (Kandel & Davies, 1982). Furthermore, although the probability of mental illness is inversely related to social class, the probability of being a psychiatric patient is lower for those with lower social status (Srole & Langner, 1979). Based on past research, then, we would expect the lower class to have the highest rates of prevalence on the mental health problem measure, no differences by class for our measure of depression, and higher prevalence among the middle class for mental health service use. We have no basis for predicting the relationship between social class and mean scale scores of mental health problems, mean number of depressive symptoms, or mean use rate of mental health services. In the absence of other evidence, we would expect that they would have either the same relationship to social class as prevalence or no relationship.

NATIONAL YOUTH SURVEY FINDINGS

Delinquency

The prevalence of serious delinquency is higher among the lower class than among the middle class (see Table 2.3). In particular, lower social class status is weakly but statistically significantly associated with felony

TABLE 2.3. Social class differences in delinquency and ADM problems.

Type of problem		Prevalence rates			Mean general offending rates (per 1,000)		
		Middle	Lower	r	Middle mean	Lower mean	r
Felony assault	1976	10.3[c]	20.0	.13[c]	192[c]	712	.11
	1980	6.6[a]	10.5	.06[a]	110[c]	386	.08
	1983	2.9[c]	9.6	.12[c]	54[b]	206	.08
Felony theft	1976	11.8	12.6	.01	338	593	.03
	1980	4.6[b]	9.9	.09[b]	168[a]	535	.06
	1983	6.3	9.3	.05	246	391	.03
Robbery	1976	2.8[b]	6.6	.08[b]	54[a]	432	.05
	1980	0.6	1.3	.03	179	49	−.04
	1983	0.0	0.2	.02	0	2	.02
Index offenses	1976	15.4[c]	23.9	.10[c]	344[c]	1288	.10
	1980	8.7[a]	13.7	.07[b]	393	703	.04
	1983	5.2[c]	11.9	.11[c]	219	362	.03
Minor assault	1976	43.8[c]	54.3	.10[c]	2900[b]	10852	.07
	1980	17.3[a]	23.8	.08[b]	723	1754	.02
	1983	7.8	6.2	−.03	147	270	.03
Minor theft	1976	21.7	19.3	−.03	898	2319	.03
	1980	16.5	12.6	−.05[a]	916	961	.00
	1983	12.3	9.4	−.05	585	799	.02
Illegal services	1976	4.6	5.2	.01	595	1412	.02
	1980	9.5	10.2	.01	861	5997	.05
	1983	6.9	9.3	.04	1029[a]	6646	.05
Public disorder	1976	47.1[b]	38.8	−.08[b]	1125	3729	.03
	1980	57.5[c]	42.8	−.14[c]	14292	8183	−.07
	1983	58.6[c]	42.4	−.16[c]	7474	7032	−.01
Vandalism	1976	31.2	35.9	.05	4151	6141	.04
	1980	16.2	14.9	−.02	557	695	.02
	1983	5.8	7.5	.03	121	193	.04
General delinquency	1976	64.6	66.0	.01	7827[b]	21099	.07
	1980	51.7	46.6	−.05	10734	16364	.03
	1983	45.7[a]	38.0	−.07[a]	8858	15547	.04
Alcohol use	1976	49.5	45.1	−.04	7156	6753	−.01
	1980	86.7[c]	77.1	−.12[c]	52272[a]	40262	−.07
	1983	92.6[c]	85.2	−.11[c]	63289	52994	−.05
Marijuana use	1976	16.4	14.0	−.03	5875	6332	.01
	1980	41.0	44.3	.03	26595	29493	.02
	1983	39.0	43.9	.05	17040[c]	40536	.11
Polydrug use	1976	4.9	4.2	−.02	1524	1204	−.01
	1980	18.5	14.2	−.06[a]	4945	5214	−.00
	1983	24.6[a]	19.1	−.06[a]	5593	9767	.04
Problem substance use	1976	NA	NA	NA	NA	NA	NA
	1980	9.5	11.2	.03	7.69	7.47	.03
	1983	5.7	9.3	.06[a]	9.01	8.98	−.00

ABLE 2.3. *Continued*

Type of problem		Prevalence rates			Mean general offending rates (per 1,000)		
		Middle	Lower	r	Middle mean	Lower mean	r
)UI/DWI	1976	NA	NA	NA	NA	NA	NA
	1980	NA	NA	NA	NA	NA	NA
	1983	52.1[b]	40.4	−.11[b]	11856[a]	24773	.07[a]
⁄ental health	1976	5.9[c]	17.7	.16[c]	37.3[c]	40.9	.21[c]
problems	1980	4.0	7.1	.06[a]	34.0[c]	36.4	.14[c]
	1983	5.2	6.2	.02	15.4[b]	16.5	.10[c]
)epression	1976	NA	NA	NA	NA	NA	NA
(symptoms)	1980	NA	NA	NA	NA	NA	NA
	1983	26.6	27.9	.01	.78	.70	−.03
⁄ental health	1976	NA	NA	NA	NA	NA	NA
service use	1980	NA	NA	NA	NA	NA	NA
	1983	10.0	6.7	−.06[a]	1470	685	.05

$p \le .05$.
$p \le .01$.
$p \le .001$.

assault in 1976, 1980, and 1983, with felony theft in 1980, and with robbery in 1976. The patterns of association for other years are the same, but not statistically significant. Social class status is significantly and inversely related to the prevalence of Index offenses for every year (including those not shown). All of the correlations are weak (.12 or smaller), indicating that the relationship, although statistically significant, is not a strong one. But where there is a statistically significant relationship, the difference between the means is often substantial, with a ratio of 2 : 1 or 3 : 1 between the lower and the middle classes.

For minor offenses, the pattern is inconsistent. For 1976 and 1980, but not 1983, minor assault prevalence is significantly higher in the lower class. Minor theft is significantly correlated (negatively) with class only in 1980. The relationship of social class to vandalism and general delinquency varies in direction from year to year, and is statistically significant only for general delinquency in 1983, for ages 18 to 24 with higher rates for the middle class. In summary, these results are generally consistent with those of past studies that suggest that there is little or no relationship between minor delinquency and social class for adolescents. The results also, however, are consistent with official statistics and more recent self-report studies in finding a significant inverse relationship between social class and more serious forms of delinquent or criminal behavior.

With few exceptions, the relationship between social class and general offending rates is not statistically significant. The general offending rates for Index offenses, minor assault, and general delinquency are significantly higher for the lower class for 1976 (and all of these results are consistent with prevalence rates), but not for 1980 or 1983, and the offending rate for public disorder offenses is significantly higher for the middle class for 1980 but not for 1976 or 1983. The most striking and consistent class difference is the consistently higher general (and individual) offending rate of felony assault for the lower class. Other than felony assault, then, it seems safest to say that there is little difference in general offending rates between lower and middle classes, even though prevalence rates for more serious offenses are higher for the lower class than for the middle class. This finding raises the possibility that offending rates among those middle-class youths who are actively involved in serious offenses may be slightly higher than those of lower-class youths who are similarly involved. The calculation of individual offending rates for 1983 from the data in Table 2.3 substantiates this result for Index offenses (mean individual offending rates of 42.1 and 30.4 for middle- and lower-class youth, respectively).

Drug Use

The prevalence of alcohol and polydrug use (Table 2.3) is consistently higher among the middle class than among the lower class. The differences are significant for alcohol use in 1976, 1980, and 1983, and for polydrug use in 1980 and 1983. For alcohol use, the use rate is also significantly higher among the middle class for 1980 and 1983, but class differences in polydrug use rates are not statistically significant. Differences in prevalence rates of marijuana are neither statistically significant nor consistent, but use rates are higher for the lower class for 1983. These results run counter to the expectation of no difference in prevalence of alcohol or polydrug use, and that if there were a difference in marijuana use, prevalence of use would be higher among the middle class. Note that, with the exception of the difference between lower- and middle-class use of marijuana in 1983, the differences tend to be small, even when they do reach statistical significance (e.g., alcohol use prevalence in 1980 and 1983).

If we focus for a moment only on the adolescent population (ages 11–17, year 1976), we find no significant differences in either prevalence or use rates by social class, as would be expected based on past literature concerning social class and drug use. It may well be that patterns of alcohol and drug use by social class shift with age or over time. It is only for the later years when some of the panel respondents have moved beyond adolescence, and particularly for 1983 when respondents are aged 18–24, that we begin to see results substantially different from those expected on the basis of past research. Finally, there appears to be little difference in problem substance use by social class. Driving under the influence of alcohol or drugs appears to be more prevalent among the middle class, but the offending rate is higher for the lower class. This finding clearly suggests that those in the middle class who drive under the influence of alcohol or drugs do so relatively infrequently, but those of the lower class who drive under the influence of alcohol or drugs do so relatively often.

Mental Health Problems

As expected, the prevalence and mean scale scores of mental health problems are higher for the lower class. With the exception of prevalence in 1983, all of the differences are statistically significant. Depression, again as expected, has no statistically significant relationship to social class; the differences in prevalence and mean number of depressive symptoms are very small, and in opposite directions in different years. Finally, there is no significant class difference in the prevalence or use rates of mental health services. The correlation between class and mental health service use is significant but very weak ($-.06$). Except for the finding relative to mental health service use, these findings are consistent with past research on the distribution of mental illness by social class.

Age, Delinquency, and ADM Problems

PAST RESEARCH

Previous studies of the relationship between age and delinquency concur that delinquent behavior peaks sometime in mid-adolescence to late adolescence, and declines thereafter (Elliott & Huizinga, 1983; Gold, 1970; Hirschi, 1969). Indeed, age structure is a fairly good predictor of trends in victimization and self-reported delinquency (Steffensmeier & Harer, 1987) as well perhaps as levels of official delinquency (Chilton & Speilberger, 1971). One weakness of prior self-report studies is that they have generally not followed adolescents (except for college students) into the young adult years (the early 20s). Based on research to date, however, we may expect rates of delinquency to increase into mid-adolescence (ages 15–17) and to decline thereafter.

According to Kandel (1980), rates of both legal and illegal drug use peak around ages 18–21 and decline thereafter. Elsewhere she qualifies this finding (Kandel, 1982) by noting that different drugs peak at different ages: alcohol and tobacco between 18 and 34, stimulants at ages 26–34, tranquilizers around age 26, and sedatives after age 50. Penning and Barnes (1982) suggest that marijuana use among adolescents increases with age, and it is unclear when it declines. For the ages (11–24) covered by the six waves of the NYS presented here, it seems most reasonable to expect an increase in the prevalence and use rates of alcohol, marijuana, and other illicit drugs as the age of the respondents increases.

What little information is available on the relationship between age and mental health problems is contradictory (Dohrenwend & Dohrenwend, 1969; Kandel & Davies, 1982; Robins et al., 1984). In the most recent study (Robins et al., 1984), the highest prevalence rates for all psychiatric disorders except drug abuse and dependence were for those aged 25 to 44. Drug abuse and dependence rates were highest for those aged 18–24. Unfortunately, few studies report rates for persons under age 18. Little (1983) concludes that the youngest ages (childhood) have usually shown the lowest rates of psychopathology, but whether psychopathology is highest in adolescence, middle age, or old age is unclear. We have no basis, therefore, to expect any particular pattern of age differences on our mental health problem measures.

NATIONAL YOUTH SURVEY FINDINGS

Delinquency

Age differences in delinquency and ADM problems are presented in Table 2.4. In 1976, for ages 11–17, the direction of the age relationship for prevalence is *positive* for every offense except vandalism and minor assault (for which the differences by age are negative but not statistically significant). By 1980, except for the relationship between age and illegal services and public disorder, all age-offense relationships were negative; in 1983 (ages 18–24), *all* offenses are negatively associated with age. About half of the age differences in Table 2.4 are statistically significant, with relatively few significant differences for more serious offenses; for

TABLE 2.4. Age differences in delinquency and ADM problems.

Type of problem		Prevalence rates			Mean general offending rates (per 1,000)		
		11/15/18	17/21/24	r	11/15/18 mean	17/21/24 mean	r
Felony assault	1976	16.2	18.8	.03	356	487	.06
	1980	10.0	7.3	−.05	239	170	−.04
	1983	9.2	5.6	−.07	314[a]	74	−.09[c]
Felony theft	1976	4.4[c]	17.8	.22[c]	92[b]	533	.15[c]
	1980	7.8	7.9	.00	544	121	−.08
	1983	10.9[a]	4.3	−.12[b]	520[a]	74	−.10[c]
Robbery	1976	3.2	4.6	.04	172	364	.05
	1980	3.9[a]	0.6	−.10[a]	196[a]	12	−.09[c]
	1983	0.9	0.0	−.06	13	0	−.06
Index offenses	1976	17.8	23.6	.07	559	995	.08[c]
	1980	14.3	9.1	−.08	770[a]	200	−.10[c]
	1983	11.0	5.6	−.09[a]	544[a]	93	−.10[c]
Minor assault	1976	45.2	42.6	−.03	2768	12733	.07
	1980	30.0[c]	6.7	−.29[c]	1100[c]	109	−.21[c]
	1983	16.7[c]	1.2	−.25[c]	908[c]	12	−.14[b]

TABLE 2.4. *Continued*

Type of problem		Prevalence rates			Mean general offending rates (per 1,000)		
		11/15/18	17/21/24	r	11/15/18 mean	17/21/24 mean	r
Minor theft	1976	9.2[c]	24.9	.21[c]	272[b]	970	.15[c]
	1980	16.5[a]	8.5	−.12[b]	1422	212	−.11[a]
	1983	16.2[a]	8.6	−.11[a]	1542[a]	228	−.10[a]
Illegal services	1976	.04[c]	10.2	.23[c]	4	3168	.06
	1980	7.0[a]	13.3	.11[a]	961	1770	.05
	1983	9.6	6.2	−.06	6677	3451	−.02
Public disorder	1976	22.5[c]	57.9	.36[c]	1217[c]	8746	.20[c]
	1980	38.9[a]	50.9	.12[b]	4170[a]	8273	.11[a]
	1983	43.2	40.7	−.02	9183[b]	3303	−.13[b]
Vandalism	1976	35.7	28.9	−.07	1434	909	−.07
	1980	23.6[c]	6.1	−.23[c]	1275[b]	139	−.13[b]
	1983	12.2[c]	0.6	−.22[c]	428[b]	6	−.12[b]
General delinquency	1976	56.4[b]	69.2	.13[b]	4658[b]	24262	.12[b]
	1980	45.7	44.2	−.01	9361	12297	.03
	1983	46.7[a]	36.0	−.11[a]	8330	13242	−.02
Alcohol use	1976	8.4[c]	81.7	.74[c]	288[c]	17533	.35[c]
	1980	66.5[c]	86.1	.22[c]	10574[c]	68394	.41[c]
	1983	83.0	88.3	.07	42847	62204	.10[a]
Marijuana use	1976	0.4[c]	39.1	.51[c]	8[c]	18213	.25[c]
	1980	30.0[c]	51.5	.22[c]	10109[c]	45818	.19[c]
	1983	41.0	40.1	−.01	28489	28259	−.00
Polydrug use	1976	0.0[c]	15.8	.31[c]	0[b]	2393	.13[b]
	1980	9.1[c]	24.2	.21[c]	3652	5933	.04
	1983	18.8	21.6	.03	9712	1765	−.07
Problem substance use	1976	NA	NA	NA	NA	NA	NA
	1980	4.4[b]	12.3	.15[b]	5.61[c]	8.55	.15[b]
	1983	9.2	4.9	−.08	8.85	8.51	−.02
DUI/DWI	1976	NA	NA	NA	NA	NA	NA
	1980	NA	NA	NA	NA	NA	NA
	1983	38.2	50.0	.12[a]	14277	16598	.02
Mental health problems	1976	11.7	14.3	.04	39.4	39.2	−.01
	1980	5.7	4.9	−.02	34.6	35.5	.05
	1983	6.6	9.3	.05	16.1	16.6	.04
Depression (symptoms)	1976	NA	NA	NA	NA	NA	NA
	1980	NA	NA	NA	NA	NA	NA
	1983	24.9	33.3	.09[a]	.62[b]	1.06	.14[b]
Mental health service use	1976	NA	NA	NA	NA	NA	NA
	1980	NA	NA	NA	NA	NA	NA
	1983	6.1[b]	15.4	.15[b]	761[a]	3356	.11[a]

[a] $p \leq .05$.
[b] $p \leq .01$.
[c] $p \leq .001$.

example, there are no significant age differences for felony assault or Index offenses in any year.

The pattern of age differences in general offending rates is similar. All except vandalism are positively associated with age in 1976, and the relationships with felony theft, Index offenses, minor theft, illegal services, public disorder, and general delinquency are statistically significant. In 1983, all offenses are negatively related to age. All except robbery, illegal services, and general delinquency are statistically significant for either the difference in means or the correlation, most often both. These patterns are consistent with the past observation that delinquency peaks in middle to late adolescence, then declines.

Of the ages in Table 2.4, age 17 is the age of highest prevalence of all offenses except illegal services (which appears to peak around age 21), and minor assault and vandalism, both of which are highest for 11-year-olds. General offending rates show a similar pattern, with vandalism peaking at age 11, felony larceny peaking at age 15, and all other offenses peaking at either age 17 or 18. Bear in mind that although the table covers the full range of ages, it does not include each age category; hence it is possible, for example, that some offenses peak at age 16 (which is not included in the table). In general, however, both prevalence and offending rates appear to peak in late adolescence and decline substantially in the twenties.

Drug Use

The associations between age and rates of alcohol, marijuana, and polydrug prevalence and use are generally positive; the only exceptions are polydrug use rate in 1983 and marijuana use prevalence in 1983, neither of which is statistically significant. The highest correlations involving demographic variables are the positive correlations between age and adolescent alcohol use (.74) and adolescent marijuana use (.51) in 1976. For 1976 and 1980, both prevalence and use rates of alcohol, marijuana, and other illicit drugs are associated with increasing age, but for 1983, when the respondents are older, only the use rate of alcohol is statistically significantly higher for older than younger respondents. Problem substance use appears to follow this same pattern, significantly higher in both prevalence and scale score for the older age group in 1980, but not significantly different by age in 1983. The correlation between DUI prevalence and age is statistically significant for 1983, but the correlation between DUI frequency and age and the differences in means, though in the expected direction, are not statistically significant. These results generally agree with the previous research suggesting that alcohol and drug use increase at least through age 20; they also suggest that in the 20s, prevalence and use rates may begin to level off.

Mental Health Problems

There is no statistically significant relationship between rates on the mental health problem measure and age for 1976, 1980, or 1983. Prevalence of depression and number of depressive symptoms and prevalence of mental health service use and use rate of mental health services both appear to be positively related to age. Since we had no basis for expecting or not expecting age differences, this result neither confirms nor contradicts expectations based on previous findings, but it does point once again to the fact that different measures of mental health problems will yield different results.

Urban Residence, Delinquency, and ADM Problems

PAST RESEARCH

Evidence collected by self-report studies on urban-rural differences, as noted earlier, includes research on various levels of population size and density and crimes ranging from trivial to serious. Slocum and Stone (1963) compared farm and nonfarm areas, and found delinquency to be associated with the latter. Dentler and Monroe's (1961) study included three areas: a middle-class suburb, a rural nonfarm area, and a farming town. No differences were found among the three areas, but it may be questioned whether any could have been expected, for none of the areas was truly urban. Clark and Wenninger (1962) studied a farm area, a lower-class nonindustrial area, an upper-class nonindustrial area, and an urban industrial area. They found the farm community to be the least delinquent of the four areas, in terms of serious rather than nuisance offenses.

Gold and Reimer (1975) provide information on the relationship between urban residence and crime. Whereas urban location refers to the place in which the crime occurs, urban residence refers to the place in which the perpetrator of the crime lives. The relationship between residence and prevalence of delinquency tends to be stronger than that between residence and seriousness of delinquency. Overall, the evidence indicates a moderate, fairly consistent relationship between urban residence and frequency of delinquency. At the same time, the relationship between urban residence and seriousness of delinquency was neither strong nor consistent. On the whole, data from both official statistics and victimization surveys (Ennis, 1967; Skogan, 1976; U.S. Department of Justice, 1983) and from both earlier and more recent self-report studies all indicate that we should expect higher prevalence and offending rates in urban areas than in suburban or rural areas.

According to Kandel (1980), the highest rates of alcohol and marijuana use occur in the cities and the suburbs, but the variation is higher among adults than among youth. Jessor (1979) also concludes that marijuana use is higher in large metropolitan areas. We may reasonably expect, therefore, that prevalence and possibly use rates will be highest among urban residents.

Urban prevalence rates of mental health problems tend to be only slightly higher than those in rural areas, and there is once again variation by type of mental health problem. Manic-depressive psychosis tends to be higher in rural areas, but schizophrenia, personality disorder, and neurosis prevalence rates are higher in urban settings (Little, 1983, p. 95). With the possible exception of depression, therefore, we may expect higher prevalence rates for mental health problems among urban residents.

NATIONAL YOUTH SURVEY FINDINGS

Delinquency

With one exception (public disorder in 1983, for which urban and rural prevalence rates are equal), prevalence rates of offenses are higher in urban than in rural areas (Table 2.5). With the exceptions of minor assault and robbery, all differences in 1976 and 1980 are statistically significant; but in 1983, the only statistically significant urban-rural differences are those for felony theft, minor theft, and illegal services. Speculating on this finding suggests two possibilities: one is that urban *background* may

TABLE 2.5. Residence differences in delinquency and ADM problems.

Type of problem		Prevalence rates			Mean general offending rates (per 1,000)		
		Urban	Rural	r	Urban mean	Rural mean	r
Felony assault	1976	22.4[c]	12.4	−.13[c]	941[c]	288	−.13
	1980	11.0[a]	6.5	−.08[a]	397	196	−.06
	1983	6.8	6.5	−.01	122	143	.01
Felony theft	1976	15.1[b]	9.1	−.09[b]	1334	475	−.05
	1980	9.7[a]	6.3	−.06[a]	622[a]	164	−.08
	1983	10.4[c]	3.4	−.14[c]	389[a]	119	−.09
Robbery	1976	7.5	4.6	−.06[a]	391	164	−.06
	1980	2.3	1.8	−.02	123	40	−.04
	1983	0.4	0.0	−.05	4	0	−.05
Index offenses	1976	26.4[c]	15.9	−.13[c]	1816[c]	513	−.13
	1980	14.1[a]	9.7	−.07[a]	803[a]	319	−.07
	1983	8.7	7.5	−.02	297	172	−.04
Minor assault	1976	53.1	50.5	−.03	10209	9190	−.01
	1980	20.8	19.8	−.02	2292	661	−.04
	1983	6.5	5.3	−.03	156	157	.00

TABLE 2.5. *Continued*

Type of problem		Prevalence rates			Mean general offending rates (per 1,000)		
		Urban	Rural	r	Urban mean	Rural mean	r
Minor theft	1976	23.0[a]	17.3	−.07[a]	3424	791	−.05[a]
	1980	16.4[b]	9.2	−.11[c]	1729	326	−.06[a]
	1983	14.0[a]	8.2	−.09[b]	928	535	−.04
Illegal services	1976	8.4[c]	3.0	−.12[c]	1630	1205	−.01
	1980	12.8[a]	7.9	−.08[b]	10236	1281	−.07[a]
	1983	10.4[a]	6.3	−.07[a]	3845	5332	.01
Public disorder	1976	43.0[a]	35.6	−.08[b]	10362	4841	−.06[a]
	1980	47.3[a]	38.6	−.09[b]	10634	7442	−.04
	1983	44.2	44.4	.00	8698	6364	−.03
Vandalism	1976	37.9[a]	30.5	−.08[b]	5740	1273	−.06[a]
	1980	17.6[a]	11.9	−.08[b]	813	485	−.05
	1983	6.9	4.4	−.05	231	216	−.00
General delinquency	1976	69.4[a]	62.1	−.08[b]	24302	16355	−.03
	1980	51.4[c]	38.7	−.13[c]	23159	7721	−.07[a]
	1983	39.6	36.8	−.03	12287	11714	−.00
Alcohol use	1976	43.2	43.1	−.00	6889	6101	−.02
	1980	79.3	74.2	−.06[a]	40962	35921	−.03
	1983	87.1	83.3	−.05	49615	52823	.02
Marijuana use	1976	20.8[c]	12.3	−.11[c]	12287[c]	3076	−.13[c]
	1980	48.8[c]	33.0	−.16[c]	44460[c]	18697	−.14[c]
	1983	50.7[c]	33.4	−.17[c]	40011[a]	20433	−.10[b]
Polydrug use	1976	6.1[b]	2.6	−.09[b]	921	1068	.01
	1980	21.0[c]	10.8	−.14[c]	8074[a]	3338	−.08[a]
	1983	24.5[a]	17.7	−.08[a]	8381	7111	−.01
Problem substance use	1976	NA	NA	NA	NA	NA	NA
	1980	11.6	7.7	−.07[a]	7.89[c]	6.40	−.07[a]
	1983	7.6	5.6	−.04	9.23[c]	7.69	−.13[c]
DUI/DWI	1976	NA	NA	NA	NA	NA	NA
	1980	NA	NA	NA	NA	NA	NA
	1983	38.6	44.7	.06	15037	12658	−.02
Mental health problems	1976	16.3	12.8	−.05	40.1	39.6	−.03
	1980	6.4	5.2	−.03	36.2[a]	35.0	−.08[a]
	1983	6.9	5.6	−.03	16.8[a]	15.8	−.10[b]
Depression (symptoms)	1976	NA	NA	NA	NA	NA	NA
	1980	NA	NA	NA	NA	NA	NA
	1983	27.7	23.0	−.05	.71	.60	−.04
Mental health service use	1976	NA	NA	NA	NA	NA	NA
	1980	NA	NA	NA	NA	NA	NA
	1983	7.9	8.5	.01	1571	962	.04

[a] $p \leq .05$.
[b] $p \leq .01$.
[c] $p \leq .001$.

matter more than (current) urban *residence* for adults as an influence in prevalence of offending; the other is that with the exception of purely economically motivated crimes (except robbery, which is also a crime of violence), for which there are greater opportunities available in urban centers than in rural areas, the urban-rural distinction may matter much less for adults than for adolescents.

With the exceptions of felony assault, minor assault, and illegal services in 1983, general offending rates are higher for urban than for rural areas. However, few of the mean differences reach statistical significance, and although more of the correlations are statistically significant, they are small; all but two (felony assault and Index offenses, both in 1976) are less than .10 in absolute value. Taken together, the prevalence and offending rate data suggest a higher prevalence and perhaps a higher offending rate for urban than rural residents, but the relationship is weak. These data do not, of course, specify where the offenses occur. It may well be that the relationship between residence and victimization, or between urban location and the occurrence of offenses, is higher than that between urban residence and commission of crime.

Drug Use

There appears to be no statistically significant difference in alcohol prevalence or use rates by urban-rural or urban-nonurban residence. Marijuana use rates and prevalence rates are statistically significantly higher for urban than for rural residents. Polydrug prevalence rates are statistically significantly higher for urban residents in all three years, and use rates are statistically significantly higher for urban residents in 1980. The data on marijuana use therefore confirm our expectation that use will be higher in urban areas than elsewhere, but the data on polydrug use provide only weak support for, and the data on alcohol do not support, the urban-rural distinction. Problem substance use is consistently and, in 1980, significantly higher in urban areas. Scale scores for problem drug use are also significantly higher for urban areas in 1983. Driving under the influence of alcohol or drugs in 1983 appears to be lower in urban than nonurban areas for prevalence and higher in urban areas for offending rate, but the differences are not statistically significant.

Mental Health Problems

The prevalence of mental health problems is not statistically significantly higher in urban areas, but the differences are in the expected direction, and the correlation between urban residence and mental health problem scale scores is significant in 1980 and 1983. Neither depression nor mental health service use appears to be significantly related to urban residence. In brief, there is no evidence from these data that the prevalence rates of mental health problems are any higher in urban areas than in rural or nonurban areas, but the scale scores indicate some evidence of more severe mental health problems in urban than in rural areas.

Summary

With the exception of age differences in alcohol and marijuana use between 11- and 17-year-olds (a difference that probably will surprise no one), none of the relationships between demographic variables and delinquency and ADM problems are strong. Most are in the expected direction, but many fail to reach statistical significance, and most, if measured by a correlation coefficient, fail to reach substantive significance as well. Mean differences, however, tell a different story for some variables.

Sex is clearly related to patterns of offending, to alcohol and drug use, and to depression and mental health service use, in ways that were anticipated on the basis of previous literature. This is especially true for prevalence rates, and less true for general offending rates, use rates, or scale scores. With regard to *race,* blacks tend to have as high or higher prevalence for serious offenses and whites have as high or higher prevalence for less serious offenses and for alcohol and polydrug use. These differences are typically not reflected in general offending rates. Blacks also have higher scale scores and prevalence rates of mental health problems except depression, for which whites have higher prevalence and mean number of depressive symptoms, and there is no difference in mental health service. use. *Social class* is related only to the more serious offenses, with the lower class having higher prevalence but not necessarily higher general offending rates than the middle class, and no systematic differences on the less serious offenses. Although the middle class appears to have higher prevalence rates of alcohol use and DUI for later years, the lower class has a higher mean general offending rate for DUI, and there appears to be little difference in marijuana use. Mental health problems (but not depression) are higher among the lower class, but mental health service use is higher among the middle class. *Age* differences are consistent with prior research indicating a curvilinear relationship between age and delinquency, with delinquency peaking in middle to late adolescence, and a positive relationship between increasing age and alcohol and drug use. Depression and mental health service use, but not mental health problems (emotional problems plus social isolation), also increase with age. There is only a weak relationship between *urban* residence and delinquency, and alcohol and drug use, and little relationship with the various mental health measures. Overall, the demographic variables are weak to moderate predictors of delinquency and ADM problems.

3
Prevalence and General Offending/Use Patterns: The Joint Occurrence of Delinquent Behavior and ADM Problems

The focus in this chapter is on the joint occurrence of delinquent behavior, alcohol and illicit drug use, and mental health problems. In this analysis we employ the delinquent and alcohol, drug, and mental health (ADM) problem typologies described earlier in Chapter 1. As in Chapter 2, the data presented in the figures and tables are for the years 1976, 1980, and 1983 and whenever these years' data do not fairly reflect the patterns of prevalence and general offending rates for all six of the study years, this observation will be noted. Data are first presented for the delinquency, drug use, and mental health problem types considered separately, then for the combined problem types.

The Prevalence of Specific Problem Types

Annual prevalence rates for each delinquent, drug use, and mental health problem type are presented in Figure 3.1. As expected, the annual prevalence rates indicate that the more serious forms of delinquency and ADM problems are relatively rare in the adolescent population. Since the panel was aged 11–17 in 1976, the data in Figure 3.1 reflect general rates in the adolescent population for that year. In 1976, 8.6% of the sample were classified as serious delinquent offenders, 3.4% as polydrug users, and 12.3% as having mental health problems. The proportion of the sample classified as serious delinquents or as having mental health problems was more than twice the proportion classified as polydrug users in 1976. Taking a slightly different approach, 60% of the sample in 1976 were classified as nondelinquent, 72.6% as nonusers of alcohol and drugs, and 87.7% as not having mental health problems.

It must be remembered that these are *annual* prevalence rates, not lifetime prevalence rates or prevalence for a population over the population's adolescent years. In this sense, the estimate that nearly 9% of adolescents were involved in serious and frequent delinquent acts in the year 1976 may be viewed as a rather high level of serious delinquency.

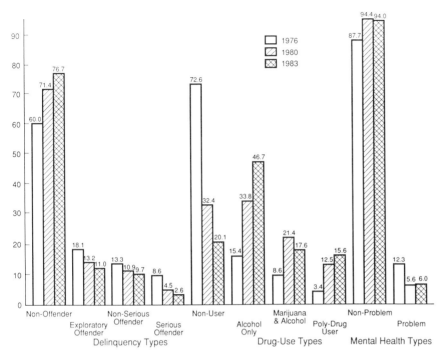

FIGURE 3.1 Prevalence Rates for Delinquent and ADM Problem Types—1976, 1980, and 1983

That 12% of youth are classified as having mental health problems may also be viewed as a relatively high annual prevalence rate. Translating these sample estimates into numerical estimates for the youth population (with .95 confidence intervals) generates an estimated 2 (± 1) million youth involved in frequent, serious delinquent acts, 1 (± .3) million youth involved in multiple illicit drug use and 3.5 (± 1.0) million youth with mental health problems in the year 1976.

By 1980 when the youth panel was aged 15–21, there were substantial changes in these prevalence rates. The annual rate for serious delinquents declined nearly 50% to 4.5% of youth; the annual rate for polydrug users increased nearly fourfold to more than 12% of youth; and the annual rate for mental health problem youth declined more than 50% to 5.6% of sample youth. Of the sample youth, 10% were classified as problem substance users in 1980.

In 1983, when the panel was aged 18–24, the annual prevalence rate for serious delinquency was down to 2.6%, a decline of 42% from 1980 and a decline of 70% from 1976. Polydrug use increased in prevalence to 15.6%, a 350% increase from 1976. The prevalence rate for mental health problems remained essentially stable, increasing only from 5.6% in 1980 to 6.0%. It is important to note that over the 8-year period from 1976 to

1983, the direction and magnitude of change in the annual prevalence of serious delinquency and polydrug use was quite different. These data, together with the data presented in Chapter 2, indicate that the dynamics of serious drug use over the adolescent and early adult years is quite different from that for serious delinquency and mental health problems.

Patterns of Prevalence and General Offending Rates by Delinquency Types

The patterns of prevalence and general offending rates for delinquent behavior by delinquency type are, at least in part, a simple reflection of the classification rules used to define these types. This is particularly true for the summary scales (General Delinquency and Index) that were used in the classification rules; that is, by definition, the prevalence of general delinquency will be 100% for all types except nondelinquents, and the prevalence of Index offenses will be 100% for serious offenders. However, this situation does not hold for the other specific scales. For this reason, we consider patterns of prevalence and general offending for each measure of delinquent behavior, drug use, and mental health problems by delinquent type. These data are presented in Table 3.1. In this section our focus is upon the prevalence and general offending rates for specific types of delinquent behavior.

In 1976, those classified as serious delinquents reported an average of 4.6 felony assaults, 5.1 felony thefts, 3.2 robberies, 10 Index offenses, and 118 total offenses. General offending rates in 1980 were similar, with 5.0 felony assaults, 7.7 felony thefts, 2.1 robberies, 11 Index offenses, and 161 total offenses. In 1983, felony assaults were down to 3.5, felony thefts were up to 11.7, robberies were down to zero (the entire sample reported a total of 5 robberies), Index offenses were down (slightly) to 9.9, and general delinquency was down slightly, to 151 offenses. Although our classification rules required a minimum of three Index offenses to be classified as a serious offender, these general offending rates are far above the minimums required. It is also important to note that serious offenders report extremely high rates of nonserious offenses as well. Compared to nonserious offenders (who by definition have 12 or more offenses per year), serious offenders report two to three times as many nonserious offenses each year.

Prevalence followed a somewhat different pattern over time. Prevalence of felony assault among serious offenders went from 89% in 1976 to 81% in 1980 and 85% in 1983. Prevalence was thus negatively associated with general offending rates for felony assault, but the variations in both were small and may represent no more than random variations in estimates. Prevalence rates for felony theft rose along with general offending rates for felony theft, and both prevalence and general offending rates for robbery declined.

Prevalence of Index offenses among those classified as serious delinquents is, by definition, 100%. Serious offenders constituted 8.6% of the sample in 1976 and only 2.6% of the sample in 1983, but accounted for more than three-fourths of all Index offenses reported in the sample each year. General offending rates for Index offenses remained stable for serious offenders, even though their numbers were declining substantially over time. In 1976 and 1980, serious offenders accounted for 62% and 50%, respectively, of *all* delinquent offenses (general delinquency). However, in 1983 they accounted for only one-third of all offenses. In sum then, prevalence rates declined over time as did offending rates for delinquency in general.

Given the pattern of prevalence and individual offending rates, the observed decline in the general offending rate for Index offenses in the total sample from 1976 to 1983 is explained primarily by a decline in the prevalence of serious offenders in the population.[1] The decline in prevalence also appears to be the explanation for the observed decline in the general delinquency offending rate, since there were *increases* in individual offending rates (the rate for active offenders) for all delinquent types (except nondelinquents).

In part as a result of the rules for constructing the delinquent types, the relationship between *general offending rates* and delinquent types is monotonic increasing for minor offenses (minor assaults, minor thefts, illegal services, public disorder, and vandalism) and general delinquency. Even though nonserious delinquents could, in principle, have higher rates of offending for minor offenses than serious delinquents, the latter have the highest offending rates for every type of offense, followed by nonserious delinquents, exploratory delinquents, and, finally, nondelinquents.

The same consistent pattern is evident in *prevalence rates* for minor thefts, illegal services, and vandalism. For public disorder in 1980, however, exploratory delinquents have the highest prevalence (by 0.2%), followed by nonserious and then serious delinquents, but the numbers are close and may reflect little more than random error. For 1976 and 1983, prevalence of public disorder follows the same pattern of offending rates, with serious delinquents highest and nondelinquents lowest. Minor

---

[1] Prevalence and general offending rates for the total sample are presented in Table 3.3. This conclusion is based on the fact that individual offending rates for Index offenses were relatively constant for serious offenders over the entire period of the study, e.g., 490 Index offenses per person in 1976, 500 in 1980, and 374 in 1983. Since serious offenders account for the vast majority of all Index offenses in the sample each year, the observed decline in general offending rates for this offense over time was primarily a result of declining prevalence rates for serious offenders.

TABLE 3.1. Prevalence and general offending/use rates[a] by delinquent type: 1976, 1980, and 1983.[b]

	1976				1980				1983			
	Nonoffender	Exploratory	Nonserious	Serious	Nonoffender	Exploratory	Nonserious	Serious	Nonoffender	Exploratory	Nonserious	Serious
Felony assault												
Prevalence	0.0	24.1	35.8	89.0	0.0	18.3	27.2	80.6	0.0	22.1	23.4	84.6
Offending rate[c]	0	24	57	460	0	18	41	501	0	22	37	346
% of total	0	8	15	77	0	8	15	77	0	16	24	60
Felony theft												
Prevalence	1.0	14.3	31.4	56.8	1.1	16.2	24.2	65.7	1.5	21.5	29.7	69.2
Offending rate	1	19	144	513	1	24	47	770	2	37	88	1174
% of total	1	5	28	65	2	7	12	79	3	9	19	68
Robbery												
Prevalence	0.0	4.2	.58	42.5	0.0	1.0	4.9	25.4	0.0	1.2	1.4	0.0
Offending rate	0	4	8	318	0	1	9	206	0	1	2	0
% of total	0	3	4	93	0	1	10	89	0	40	60	0
Index offenses												
Prevalence	0.0	32.2	46.5	100.0	0.0	26.9	40.1	100.0	0.0	30.7	31.7	100.0
Offending rate	0	32	77	995	0	27	64	1140	0	31	52	990
% of total	0	6	10	84	0	6	11	83	0	10	15	75
Minor assault												
Prevalence	27.7	79.8	84.5	93.2	8.9	46.2	45.7	73.1	3.0	18.4	17.9	30.8
Offending rate	43	254	1844	5093	14	117	244	1513	4	39	68	277
% of total	3	6	32	58	8	13	22	57	16	20	31	34
Minor theft												
Prevalence	5.9	29.0	48.2	61.0	3.8	33.0	40.7	68.7	4.2	25.2	34.5	53.8
Offending rate	8	58	366	1204	5	90	418	1069	6	82	334	1077
% of total	3	6	29	62	4	11	42	44	6	12	44	38
Illegal services												
Prevalence	0.7	5.2	13.3	26.4	1.5	23.4	37.7	56.7	0.6	19.6	42.1	56.4
Offending rate	1	14	128	1104	3	77	1282	6640	1	77	1699	7231
% of total	0	2	15	82	1	2	31	66	0	2	45	52
Public disorder												
Prevalence	21.0	67.0	78.2	80.1	33.5	84.2	84.0	80.6	36.3	82.8	86.2	89.7
Offending rate	112	338	1659	3606	229	1437	3807	5942	288	994	3233	3982
% of total	10	9	33	47	16	18	40	26	29	15	42	14
Vandalism												
Prevalence	20.7	47.2	59.7	76.7	6.1	31.5	34.0	71.2	1.9	13.5	22.8	51.3
Offending rate	57	148	299	2033	18	83	129	571	3	31	57	497
% of total	12	10	14	64	21	17	22	40	10	14	23	53

General delinquency												
Prevalence	41.7	100.0	100.0	100.0	26.8	100.0	100.0	100.0	22.3	100.0	100.0	100.0
Offending rate	73	549	3534	11751	48	567	5670	16142	39	575	7264	15100
% of total	3	6	29	62	2	5	42	50	2	5	59	33
Alcohol use												
Prevalence	34.3	58.3	66.4	73.3	75.0	94.9	96.9	94.0	85.4	97.5	96.6	97.4
Use rate	298	683	1567	2781	2718	6586	10136	12075	4360	8617	10884	15964
% of total	24	16	28	32	44	20	25	12	58	16	18	7
Marijuana use												
Prevalence	8.2	22.8	36.3	39.7	32.7	65.5	72.2	85.1	34.5	66.9	72.4	92.3
Use rate	166	839	1823	2740	1081	4939	9933	14001	1723	3834	11412	16495
% of total	14	21	33	32	25	21	34	20	40	13	34	13
Polydrug use												
Prevalence	1.9	5.9	11.6	20.0	8.0	24.4	47.5	55.2	12.8	38.0	53.8	76.9
Use rate	68	26	231	406	116	480	1876	4352	273	1236	2237	10046
% of total	37	4	28	31	15	12	38	36	25	16	26	32
Problem Substance use												
Prevalence	Not available in 1976	Not available in 1976			2.9	19.8	28.4	54.5	3.2	13.0	26.2	43.6
Mean scale score	Not available in 1976	Not available in 1976			5.90	10.40	11.83	15.52	7.33	12.45	14.89	22.60
DWI/DUI												
Prevalence	Not available in 1976	Not available in 1976			Not available in 1980	Not available in 1980			37.5	58.3	72.4	74.2
Offending rate	Not available in 1976	Not available in 1976			Not available in 1980	Not available in 1980			936	1713	7341	9942
% of total	Not available in 1976	Not available in 1976			Not available in 1980	Not available in 1980			35	10	41	15
Mental health problems												
Prevalence	9.2	12.7	14.2	27.6	4.5	8.7	2.5	21.2	3.7	10.4	11.7	25.6
Mean scale score	28.14	40.31	41.46	44.70	34.53	37.24	36.52	42.79	15.53	17.26	17.96	21.08
Depression												
Prevalence	Not available in 1976	Not available in 1976			Not available in 1980	Not available in 1980			24.8	33.7	31.0	33.3
Mean no. of symptoms	Not available in 1976	Not available in 1976			Not available in 1980	Not available in 1980			.66	.93	.86	1.05
% of total	Not available in 1976	Not available in 1976			Not available in 1980	Not available in 1980			70	14	12	4
Mental health service use												
Prevalence	Not available in 1976	Not available in 1976			Not available in 1980	Not available in 1980			6.9	6.1	13.8	10.3
Mean no. of uses	Not available in 1976	Not available in 1976			Not available in 1980	Not available in 1980			.85	.44	1.29	.33 NS
% of total	Not available in 1976	Not available in 1976			Not available in 1980	Not available in 1980			79	6	15	1

[a] Rates per 100 persons.

[b] All differences by type are statistically significant ($p \le .05$) unless otherwise indicated (i.e., NS).

[c] Percentage of total offenses committed by those in the category.

assault in 1976 follows the typical pattern (serious highest, then nonserious, exploratory, and nonoffenders) but in 1980 and 1983 the prevalence of minor assault is slightly higher for exploratory offenders than for nonserious offenders. The figures are close—both about 46% in 1980 and 18% in 1983—and for both years serious offenders have the highest prevalence and nonoffenders the lowest. It is worth recalling that the minor assault scale had the lowest reliability and the highest proportion of trivial offenses reported of all the offense scales. For general delinquency, prevalence is 100% by definition for all but nonoffenders.

Significance tests for differences among the delinquent types for prevalence (chi-square) and general offending rates (F) indicate that all of the differences among types are statistically significant at the .01 level or better. For minor as well as Index crimes, nonoffenders consistently had the lowest prevalence rates and (by definition) the lowest offending rates. With almost equal consistency, serious offenders had the highest rates of both prevalence and offending, with nonserious and exploratory offenders usually following in that order. The small group of serious offenders does appear to be a truly serious and high-frequency group of offenders, and their self-reported levels of criminal behavior are quite similar to those reported by youth on probation (Krisberg & Austin, 1983) and an adult prison population (Chaiken & Chaiken, 1982; Petersilia, Greenwood, & Lavin, 1978).

Delinquency Types and Drug Use

Although there is no necessary relationship (by definition) between the delinquency typology and use of alcohol, marijuana, or other illicit drugs, there is a clear, monotonic relationship between delinquency type and use rates of alcohol, marijuana, and multiple illicit drugs for all three years. Serious offenders have the highest rates of consumption of alcohol, marijuana, and other illicit drugs; nonserious offenders are next, followed by exploratory offenders and, with the lowest use rates, nonoffenders. The same pattern holds for prevalence of marijuana and multiple illicit drug use, and for alcohol in 1976. For 1980 and 1983, however, there is little difference in the prevalence of alcohol use among serious, nonserious, and exploratory offenders, but nonoffenders consistently have the lowest prevalence of alcohol use.

Problem use of alcohol, marijuana, and other drugs has much the same relationship to the delinquency types as general use of those substances. Serious offenders have the highest prevalence rates and mean scale scores for problem substance use, followed in turn by nonserious offenders, exploratory offenders, and nonoffenders. This pattern holds for both 1980 and 1983. Driving while intoxicated or under the influence of alcohol, marijuana, or other drugs also follows this pattern.

The prevalence and use rates of alcohol and multiple illicit drugs increases consistently over the 8 years covered by waves 1–6. Marijuana use and prevalence rates increase from 1976 to 1980, but appear to remain stable from 1980 to 1983. In part, this result may reflect a general period decline in marijuana use beginning about 1980 (Flanagan & McGarrell, 1986, p. 331) coupled with a trend toward increasing use with increasing age. In general, delinquent types were clearly differentiated by use of both conventional and illicit drugs. The increase in the general prevalence rates for drug use between 1976 and 1983 was reflected in the drug use prevalence rates of *all* delinquency types. The increase did not occur disproportionately among the serious delinquents. Despite the general increase in substance use, *problem* substance use decreased in prevalence from 1980 to 1983. The increase in mean scale score is probably an artifact of the different methods that were used to construct the scale in 1980 (trouble associated with alcohol, with other drugs including marijuana) and 1983 (trouble associated with alcohol, with marijuana, with other drugs excluding marijuana). Overall, substance use increased but problem substance use decreased from 1980 to 1983.

Delinquency Types and Mental Health Problems

Both prevalence of mental health problems and mean mental health problem scale scores are significantly related to the delinquency types. Serious offenders have the highest prevalence of mental health problems and nonoffenders the lowest (except in 1980, when nonserious offenders report the lowest prevalence of mental health problems). Similarly, the mean mental health problem scale scores are highest for serious offenders and lowest for nonoffenders in all three years. For 1976 and 1983, the relationship is monotonic, but for 1980, nonserious offenders have the lowest prevalence and the second lowest mean scale score. In all 3 years, differences between exploratory and nonserious offenders are small. Overall, the prevalence of mental health problems appears to follow the same general pattern across types as was observed for delinquent behavior and alcohol and drug use.

For depression, available only in 1983, nonoffenders again have the lowest prevalence and the lowest mean number of symptoms. Nonserious offenders score second lowest on both measures. Exploratory offenders have the highest prevalence, but serious offenders (with prevalence almost equal to that of exploratory offenders) have the highest mean number of symptoms. The pattern for depression is similar to that for alcohol use, with nonoffenders clearly being the least affected, but with little distinction among the other three delinquency types.

Mental health service use[2] has a pattern different from depression and mental health problems. Nonserious offenders have the highest prevalence and mean frequency of use of professional mental health services. Serious offenders have the next highest prevalence, followed by nonoffenders and exploratory offenders. Serious offenders, however, have the *lowest* mean frequency of mental health service use. Nonoffenders have the second-highest mean frequency of use, followed by exploratory offenders.

Bear in mind that with mental health service use, we are not measuring symptoms or indications of mental health problems as such, but *responses* to mental health problems. Whether a person seeks professional help may be related to factors other than the nature or extent of the problem (access to services, ability to pay, stigma associated with being mentally ill). Given their high delinquency offending rates, high polydrug use and problem use rates, and high proportions with mental health problems, it might well be argued that serious delinquents are underusing mental health services. Also note that there is no statistically significant difference among the delinquency types in mean frequency of use, but differences in prevalence are statistically significant. In these different patterns of relationships between delinquency types and the three mental health problem indicators, we have the first (but not the only) indication that mental health problems are differentially distributed across delinquent types.

Patterns of Alcohol, Marijuana, and Polydrug Use by Drug Use Types

By definition of our substance use types, those classified as users of a particular substance have a 100% prevalence rate for that particular substance. Also by definition, those who are not classified as users of a particular substance but as nonusers, or users of a substance "lower" on

---

[2] In this book, we use a measure of mental health service use that differs from that used in earlier papers (Elliott et al., 1985; Elliott & Huizinga, 1984). The present measure involves utilization only of professional mental health services (mental health clinics, physicians, psychiatrists, etc.), and not nonprofessional services (friends, clergy, herbalists, etc.). For details on the contents of the index of mental health service utilization, its psychometric properties, and its relationship to other mental health measures see Appendix A and Chapter 1.

the drug typology, have low prevalence and use rates for that substance. It is clear from Table 3.2, however, that polydrug users have extremely high prevalence rates of alcohol and marijuana use, and marijuana users have extremely high prevalence rates of alcohol use (all over 95% for alcohol, about 90% for marijuana use by polydrug users). More dramatically, the use rate for all three substances (alcohol, marijuana, multiple illicit drugs) is highest for polydrug users, then for marijuana users, alcohol users, and lowest for nonusers, for all 3 years. The drug use typology thus forms an ascending scale from nonuse to extensive use; and as variety of use increases, so does frequency of use for all substances used.

There are several important observations about use rates by drug type. Not only did the prevalence rate for each drug type (and each drug substance) increase rather dramatically between 1976 and 1980, the general use rate for all drug substances taken as a whole also increased over fourfold during this 5-year period. The use rates of marijuana and other illicit drugs increased 80% and 40%, respectively, among those in the polydrug use category. The alcohol use rate doubled for each drug use type. By 1980, multiple illicit drug users in the NYS reported an average (per person) of 123 alcohol use occasions, 167 marijuana use occasions, and 44 other illicit drug use occasions during that year. Not only were more youth using each drug substance in 1980 than in 1976, but those using these drugs were using them much more frequently.

From 1980 to 1983, alcohol prevalence and use rates continued to increase. The increase in the proportion of those classified as alcohol (only) users may be attributable in part to the fact that many in the sample attained legal age for consumption of alcohol. The proportion of the sample classified as marijuana users (as opposed to nonusers, alcohol users, or polydrug users) declined slightly, but was accompanied by a slight increase in the proportion classified as polydrug users. Taken together, these two types (marijuana and polydrug users) remained constant from 1980 to 1983, as did the combined proportion of nonusers plus alcohol users.

The prevalence and use rates of marijuana remained nearly constant between 1980 and 1983, possibly reflecting countervailing trends of increased substance use with age and decreased age-specific substance use over time. (Although the proportion classified as marijuana users declined, recall that polydrug users, for whom prevalence rates increased during this same period, also use marijuana). Both polydrug prevalence and use rates increased. As noted earlier, the prevalence of problem substance use decreased, and although mean scale scores may be compared across types within a given year, comparison between years is problematic as the measures changed. The scale score and prevalence rate of problem substance use is highest for polydrug users, followed by marijuana users and alcohol users, and lowest for nonusers.

TABLE 3.2. Prevalence and general offending/use rates[a] by drug user type: 1976, 1980, and 1983.[b]

	1976				1980				1983			
	Nonuser	Alcohol	Marijuana	Polydrug	Nonuser	Alcohol	Marijuana	Polydrug	Nonuser	Alcohol	Marijuana	Polydrug
Felony assault												
Prevalence	12.7	18.3	33.8	51.7	4.1	5.2	13.5	24.2	1.0	4.6	11.4	16.7
Offending rate	36	56	118	181	8	15	38	110	1	7	19	54
% of total[c]	51	17	20	12	9	17	27	47	1	21	22	56
Felony theft												
Prevalence	6.3	18.6	32.4	55.2	2.3	4.4	13.5	27.3	2.0	3.4	9.8	28.3
Offending rate	14	97	137	869	4	9	44	243	3	8	29	226
% of total	16	22	18	44	3	7	21	70	1	9	11	79
Robbery												
Prevalence	4.0	5.7	6.8	22.4	0.8	0.4	2.8	6.4	0.7	0.1	0.0	0.4 NS
Offending rate	14	77	32	122	11	1	8	36	1	0	0	1 NS
% of total	35	41	10	14	35	5	16	44 NS	40	20	0	40
Index offenses												
Prevalence	15.3	24.8	41.5	58.6	5.6	6.7	20.1	32.3	2.0	6.0	12.5	23.5
Offending rate	54	148	205	597	21	19	70	268	3	8	33	155
% of total	39	23	18	20	11	10	24	54	2	12	17	70
Minor assault												
Prevalence	45.4	59.5	65.3	72.4	17.2	19.0	23.3	29.9	3.0	6.2	5.3	15.7
Offending rate	513	1238	1207	2645	54	56	100	496	4	18	17	60
% of total	49	25	14	12	14	16	18	52	4	39	14	43
Minor theft												
Prevalence	12.6	33.7	49.3	50.0	4.6	10.7	23.2	36.4	4.0	6.7	14.4	27.0
Offending rate	97	248	305	898	9	28	201	428	9	29	49	321
% of total	43	23	16	18	3	9	39	49	2	18	12	68
Illegal services												
Prevalence	0.9	1.1	27.4	60.3	0.6	1.0	18.8	50.0	0.7	0.3	14.4	35.3
Offending rate	1	5	518	1962	3	3	122	3382	101	1	120	2228
% of total	1	1	39	59	0	0	6	94	5	9	5	90
Public disorder												
Prevalence	28.8	71.2	85.0	84.5	15.8	49.9	69.3	87.7	12.4	45.8	62.9	82.0
Offending rate	249	660	2272	5193	98	474	1237	4601	41	437	768	2564
% of total	28	16	30	27	3	15	26	56	1	27	18	53
Vandalism												
Prevalence	30.6	40.5	56.8	62.1	9.7	12.3	19.7	31.2	1.7	3.9	8.0	19.0
Offending rate	150	291	1101	719	32	40	97	153	4	16	23	76
% of total	40	16	35	9	16	21	33	30	4	31	17	48

General delinquency											
Prevalence	55.9	87.0	90.3	91.4	41.7	66.0	84.9	16.8	34.0	51.9	77.6
Offending rate	867	2282	4001	8400	509	1350	7169	227	479	974	4919
% of total	39	22	21	18	12	20	62	4	19	14	63
Alcohol use											
Prevalence	26.6	100.0	95.3	96.6	100.0	97.8	98.9	44.0	100.0	97.7	98.7
Use rate	53	1980	2808	4595	3985	7222	12289	86	5608	7347	11819
% of total	5	41	33	21	30	35	35	0	45	22	32
Marijuana use											
Prevalence	3.4	20.5	100.0	89.7	23.6	100.0	97.9	5.7	22.5	100.0	90.6
Use rate	7	45	4396	9288	50	4837	16736	9	41	7130	12808
% of total	1	1	54	45	1	33	66	0	1	38	61
Polydrug Use											
Prevalence	0.4	1.9	16.2	100.0	2.0	16.0	100.0	1.0	4.4	20.5	100.0
Use rate	1	4	32	3131	4	25	4372	2	8	38	5229
% of total	1	1	3	96	0	1	99	0	0	1	99
Problem Substance use											
Prevalence	Not available in 1976	Not available in 1976			7.5	13.8	37.4	0.3	3.3	11.7	24.9
Mean scale score	Not available in 1976	Not available in 1976			3.66	11.79	14.90	2.64	7.11	12.82	18.88
DWI/DUI											
Prevalence	Not available in 1976	Not available in 1976			Not available in 1980			2.5	41.0	60.2	89.1
Offending rate	Not available in 1976	Not available in 1976			Not available in 1980			7	353	2472	8548
% of total	Not available in 1976	Not available in 1976			Not available in 1980			0	8	25	67
Mental health problems											
Prevalence	10.8	12.5	19.0	26.3	4.8	4.7	10.2	5.0	4.0	7.2	11.6
Mean scale score	39.00	39.84	41.42	45.33	34.56	36.52	39.02	15.56	15.42	16.88	18.21
Depression											
Prevalence	Not available in 1976	Not available in 1976			Not available in 1980			21.0	25.3	26.5	39.1
Mean # symptoms	Not available in 1976	Not available in 1976			Not available in 1980			.51	.68	.71	1.12
% of total	Not available in 1976	Not available in 1976			Not available in 1980			14	44	17	24
Mental health service use											
Prevalence	Not available in 1976	Not available in 1976			Not available in 1980			7.7	5.6	9.5	12.4
Mean # uses	Not available in 1976	Not available in 1976			Not available in 1980			.44	.74	1.15	2.24
% of total	Not available in 1976	Not available in 1976			Not available in 1980			9	37	21	33

[a] Rates per 100 persons.

[b] All difference by type are statistically significant ($p \leq .05$) unless otherwise indicated (i.e., NS).

[c] Percentage of total offenses committed by those in the category.

Drug Use Types and Delinquent Behavior

There is a strong and consistent relationship between the prevalence and offending rates of delinquent behavior and the drug use types. Drug use types are clearly differentiated on the basis of their involvement in all types of delinquent behavior, and, with two exceptions, polydrug users report the highest prevalence and general offending rates and nonusers the lowest. The two exceptions are robbery in 1983, for which there were too few cases (5 robberies) for a clear pattern to emerge, and illegal services in 1983, for which alcohol users report lower prevalence and general offending rates than nonusers. For most other offenses, there is a clear ordering from polydrug users to marijuana users to alcohol users to nonusers for both prevalence and general offending rates, but on a few offenses (prevalence and general offending rate of minor assault in 1983, offending rates on robbery and minor assault in 1976) alcohol users have higher rates than marijuana users.

In 1980, 12.5% of the sample were classified as polydrug users, and this group accounted for 47% of all felony assaults, 70% of all felony thefts, 44% of all robberies, 54% of all index offenses, and 62% of all offenses included in the general delinquency measure. In 1983 the polydrug users constituted 15.6% of the total sample and accounted for 56% of felony assaults, 79% of felony thefts, 40% of all robberies, 70% of all Index offenses, and 63% of general delinquency. For most offenses, the slight increase in the proportion classified as polydrug users was accompanied by a small increase in the proportion of offenses accounted for by this type.

There are several specific findings that deserve highlighting. First, the felony theft general offending rate for polydrug users in 1976 is as great as that for serious delinquents (8.7% vs. 5.1%, $p=$NS) and the prevalence rates are very similar (55% vs. 57%). Although this pattern is not observed in 1980 or 1983, polydrug users (12.5%) do account for 70% of all felony thefts in 1980 and 79% of felony thefts in 1983; and while constituting only 3.4% of youth in 1976, they account for 44% of all felony thefts that year. It is clear that multiple illicit drug users account for a highly disproportionate number of felony thefts in both years.

Patterns of illegal services crimes also appear unusual. It should be noted however that two offenses, selling marijuana and other illicit drugs, account for the majority (over 90%) of all illegal service offenses reported each year. (The other offense in this category is prostitution.) Both the prevalence and general offending rates for illegal services are higher for multiple illicit drug users than serious delinquents in 1976, and this small group (3.4%) of drug users accounts for nearly 60% of all illegal service crimes. This result reflects a very high association between polydrug use and selling drugs. For 1980 and 1983 neither the prevalence nor the general offending rate is as high for polydrug users as for serious delinquents. Still, 94% of all reported drug sales and prostitution in 1980 and 89% in 1983 involved polydrug users. Virtually no drug sales were reported by nondrug users or alcohol users in 1976 or 1980. The high offending rate of nonusers for illegal services in 1983 is wholly attributable to a single respondent who, though reporting no personal use of alcohol, marijuana, or other drugs, reported selling marijuana almost daily (300 times) in 1983.

An examination of public disorder offense rates reveals a pattern similar to that observed for illegal services. Both prevalence and offending rates are higher in 1976 and the prevalence rate is higher in 1980 for polydrug users compared to serious delinquent offenders (note that these types are not independent). By 1983, however, serious delinquent offenders have higher prevalence and offense rates for public disorder than do polydrug users. Illicit drug use is thus linked very strongly to serious theft, illegal service offenses (primarily drug sales) and, at least during adolescence, to public disorder crimes.

It is also interesting to note the rather dramatic decline over time in delinquency rates, both serious and nonserious, for those in the nonuser category. In 1976, 15% of nonusers report Index offenses, compared to 6% in 1980 and 2% in 1983. Likewise, in 1976, 56% of nonusers report some delinquency (General Delinquency scale), compared to 28% in 1980 and 17% in 1983. As the youth panel moves into mid-adolescence and then late adolescence, when alcohol use becomes normative, those individuals who are classified as nonusers have increasingly lower rates of delinquency. This finding suggests that dropping out of the nonuser class may be associated with prior delinquency, an observation which is confirmed in Chapter 5.

Drug Use Types and Mental Health Problems

Polydrug users consistently have the highest prevalence of mental health problems and the highest mental health problem scale scores (Table 3.3). Rank on scale scores is fairly consistent, with polydrug users followed by marijuana users, then alcohol users, then nonusers except for 1983, when alcohol users and nonusers are reversed (but almost equal). Prevalence of mental health problems is lowest among nonusers in 1976 but lowest among alcohol users in 1983, perhaps reflecting a shift in age-specific norms regarding alcohol use. In 1980, prevalence of mental health problems is lowest (by 0.1%) among marijuana users, then alcohol users, then nonusers but the differences are so small as to render the three groups practically equal. For nonusers and alcohol users, prevalence rates of mental health problems decline monotonically over time, but for marijuana and polydrug users they decline and then increase. Because of

TABLE 3.3. Prevalence and general offending/use rates[a] by mental health problem type: 1976, 1980, and 1983.[b]

	1976			1980			1983		
	Nonproblem	Problem	Total sample	Nonproblem	Problem	Total sample	Nonproblem	Problem	Total sample
Felony assault									
Prevalence	15.2	28.4 NS	11.8	8.2	20.5	9.0	5.6	28.4	7.0
Offending rate	48	70	51	23	124	29	13	53	15
% of total[c]	83	17	100	76	24	100	79	21	100
Felony theft									
Prevalence	11.0	20.5 NS	12.2	7.9	18.1	8.5	7.4	20.2 NS	8.2
Offending rate	64	89	67	32	236	44	40	115	45
% of total	84	16	100	70	30	100	85	15	100
Robbery									
Prevalence	4.1	12.4 NS	5.2	1.5	7.2	1.8	0.3	0.0 NS	0.3
Offending rate	26	52	29	8	43	10	0	0 NS	0
% of total	78	22	100	77	23	100	100	0	100
Index offenses									
Prevalence	18.2	37.5	20.6	11.4	26.5	12.4	7.7	31.4	9.1
Offending rate	93	163	101	47	305	62	29	124	34
% of total	80	20	100	72	28	100	79	21	100
Minor assault									
Prevalence	49.3	57.3 NS	50.4	20.2	28.9 NS	20.7	6.3	14.8 NS	6.8
Offending rate	691	1244	756	74	892	120	21	39	22
% of total	80	20	100	59	41	100	89	11	100
Minor theft									
Prevalence	19.9	23.8 NS	20.4	14.1	24.1	14.6	9.8	25.0	10.7
Offending rate	124	471	166	95	351	109	68	175	74
% of total	65	35	100	72	18	100	86	14	100
Illegal services									
Prevalence	4.4	12.3	5.3	10.4	16.9 NS	10.8	7.4	22.5 NS	8.3
Offending rate	77	382	113	231	4170	450	336	1211	388
% of total	60	40	100	48	52	100	81	19	100
Public disorder									
Prevalence	41.0	48.8 NS	41.1	46.8	65.1	47.7	46.9	62.5	47.8
Offending rate	595	1983	653	905	3230	1033	691	1680	748
% of total	80	20	100	83	17	100	87	13	100
Vandalism									
Prevalence	33.9	46.7 NS	35.5	14.8	25.6	15.4	6.1	12.5 NS	6.5
Offending rate	287	175	273	56	205	64	24	38	24
% of total	92	8	100	82	18	100	91	9	100

General delinquency									
Prevalence	63.5	74.9	64.9	47.0	59.0	47.7	39.1	62.8	40.4
Offending rate	1442	2900	1611	1027	8199	1450	1081	3108	1197
% of total	22	78	100	68	32	100	85	15	100
Alcohol use									
Prevalence	45.7	51.0 NS	46.3	80.8	80.7 NS	80.9	88.0	91.0 NS	88.2
Use rate	686	1208	748	4426	4555 NS	4452	5680	7403 NS	5775
% of total	80	20	100	94	6	100	92	8	100
Marijuana use									
Prevalence	16.3	24.8	17.3	43.4	50.6 NS	43.8	42.1	65.2	43.4
Use rate	610	1554	723	2890	7589	3148	3013	7469	3274
% of total	74	26	100	87	13	100	86	14	100
Polydrug use									
Prevalence	4.6	10.5	5.4	16.0	26.5	16.6	20.6	36.0	21.4
Use rate	72	378	110	441	2482	554	721	2492	825
% of total	58	42	100	75	25	100	82	18	100
Problem substance use									
Prevalence	Not available in 1976	Not available in 1976		9.6	21.7	10.2	6.8	20.7	7.6
Mean scale score	Not available in 1976	Not available in 1976		3.48	9.69	7.60	8.76	13.85	9.05
DWI/DUI									
Prevalence	Not available in 1976	Not available in 1976		Not available in 1980	Not available in 1980	Not available in 1980	44.9	45.6 NS	49.4
Offending rate	Not available in 1976	Not available in 1976		Not available in 1980	Not available in 1980	Not available in 1980	1997	1854 NS	1986
% of total	Not available in 1976	Not available in 1976		Not available in 1980	Not available in 1980	Not available in 1980	94	6	100
Mental health problems									
Prevalence	0.0	100.0	12.3	0.0	100.0	5.6	0.0	100.0	6.0
Mean scale score	37.66	53.10	39.56	34.48	52.20	35.46	15.31	29.29	16.14
Depression									
Prevalence	Not available in 1976	Not available in 1976		Not available in 1980	Not available in 1980		24.6	61.8	26.8
Mean # symptoms	Not available in 1976	Not available in 1976		Not available in 1980	Not available in 1980		.63	2.15	.72
% of total	Not available in 1976	Not available in 1976		Not available in 1980	Not available in 1980		82	18	100
Mental health service use									
Prevalence	Not available in 1976	Not available in 1976		Not available in 1980	Not available in 1980		6.4	29.5	8.2
Mean # uses	Not available in 1976	Not available in 1976		Not available in 1980	Not available in 1980		.63	7.05	.96
% of total	Not available in 1976	Not available in 1976		Not available in 1980	Not available in 1980		62	38	100

[a] Rates per 100 persons.

[b] All difference by type are statistically significant ($p \leq .05$) unless otherwise indicated (i.e., NS).

[c] Percentage of total offenses committed by those in the category.

the change in measuring mental health problems in 1983, we cannot be certain whether this result is a measurement artifact, reflective of an age-specific shift in norms regarding experimental drug use, or a more general shift in societal norms.

Depression has a clear monotonic relationship with drug use type for 1983, with polydrug users reporting the highest prevalence and frequency of depressive symptoms, followed by marijuana users, alcohol users, and nonusers. The prevalence and mean frequency of depressive symptoms are slightly higher among polydrug users than among serious delinquent offenders. Mental health service use follows a similar pattern, except that prevalence of mental health service use is lower among alcohol users than among nonusers. Mean frequency of mental health service use, however, is higher among alcohol users than among nonusers. Polydrug users have by far the highest mean frequency of mental health service use, nearly twice that of the next highest group (nonserious offenders). Clearly, there is a link between drug use patterns and mental health problems.

Patterns of Prevalence and General Offending by Mental Health Problem Type

There are two important ways in which the mental health problem typology differs from the delinquent offense and drug use typologies. First, the mental health typology is not inclusive of the full range of potential mental health problems. Second, even disregarding its lower inclusiveness, the mental health typology is cruder than the other two typologies. Instead of a series of four categories representing increasing levels of seriousness, the mental health problem typology is dichotomous; instead of being based on a specified number of incidents with specific levels of seriousness (in terms of legal and normative violation), it is based on an attitudinal scale score with less than an interval level of measurement. Based on these qualifications we may expect some attenuation in the relationships of other variables with the mental health problem typology as compared to the delinquent offense and drug use typologies.

Individuals classified as having mental health problems have mean mental health problem scale scores 1.4 to 1.9 times as large as those not classified as having mental health problems. They also have significantly higher prevalence and mean number of symptoms of depression, and prevalence and mean frequency of mental health service utilization as those not classified as having mental health problems. In terms of prevalence, those classified as having mental health problems are 2.5 times as likely to report depressive symptoms and 4.6 times as likely to have used professional mental health services as those not so classified.

People classified as having mental health problems have an average of 3.4 times as many symptoms of depression and are more than 11 times as likely to receive professional mental health services as those people who are not. Although the three mental health measures are conceptually distinct, it is clear that there is substantial overlap between our mental health problem typology and the other two mental health problem indicators.

Mental Health Problem Types and Delinquent Behavior

Mental health problems are significantly related to the prevalence of felony assault, felony theft, robbery (except for 1983), and Index offenses, usually with ratios of about 2 : 1 between mental health problem and nonproblem respondents. The relationship of mental health problems to general offending rates is not as clear. Those subjects with mental health problems have significantly higher offending rates for Index offenses in 1976, 1980, and 1983, and for felony assault in 1980, and 1983, but for robbery and felony theft only in 1980. They have significantly higher prevalence and offending rates for general delinquency and public disorder for all three years, but their pattern on other offenses varies.

For minor assaults, individuals with mental health problems have significantly higher prevalence rates but not general offending rates in 1976 and 1983, and higher general offending rates but not prevalence rates in 1980. For minor thefts, only the general offending rate is significantly higher in 1976, only the prevalence rate is higher in 1983, and both prevalence and offending rates are higher in 1980 for those subjects with mental health problems. Individuals classified as having mental health problems showed significantly higher prevalence and general offending rates on illegal services in 1976, higher offending rates but not prevalence rates in 1980, and higher prevalence but not significantly higher offending rates in 1983. For vandalism, the general offending rate is significantly *lower* in 1976 for subjects classified as having mental health problems; the general offending rate in 1980 and prevalence rates in both 1980 and 1983 are higher for those individuals classified as having mental health problems.

One conclusion to be drawn from these relationships is that mental health problems are related to delinquent behavior generally but may not be related to specific types of delinquent behavior. Second, with the exception of vandalism in 1980 and robbery in 1983, individuals with mental health problems consistently, if not always significantly, have higher offending and prevalence rates than those without mental health problems. The general pattern is clearly one which indicates that mental health problems are associated with delinquent behavior, but it is equally clear, at least with the present, limited measure of mental health problems, that this relationship is much weaker than the relationship between drug use and delinquency. Finally, only the more general summary scales (Index and General Delinquency) and one of the two offense category scales (Public Disorder) have a consistent relationship with mental health problem type. The less general offense-specific scales have a relationship with mental health problem type that is not consistent over time. It is thus possible that those with mental health problems are prone to getting into trouble, but the crudeness of the mental health measure renders this finding difficult to detect except with broad, summary measures of delinquent behavior.

Mental Health Problem Type and Alcohol, Marijuana, and Polydrug Use

Being classified as having mental health problems is not significantly related to prevalence of alcohol use in any of the three years (1976, 1980, 1983), nor is it related to the use rate of alcohol except in 1976. People with mental health problems have significantly higher use rates of marijuana for all three years, and higher prevalence of marijuana use except in 1980. Having mental health problems is consistently associated with polydrug prevalence and use rates, and with prevalence and scale scores of problem substance use in 1980 and 1983. There appears to be no relationship, however, between mental health problem type and prevalence or offending rate of DUI, a fact which is surprising in light of the association between mental health problems and more serious forms of substance use. It thus appears that mental health type is closely associated with more serious forms of drug use (polydrug use and problem substance use) but not with alcohol use or DUI.

The relationship of delinquent behavior and drug use to mental health problem type is not nearly so strong or consistent as the relationship of delinquency and drug use (types and behavior) to each other. In part this finding may be a result of the crudeness of our measurement of mental health problems, yet despite this crudeness of measurement, a clear relationship emerged between mental health problem type and more serious forms of drug use. One possible conclusion is that mental health problems may be more related to certain types of problem behavior (multiple illicit drug use, problem substance use, public disorder) than to others, but that mental health problems are still at least weakly related to delinquency and drug use in general.

Serious Offender, Polydrug User, and Mental Health Problem Types

Before considering the general patterns of delinquency and ADM problems by joint types, it is appropriate to consider the prevalence of various combinations of the most serious delinquent and ADM problem types in the adolescent population. These serious joint types are presented in Figures 3.2 and 3.3.

Only 0.5% of the sample, a total of eight cases, fall into the serious delinquent–polydrug user–mental health problem category in 1976, 0.6% in 1980, and 0.5% in 1983 (see Figure 3.2). Serious delinquent polydrug users (mental health problem plus nonproblem) constituted 0.8% of the sample in 1976, 2.1% in 1980, and 1.8% in 1983. Serious delinquents with mental health problems account for 2.3% of the sample in 1976, 0.9% in 1980, and 0.7% in 1983. Polydrug users with mental health problems represented 0.9% of the sample in 1976, 1.3% in 1980, and 1.7% in 1983. These figures reflect the joint dynamics of declining serious delinquency, increasing multiple illicit drug use, and first decreasing and then stabilizing mental health problem prevalence as the sample gets older, from 1976 to 1983. Although the numbers and percentages in the two-way classifications vary from year to year, the number and percentages in the combined serious delinquent–polydrug user–mental health problem category remains relatively stable over the entire 8-year period.

Because of the small numbers reporting serious delinquency, polydrug use, and mental health problems, the number of cases in some cells of the joint distribution is too small to yield reliable estimates of prevalence and offending rates–use rates–mean scale scores. This is frequently a problem even for the bivariate joint classification (for example, joint delinquency–drug use types) in 1983. For the sake of completeness, we present the full, trivariate, delinquency–drug use–mental health joint distribution for all three years in Appendix C, but we urge caution in interpreting results involving cells with small numbers of cases.

Changing our base from the total sample to the sample of serious offenders (see Figure 3.3), we find that the proportion of serious offenders who are polydrug users (combining PD and PD&MH types in Figure 3.3) is only 16% in 1976, but 49% in 1980 and 70% in 1983. The proportion of marijuana users among the serious offenders increases from 18% to 29% from 1976 to 1980, then declined to 23% in 1983 (Appendix C). The proportion of both alcohol user and nonuser types among the serious offenders declines consistently from 1976 to 1980, and by 1983 there are no nonusers among the serious offenders. Over time, then, there appears to be a convergence between serious offending and illegal drug use. If we consider marijuana use as well as polydrug use, then by 1983 92% of the serious offenders reported use of some illegal drug (marijuana or other illicit drugs).

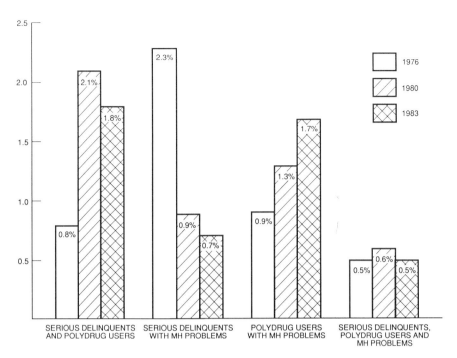

FIGURE 3.2 Multiple Problem Youth: Prevalence Rates 1976, 1980, and 1983

Among the polydrug users, 40% are serious offenders in 1976, 17% in 1980, and only 12% in 1983. This finding contrasts sharply with the apparent convergence based on an examination of drug users within the serious delinquency classification. If we combine marijuana and polydrug users, the proportion of them who are serious delinquents goes from 24% for 1976 to 10% for 1980, and 7% in 1983, still a declining trend (see Appendix C). Combining these results with those based on analysis of the serious offender category again leads us to the interaction of two countervailing trends. On the one hand, the prevalence and frequency of drug use increases as the sample gets older over time, both for the sample in general and for the serious offenders in particular. On the other hand, delinquency decreases over time for the sample in general and for users of illegal substances. This trend is clearly borne out by the data in Tables 3.4–3.6 and Appendix C.

Using serious offenders again as a base, 28% of the serious offenders are classified as having mental health problems in 1976, 22% in 1980, and 26% in 1983. Although there is some fluctuation, there is no clear trend in the relationship between mental health problems and delinquent behavior over time. However, there is a clear increasing trend in the percentage of serious offenders who are both polydrug users and have mental health

SO = Serious Offender PD = Polydrug User MH = Mental Health Problems

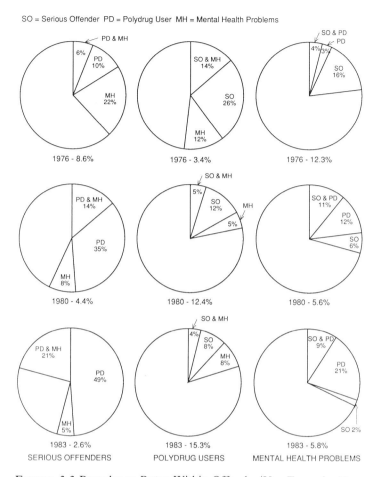

FIGURE 3.3 Prevalence Rates Within Offender/Use Types by Year

problems, with 6% evidencing both problems in 1976, 14% in 1980, and 21% in 1983. With advancing age, those who are serious offenders are increasingly likely to be multiple problem youth. Thus 38% of serious offenders in 1976 reported other serious problem behaviors and this rate increased to 75% among serious offenders in 1983. This suggests either a selective dropout (i.e., multiple problem youth have longer delinquent careers) or a tendency for multiple problem youth to initiate serious delinquency later in the lifespan (or both), and given the general decline in serious offending, the former appears to be more likely.

Returning to polydrug users as a base, the percentage of polydrug users classified as having mental health problems is 26% in 1976, 10% in 1980, and 12% in 1983. This trend reflects the more general trend in the sample (see Tables 3.1–3.3). Looking at the trends in mental health classification for serious offenders and polydrug users at the same time, it is evident that, *relative to trends in mental health problems in the sample,* there is an increasing likelihood over time of finding those with mental health problems among the serious offenders, but little change (perhaps even a slight decrease) in the likelihood of finding those with mental health problems among the polydrug users. This relationship, which receives further confirmation in Chapter 7, suggests either that early use of drugs is associated with mental health problems, but the relationship weakens with age, or that mental health problems and drug use may be alternative responses to a similar set of causes, and that behavior is more likely to crystallize around one of the two as the respondents get older. This same declining trend is observed for polydrug users with both mental health and serious delinquency problems, with the rate in 1983 (4%) being approximately one-third the rate in 1976 (14%). In general then, early use of multiple illicit drugs appears to be associated with both serious delinquency and mental health problems, but this relationship is attenuated with age. Either those who initiate polydrug use early desist in their serious offending and resolve their mental health problems over time or those who initiate the use of illicit drugs later in the lifespan are less likely to be multiple problem youth (or both). In any case, 80% of polydrug users in 1983 (ages 18 to 24) report no serious levels of delinquency or mental health problems compared with 48% in 1976 (ages 11 to 17).

Using those subjects with mental health problems as our base, the proportion who are serious offenders declines from 20% in 1976 to 17% in 1980 and 11% in 1983. These percentages are all still higher than the percentage of those in the total sample who are classified as being serious offenders. The proportion of those with mental health problems who are polydrug users increases from 7% for 1976 to 23% for 1980 to 30% for 1983. These percentages are also higher than the percentage of individuals in the total sample who report being polydrug users each year. Still, the decrease in delinquent behavior and the increase in polydrug use reflect trends in the sample as a whole. The percentage of those with mental health problems who are both serious delinquents and polydrug users increases from 1976 (4%) to 1980 (11%), but then declines between 1980 and 1983 (9%). Overall, the proportion of those with mental health problems who report other serious levels of problem behavior is relatively constant over time (68% to 73%).

Prevalence and General Offending/Use Rates for Joint Delinquent–Drug Use–Mental Health Types

Tables 3.4, 3.5, and 3.6 present the prevalence and offending/use rates for delinquent behavior and ADM problems by joint delinquency–drug use–mental health types. These tables focus upon the most serious types and do not include all of the possible breakdowns resulting from a cross-tabulation of all three typologies. The full set of prevalence and general offending/use rates for all combinations of types are presented in Appendix C. Tables 3.4–3.6 highlight the major findings discussed below, but the reader is encouraged to examine the more complete set of tables to verify the summary presented here. In the event the trends presented in Tables 3.4–3.6 do not fairly represent the trends across all combinations of multiple types, we will note this in the discussion when making generalizations. The discussion of the three-way classifications presented here is purely descriptive. More sophisticated analyses involving the correlations between types of behavior, the sequencing of behaviors, and the extent to which the onset of one increases the risk of onset for the others, are presented in later chapters.

DELINQUENT TYPES AND DRUG USE–MENTAL HEALTH SUBTYPES

In Tables 3.4–3.6, prevalence and general offending rates are presented for two classes of delinquent behavior—Index offenses and general delinquency. Because Index and general delinquency scales are summary scales included in the definition of serious offenders, the prevalence rates for all drug and mental health subtypes is 100% for those offenses. Prevalence rates for the other offense-specific scales are not constrained by the type definition, and rates for these offenses are found in Appendix C.

As indicated in Tables 3.4–3.6, among serious delinquents, polydrug users have the highest prevalence and general offending rates of all of the drug subtypes. This generalization holds for many, but not all offense-specific scales. However, this trend is clearly indicated in the summary scales presented in these tables. Serious delinquent–polydrug users account for a disproportionately large share of all serious and total delinquent acts. In 1976, they constituted 1.4% of the adolescent sample and accounted for 20% of all reported Index crimes and 16% of total reported crimes; by 1983 they still constituted less than 2% (1.8%) of the sample but accounted for 62% of all reported Index crimes and 30% of total reported crimes. They also accounted for 46% to 62% of all illegal service crimes, which are primarily drug scales.

Although it is not shown in Tables 3.4–3.6, this same pattern of differences by drug subtype is observed for nonserious delinquent offenders. It is *not* observed for exploratory or nondelinquent types. It should also be noted that there is no consistent pattern of differences in prevalence or general offending rates among other drug use types within the serious or nonserious offender classification. For example, among serious offenders, Index offense rates are highest for the alcohol use

TABLE 3.4. Prevalence (P) and general offending/use rates[1] (R)[a] for multiple problem types: 1976.

Offender/user type	Sample		Index			General delinquency			Mental health problems	
	N	(%)	P	R	% of total[b]	P	R	% of total[b]	P	X̄[c]
Serious delinquent	144	(8.6)	100.0	995	85	100.0	11751	62	27.6	44.70
Polydrug user	23	(1.4)	100.0	1430	20	100.0	18626	16	34.8	47.94
MH problems	8	(0.5)	100.0	788	4	100.0	9763	3	100.0	54.33
No MH problems	15	(0.9)	100.0	1773	16	100.0	23353	13	0.0	44.53
Marijuana user	26	(1.5)	100.0	965	15	100.0	14115	13	26.9	41.88
MH problems	7	(0.4)	100.0	900	4	100.0	5471	1	100.0	49.71
No MH problems	19	(1.1)	100.0	989	11	100.0	17300	12	0.0	39.00
Alcohol user	33	(2.0)	100.0	1054	20	100.0	8382	9	18.2	44.27
MH problems	6	(0.4)	100.0	867	3	100.0	1517	<1	100.0	55.50
No MH problems	27	(1.6)	100.0	1096	17	100.0	9908	9	0.0	41.78
Nonuser	62	(3.7)	100.0	808	30	100.0	10256	23	30.6	44.91
MH problems	19	(1.1)	100.0	584	7	100.0	10756	7	100.0	53.91
No MH problems	43	(2.5)	100.0	907	23	100.0	10035	16	0.0	40.94
MH problems	40	(2.4)	100.0	723	18	100.0	8247	12	100.0	53.50
No MH problems	104	(6.2)	100.0	1096	67	100.0	13250	50	0.0	41.32

Polydrug user	N	(%)	Marijuana			Polydrug			Mental health problems	
			P	R	% of total[b]	P	R	% of total[b]	P	X̄[c]
Polydrug user	57	(3.4)	89.7	9288	45	100.0	3131	97	26.3	45.33
Serious delinquent	23	(1.4)	91.3	11430	22	100.0	2505	31	34.8	47.59
MH problems	8	(0.5)	87.5	10675	7	100.0	4163	18	100.0	53.33
No MH problems	15	(0.9)	93.3	11833	15	100.0	1620	13	0.0	44.53
Nonserious	15	(0.9)	93.3	9160	12	100.0	3320	27	26.7	44.13
MH problems	4	(0.2)	100.0	16875	6	100.0	2325	5	100.0	50.50
No MH problems	11	(0.7)	90.9	6355	6	100.0	3682	22	0.0	41.82
Exploratory	8	(0.5)	100.0	9238	6	100.0	750	3	0.0	39.13
MH problems	0	(0.0)	NA	NA	NA	NA	NA	NA	NA	NA
No MH problems	8	(0.5)	100.0	9238	6	100.0	750	3	0.0	39.13
Nondelinquent	11	(0.7)	72.7	5845	5	100.0	6091	36	27.3	46.00
MH problems	3	(0.2)	66.7	7833	2	100.0	11633	19	100.0	57.00
No MH problems	8	(0.5)	75.0	5100	3	100.0	4013	17	0.0	41.88
MH problems	15	(0.9)	86.7	11760	15	100.0	5167	42	100.0	53.31
No MH problems	42	(2.5)	90.5	8622	30	100.0	2450	55	0.0	42.29

[a] Per 100 persons.
[b] Percentage of total offenses in NYS sample.
[c] Mean scale score.

TABLE 3.5. Prevalence (P) and general offending/use rates (R)[a] for multiple problem types: 1980.

Offender/user type	Sample		Index			General delinquency			Problem substance use		Mental health problems	
	N	(%)	P	R	% of total[b]	P	R	% of total[b]	P	$\bar{X}^3$	P	$\bar{X}^3$
Serious delinquent	66	(4.4)	100.0	1140	83	100.0	16142	50	54.5	15.52	21.2	42.79
Polydrug user	32	(2.1)	100.0	1428	51	100.0	25400	38	75.0	18.53	28.1	44.25
MH problems	9	(0.6)	100.0	2178	22	100.0	59267	25	100.0	22.11	100.0	53.67
No MH problems	23	(1.5)	100.0	1135	29	100.0	12148	13	65.2	17.13	0.0	40.57
Marijuana user	19	(1.3)	100.0	879	19	100.0	6700	6	57.9	17.00	15.8	43.21
MH problems	3	(0.2)	100.0	1400	5	100.0	15867	2	66.7	13.67	100.0	53.00
No MH problems	16	(1.1)	100.0	781	14	100.0	4981	4	56.3	17.63	0.0	41.38
Alcohol user	6	(0.4)	100.0	850	5	100.0	10017	3	50.0	12.17	16.7	40.00
MH problems	1	(0.1)	100.0	300	<1	100.0	2400	<1	0.0	7.00	100.0	50.00
No MH problems	5	(0.3)	100.0	960	5	100.0	11540	3	60.0	13.20	0.0	38.00
Nonuser	9	(0.6)	100.0	878	8	100.0	4867	2	0.0	3.10	11.1	38.56
MH problems	1	(0.1)	100.0	300	<1	100.0	400	<1	0.0	5.00	100.0	46.00
No MH problems	8	(0.5)	100.0	950	8	100.0	5425	2	0.0	2.86	0.0	37.63
MH problems	14	(0.9)	100.0	1743	27	100.0	41700	28	78.6	18.00	100.0	52.72
No MH problems	52	(3.5)	100.0	981	56	100.0	8850	22	51.9	14.71	0.0	40.12

	N	(%)	Marijuana			Polydrug			Problem substance abuse		Mental health problems	
			P	R	% of total[b]	P	R	% of total[b]	P	$\bar{X}^c$	P	$\bar{X}^c$
Polydrug user	185	(12.4)	97.9	16736	66	100.0	4372	99	37.4	14.90	10.2	39.02
Serious delinquent	32	(2.1)	100.0	23281	16	100.0	9090	35	75.0	18.53	28.1	44.25
MH problems	9	(0.6)	100.0	28989	6	100.0	16500	18	100.0	22.11	100.0	53.67
No MH problems	23	(1.5)	100.0	21048	10	100.0	6191	17	65.2	17.13	0.0	40.57
Nonserious	65	(4.4)	96.9	19645	27	100.0	4697	38	41.5	15.06	4.6	37.42
MH problems	3	(0.2)	100.0	48800	3	100.0	15233	6	100.00	18.00	100.0	52.00
No MH problems	62	(4.2)	96.8	18234	24	100.0	4187	32	38.7	14.92	0.0	36.71
Exploratory	36	(2.4)	100.0	15770	12	100.0	2562	11	38.6	15.78	8.3	40.44
MH problems	3	(0.2)	100.0	20333	1	100.0	2600	1	100.0	25.67	100.0	47.00
No MH problems	33	(2.2)	100.0	15355	11	100.0	2558	10	33.3	14.88	0.0	39.85
Nondelinquent	52	(3.5)	96.2	9794	11	100.0	2277	14	13.5	11.81	7.7	36.74
MH problems	4	(0.3)	100.0	1800	<1	100.0	900	<1	25.0	13.25	100.0	54.00
No MH problems	48	(3.2)	95.8	10460	11	100.0	2392	14	12.5	11.69	0.0	35.30
MH problems	19	(1.3)	100.0	25026	10	100.0	10821	26	84.2	20.16	100.0	52.42
No MH problems	166	(11.1)	97.6	15804	56	100.0	3622	73	33.7	14.28	0.0	37.46

[a] Per 100 persons.
[b] Percentage of total offenses in NYS sample.
[c] Mean scale score.

TABLE 3.6. Prevalence (P) and general offending/use rates (R)[a] for multiple problem types: 1983.

Offender/user type	Sample		Index			General delinquency			Problem substance use	
	N	(%)	P	R	% of total[b]	P	R	% of total[b]	P	$\bar{X}$[c]
Serious delinquent	39	(2.6)	100.0	990	75	100.0	15100	33	43.6	22.60
Polydrug user	27	(1.8)	100.0	1185	62	100.0	20360	30	44.4	25.53
MH problems	8	(0.5)	100.0	975	15	100.0	7788	3	50.0	26.59
No MH problems	19	(1.3)	100.0	1274	47	100.0	25653	27	42.1	25.09
Marijuana user	9	(0.6)	100.0	633	11	100.0	3189	1	44.4	17.47
MH problems	2	(0.1)	100.0	350	1	100.0	1500	<1	50.0	17.50
No MH problems	7	(0.5)	100.0	714	10	100.0	3671	1	42.9	17.46
Alcohol user	3	(0.2)	100.0	300	2	100.0	3500	1	33.3	11.50
MH problems	0	(0.0)	NA	NA	NA	NA	NA	NA	NA	NA
No MH problems	3	(0.2)	100.0	300	2	100.0	3500	1	33.3	11.50
Nonuser	0	(0.0)	NA	NA	NA	NA	NA	NA	NA	NA
MH problems	0	(0.0)	NA	NA	NA	NA	NA	NA	NA	NA
No MH problems	0	(0.0)	NA	NA	NA	NA	NA	NA	NA	NA
MH problems	10	(0.7)	100.0	850	16	100.0	6530	4	50.0	24.77
No MH problems	29	(2.0)	100.0	1038	59	100.0	18055	29	41.4	21.84

	Sample		Marijuana			Polydrug			Problem substance use	
	N	(%)	P	R	% of total	P	R	% of total²	P	X̄c
Polydrug user	228	(15.3)	90.6	12808	61	100.0	5229	99	24.9	18.88
Serious delinquent	27	(1.8)	92.6	20841	11	100.0	14608	32	44.4	25.53
MH problems	8	(0.5)	100.0	14950	2	100.0	4663	3	50.0	26.59
No MH problems	19	(1.3)	89.5	23321	9	100.0	18795	29	42.1	25.09
Nonserious	65	(4.4)	95.4	19660	26	100.0	4957	26	40.0	20.18
MH problems	7	(0.5)	100.0	20571	3	100.0	8514	5	57.1	26.79
No MH problems	58	(3.9)	94.8	19550	23	100.0	4528	21	37.9	19.38
Exploratory	51	(3.4)	90.2	8459	8	100.0	3906	16	15.7	17.83
MH problems	7	(0.4)	100.0	16357	2	100.0	4886	3	28.6	20.04
No MH problems	44	(3.0)	88.6	7202	6	100.0	3750	13	13.6	17.48
Nondelinquent	85	(5.7)	87.0	8277	14	100.0	3542	24	12.9	16.49
MH problems	4	(0.2)	100.0	26675	2	100.0	22850	7	25.0	19.69
No MH problems	81	(5.5)	86.4	7368	12	100.0	2588	17	12.3	16.33
MH problems	26	(1.7)	100.0	18646	9	100.0	8558	18	42.3	23.82
No MH problems	202	(13.6)	89.6	12330	50	100.0	4923	80	22.8	18.28

TABLE 3.6. Continued

Offender/user type	Mental health problems		Depression		Mental health service use			DUI		
	P	$\bar{X}^c$	P	$\bar{X}^d$	P	R	% of total[b]	P	R	% of total[b]
Serious delinquent	25.6	21.08	33.3	1.05	10.3	33	1	74.2	9942	15
Polydrug user	29.6	11.97	40.7	1.33	14.8	54	1	85.2	12464	14
MH problems	100.0	14.38	50.0	1.63	12.5	14	<1	87.5	6263	2
No MH problems	0.0	10.96	36.8	1.21	15.8	71	1	82.4	15076	12
Marijuana user	22.2	10.22	22.2	.56	0.0	0	0	44.4	350	<1
MH problems	100.0	16.50	100.0	2.50	0.0	0	0	0.0	0	0
No MH problems	0.0	8.43	0.0	.00	0.0	0	0	57.0	450	<1
Alcohol user	0.0	7.67	0.0	.00	0.0	0	0	0.0	0	0
MH problems	NA	NA	NA	NA	NA	NA	NA	NA	NA	NA
No MH problems	0.0	7.67	0.0	.00	0.0	0	0	0.0	0	0
Non-User	NA	NA	NA	NA	NA	NA	NA	NA	NA	NA
MH problems	NA	NA	NA	NA	NA	NA	NA	NA	NA	NA
No MH problems	NA	NA	NA	NA	NA	NA	NA	NA	NA	NA
MH Problems	100.0	14.80	60.0	1.80	10.0	11	<1	70.0	501	2
No MH Problems	0.0	10.01	24.1	.79	10.4	47	1	67.7	9986	12

	Mental health problems		Depression		Mental health service use			DUI		
	P	$\bar{X}^c$	P	$\bar{X}^d$	P	R	% of total[b]	P	R	% of total[b]
Polydrug user	11.6	18.21	39.1	1.12	12.4	224	27	89.1	8548	67
Serious delinquent	29.6	11.97	40.7	1.33	14.8	54	1	85.2	12464	14
MH problems	100.0	14.38	50.0	1.63	12.5	14	<1	87.5	6263	2
No MH problems	0.0	10.96	36.8	1.21	15.8	71	1	82.4	15076	12
Nonserious	10.8	9.08	35.4	.99	16.9	200	9	90.8	13768	34
MH problems	100.0	14.43	57.1	2.86	57.1	1400	7	83.3	3217	1
No MH problems	0.0	8.31	32.8	.76	12.1	55	2	91.3	15041	33
Exploratory	13.7	9.33	43.1	1.06	5.9	104	4	76.5	4710	7
MH problems	100.0	14.57	71.4	2.00	14.3	250	1	100.0	5000	1
No MH problems	0.0	8.50	38.6	.91	4.5	81	3	71.6	4664	6
Nonoffender	4.7	8.39	37.6	1.20	10.6	197	13	95.3	4568	11
MH problems	100.0	13.50	50.0	2.50	25.0	500	2	66.7	1000	<1
No MH problems	0.0	8.14	37.0	1.14	9.9	182	11	96.0	4744	11
MH Problems	100.0	14.31	57.7	2.19	26.9	525	10	88.5	4293	4
No MH Problems	0.0	8.53	36.1	.99	9.9	113	17	88.1	8655	62

[a] Per 100 persons.
[b] Percentage of total offenses in NYS sample.
[c] Mean scale score.
[d] Mean number of symptoms.

subtype for 1976; there are no substantive differences in rates between alcohol, marijuana, and nonuser subtypes for 1980; and marijuana users report the next highest rate for 1983. There is also no consistency in the pattern of general delinquency offending rates by marijuana use, alcohol use, or nonuser subtypes over time. Whereas drug use subtype appears to specify offending rates within the serious and nonserious offender types, this specification applies only to polydrug versus other drug use types.

The effect of mental health problems on prevalence and general offending rates within delinquent offender types and across drug use subtypes, is unclear. When considering the effect on prevalence for offense-specific scales (where prevalence is unconstrained) there is no consistency from offense to offense in any year; nor is there any consistency in the effect on a particular offense across years. With respect to general offending rates, there is a consistent effect across offenses each year (i.e., either higher or lower) but this effect is not consistent across years. For example, 1976 general offending rates for Index and general delinquency (and seven of the ten offense-specific scales) are substantially lower for those serious offenders classified as having mental health problems. The effect on general offending rates in 1980 is the reverse and in 1983 the direction of the effect is similar to that in 1976. Overall, then, there is no consistent pattern to differences by mental health problem status within delinquent offender types over time. If the presence of mental health problems has an independent effect on prevalence or general offending rates, the effect changes over time. This conclusion seems unlikely.

It is interesting to note that our earlier finding about polydrug use being associated with higher prevalence and offending rates within serious and nonserious offender types holds for youth classified as having no mental health problems, but it does *not* hold for those classified as having mental health problems in 1976. However, this polydrug specification finding does hold for both mental health types for 1980 and 1983.

In general, the prevalence of mental health problems is highest for polydrug user subtypes within each delinquent type (the one exception involves nonserious delinquents in 1983, among whom marijuana users show slightly higher prevalence rates). This trend is clearly indicated for the serious delinquent type in Tables 3.4–3.6. Once again, there is no consistent trend across other drug use subtypes within delinquent types.

Problem substance use prevalence is also highest for polydrug user subtypes within each delinquent type. Further, within polydrug user subtypes (for all delinquency types), higher prevalence rates are observed for individuals who have mental health problems than for those who do not. Thus, the highest problem substance use prevalence rates each year are found among serious delinquents who are polydrug users who have mental health problems. The highest problem substance use mean scores are also found in this most serious three-way subtype.

Turning to depression, mental health service use rates, and DUI rates, which are available only for 1983, the highest prevalence rates for all three outcomes are observed for the polydrug user subtype within the serious delinquent type. With only one exception (the exploratory delinquent type for mental health service use) this finding holds not only for serious delinquents, but for *all* delinquency types; that is, within each delinquency type, the highest prevalence rates for depression, mental health service use, and DUI are observed for polydrug user subtypes. The pattern across the other drug subtypes is unclear.

DRUG TYPES AND DELINQUENCY–MENTAL HEALTH SUBTYPES

Within the polydrug user type, there is some slight variation in marijuana prevalence rates by delinquent and mental health subtypes every year. This variation is most apparent in 1976 for nonoffenders, where the prevalence rate 72.7% is substantially lower than for other delinquent subtypes (all above 90%). Within the subtype, the rate is even lower (66.7%) for those with mental health problems, but the N in this cell is too small for a reliable estimate. Although the differences are not as great for 1980 or 1983, this same trend holds.

In general, exceptions to the unidimensional or hierarchical assumption about substance use such as that noted above typically involve nondelinquent youth or those in the exploratory delinquent type.

In Tables 3.4–3.6, marijuana and polydrug use rates are highest for serious delinquent and lowest for nondelinquent subtypes within the polydrug type each year (except for the 1976 polydrug use rate where this pattern is essentially reversed). Although there are some exceptions, in general, the systematic ordering of drug use rates by delinquent subtype (with highest rate for serious delinquents and lowest rates for nondelinquents) holds for *each* drug use type.

There is also a consistent difference in the marijuana and polydrug use rates by mental health problem type, with higher use rates for those with mental health problems. This difference does not hold for rates of alcohol use, however. Further, within particular drug and delinquency subtypes, there are a number of exceptions to the general finding that those with mental health problems have higher use rates, although this is still the most typical finding.

Among polydrug users, those who are serious delinquents have the highest prevalence rates for mental health problems. With two exceptions (alcohol and nonuser types in 1983), this same finding holds for all drug use types each year. The ordering of other delinquency subtypes by prevalence of mental health problems is not consistent or systematic for any drug use type. Essentially the same pattern holds for mean mental health scale scores.

The prevalence of problem substance use also varies systematically by delinquency subtype and mental health problem subtype within the polydrug user type (Tables 3.5 and 3.6). This pattern is also observed within the other drug use types as well (see Appendix C). In 1980, 84% of polydrug users classified as having mental health problems were also problem substance users, compared with only a third of polydrug users who were classified as not having mental health problems. The difference by mental health subtype among polydrug users was still substantial in 1983, but the absolute levels of prevalence were substantially lower (42% and 22%). Although the numbers in the three-way classification cells in Table 3.5 and 3.6 are very small, they are nevertheless consistently and systematically ordered by seriousness of delinquency and mental health problem subtypes. This same consistency in ordering across all delinquent and mental health subtypes is observed for problem substance use mean scores. This same pattern of prevalence and mean scale scores is generally found in the other drug use types, but there are some exceptions.

There is no systematic ordering by delinquency subtype in the prevalence rates for depression, mental health service use, or DUI. Among polydrug users, the highest depression prevalence rate occurs for those who are exploratory offenders; the highest prevalence of mental health service use is for nonserious offenders; and the highest prevalence of DUI is for nondelinquents. Although both drug type and delinquency type were related to these three outcomes when considered separately (see Tables 3.1 and 3.2), the pattern of relationships by delinquent subtypes within drug use types is unclear. This generalization applies to mean numbers of symptoms or frequency measures as well.

As expected, the mental health problem classification is related to the prevalence and symptom/use rates for depression and mental health service use independently of drug use type (i.e., within each drug use type). Mental health problem type is not related to DUI prevalence, but it is related to the DUI offending rate among polydrug, marijuana, and alcohol drug types, with those classified as non–mental health problem subtypes reporting higher DUI offending rates.

To summarize findings from the joint distribution tables:

1. Each problem behavior typology has a clear and consistent impact on the specific problem behavior upon which it is based, even controlling for the other two problem behavior typologies.

2. Within the delinquency types: (a) Polydrug users tend to have higher rates of offending and (among those without mental health problems) the highest mental health problem scale scores, as well as the highest prevalence and number of symptoms of depression. They also have higher rates (prevalence and offending/use) of problem substance use, mental health service use and DUI. (b) Among serious and nonserious offenders, those classified as having mental health problems have the

lowest rates of DUI and the highest rates of problem substance use but there were no other consistent differences in delinquency or substance use by mental health subtype.

3. Within substance user types: (a) Serious delinquents have the highest mental health problem prevalence and scale scores. Serious offenders also have the highest rates of alcohol use (and nonoffenders the lowest), and, with some exceptions, the same pattern is evident for marijuana and polydrug users. This same pattern was observed for problem substance use prevalence rates and mean scale scores. (b) Those classified as having mental health problems tend to have higher prevalence and use rates–scale scores for marijuana use, polydrug use, and problem substance use. This pattern was not consistent within delinquent subtypes (i.e., in the three-way classifications), however, except for rates of problem substance use. Having mental health problems was also related to rates of depression and mental health service utilization, but not to DUI prevalence. Among polydrug, marijuana and alcohol use types, having mental health problems was associated with lower DUI offending rates.

4. Within mental health types: (a) For those with no mental health problems, increasing seriousness or variety of drug use is generally associated with higher prevalence and offending rates on delinquent offenses, but this pattern is less evident when simultaneously controlling for offender type. The pattern for those with mental health problems is less clear. (b) Polydrug users without mental health problems tend to have higher mental health problem scale scores, depression, DUI, and problem substance use than other drug use types without mental health problems, but the relationship among those with mental health problems is again unclear. (c) More serious delinquents with no mental health problems tend to have higher mental health problem scale scores than other delinquency types with no mental health problems, but there is no clear pattern for depression or mental health service use and no clear pattern of relationship between offender type and mental health problem scale scores for those *with* mental health problems. Alcohol and marijuana use tends to be higher for serious delinquents and lower for nondelinquents among those without mental health problems, but the pattern for polydrug use is less clear.

From these results, it appears that the presence of mental health problems attenuates or confounds relationships between drug use and delinquency for serious offenders and polydrug users. Although mental health problems do not appear to be strongly related to the use of drugs generally, they do appear to be inversely related to problem drug use and DUI. Regardless of the presence or absence of mental health problems, polydrug users have the highest rates of problem drug use and DUI (as well as drug use in general) and the highest rates of self-reported delinquency. Also, regardless of mental health problem type, serious delinquents have the highest rates of alcohol, marijuana, and polydrug use, as well as the highest rates of delinquency. It appears, then, that delinquency and drug use may be more closely related to one another than either is to mental health problems. This pattern receives further confirmation in later chapters, particularly in Chapter 6.

4
Age, Period, and Cohort Effects

The National Youth Survey sample is drawn from seven cohorts, aged 11–17 in the first year of data collection (1976) and aged 18–24 in the most recent year for which data are presently available. The oldest cohort was born in 1959, near the peak of the postwar baby boom; the youngest was born in 1965, a year in which total fertility rates had declined back to their 1946 levels (Easterlin, 1987), thereby marking the end of the baby boom. Table 4.1 presents age and cohort statistics for the National Youth Survey's seven cohorts.

Total fertility rates over the period 1959–1965 show a steady decline. This decline reflects an increase in the number of women of child-bearing age as well as the number of births to those women from 1959 to 1961. From 1961 to 1965, both total fertility rate and total number of births decline. Total births (and therefore absolute cohort size) are highest for the fifth (1961) cohort and lowest for the first. Average annual parity (or birth order) is highest for cohort 4 (1962) and lowest for cohort 1.

The data in Table 4.1 form a basis for discussing age, period, and cohort trends in delinquency, drug use, and mental health problems. As Glenn (1977) explains, the separation of age, period, and cohort effects in sample survey research is problematic because of sampling variability, cohort attrition, and the confounding of age, period and cohort effects. In some cases, however, it is possible to ascertain which of the three is responsible for changes over time, particularly if we examine the data in light of two hypotheses: the Maturational Reform hypothesis and the Easterlin hypothesis.

The Easterlin hypothesis has been applied to illegal behavior, alcohol, and drug use, suicide, divorce, and unemployment—in short, to a wide range of social problems (Easterlin, 1987). Easterlin asserts that the size of a cohort tends to be inversely related to the relative income of that cohort (relative, specifically, to aspirations, which are largely determined and measured in terms of parental income). More generally, resources are scarcer for larger cohorts than for smaller ones (see also Harter, 1977;

TABLE 4.1. Fertility, cohort size, and average birth order, 1959–1965 (national population).

Cohort number	Year of birth	Age in 1976	Total fertility rate in year of birth	Total births[a] in year of birth	Average parity in year of birth
1	1965	11	2.93	3,760	2.84
2	1964	12	3.21	4,027	2.92
3	1963	13	3.33	4,098	2.96
4	1962	14	3.47	4,167	3.00
5	1961	15	3.63	4,268	2.99
6	1960	16	3.65	4,258	2.98
7	1959	17	3.71	4,245	2.94

Sources: From *Historical Statistics of the United States, Colonial Times to 1970*, U.S. Bureau of the Census, 1975, Washington, DC: U.S. Government Printing Office; see also "Family Configuration and Intelligence," by R.B. Zajonc, 1976, *Science, 192*, pp. 227–236, and *Birth and Fortune* (2nd ed.) by R.A. Easterlin, 1987, Chicago: University of Chicago Press.

[a] In thousands.

Jones, 1980). Resources include not only income (in adult life), but also classroom space, parental attention, and assistance from teachers in childhood. It is not only absolute cohort size that is important, but also the size of the children's cohort relative to the size of earlier cohorts, particularly the cohort of the parents (Ahlburg & Schapiro, 1984; Harter, 1977).

The greater scarcity of resources for larger cohorts leads to higher levels of psychological and emotional stress, generated by the competition for (and, in proportionally more cases for larger cohorts, the failure to obtain) parental attention, employment, and so forth. This stress in turn leads to increases in a variety of social problems. The Easterlin hypothesis is thus a variant of strain theory, and Easterlin explicitly cites Durkheim (1951) and Merton (1968) regarding anomie. Easterlin is concerned with *macrosocial* variations, with differences between cohorts in *aggregate rates,* not with individual or microsocial patterns of behavior. In this respect it returns to the anomie theories of Durkheim and Merton, in contrast to the more social-psychologically oriented strain theories (e.g., Cloward & Ohlin, 1960) of the more recent past.

The Maturational Reform hypothesis arises from the empirical generalization that illegal behavior increases in early adolescence, is highest in middle to late adolescence, and then declines in early adulthood. This pattern holds true whether official statistics or self-report data are used (Blumstein et al., 1986, pp. 41–42; Jensen & Rojeck, 1980, pp. 70–71, 102) and forms the basis for the analysis of age structure and crime (Chilton & Spielberger, 1971; Steffensmeier & Harer, 1987). A number of different explanations have been suggested for this apparent pattern of maturational reform or "aging out" of delinquency.

Matza (1964) suggests that the increase in delinquent behavior during adolescence arises from uncertainties about roles and misinformation about the attitudes of peers, a condition of normlessness (in the Durkheimian sense of anomie) that is resolved with the completion of the transition from childhood (through adolescence) to adulthood. Briar and Piliavin (1965) suggest that the declining illegal behavior of late adolescence and early adulthood is a result of increased commitment to conventional institutions and to behavioral conformity. Greenberg (1977) explains the variations in delinquency with age by a combination of elements of strain and control theory, whereas Hirschi and Gottfredson (1983) assert that age has a direct effect on crime, independent of other theoretically important variables. Regardless of which (if any) of these explanations we accept, the inverted U-shaped pattern of delinquency is to be expected.

The Maturational Reform hypothesis would lead us to expect rates of delinquency to increase in early adolescence (11 or 12 to 15), peak in middle to late adolescence (15–18), and decline with the onset of adulthood, sometime after ages 18–21 (Farrington, 1986; Gold, 1970; Hirschi, 1969). A similar pattern appears to be characteristic of alcohol and drug use, but both initiation and age of maximum involvement occur later for alcohol and drug use than for other types of delinquency (see Chapter 5). According to Kandel (1980), rates of both legal and illegal drug use peak around ages 18–21 and decline thereafter, and our own results in Chapter 3 are consistent with this pattern. No such curvilinear pattern of association with age is expected for mental health problems. According to the Easterlin hypothesis, we should expect higher rates of delinquency, alcohol use, drug use, and mental health problems for the larger cohorts (5, 6, and maybe 7 and 4) or perhaps for those cohorts with higher average birth order (4, 5, 6, and maybe 3) and lower rates for the smaller, low-birth-order cohorts (1, 2, and maybe 3 or 7).

A third expectation results from the empirical generalization that, although FBI Uniform Crime Report data show stable or increasing rates of crime, both victimization and self-report data show stable decreasing period trends (Menard, 1987; O'Brien, 1985; Steffensmeier & Harer, 1987). This finding is true in particular for age-specific trends (Gold & Reimer, 1975; Menard, 1987), and it suggests that we may expect stable or declining short-term, age-specific trends in delinquent behavior. Data on high school seniors from 1975 to 1983 (Johnston, O'Malley, & Bachman, 1984) indicate an upward trend in alcohol and marijuana use from 1975 to 1979, but a generally declining trend thereafter. We may therefore expect NYS data to parallel this curvilinear trend for alcohol and marijuana. The data from Johnston et al. reflect mixed trends for those substances included in our polydrug measure, so we have no basis for expectations regarding age-specific trends in polydrug use, and we have no basis for expecting particular age-specific trends in mental health problems other than those implied by the Easterlin hypothesis and attributable to cohort rather than period effects.

TABLE 4.2. General delinquency.

Age	1976	1977	1978	1979	1980	1983	Age-specific mean
				Prevalence rate			
12	62	54					58
13	65	55	51				57
14	68	60	56	52			59
15	69	68	56	53	46		58
16	67	70	62	56	49		61
17	69	59	61	57	52		60
18		53	54	56	51	47	52
19			50	49	46	43	47
20				51	45	45	44
21					44	43	44
(22–24)						(34)	(34)
			General offending rate (per thousand)				
12	18,373	5,398					11,886
13	18,970	9,819	5,834				11,541
14	15,468	17,210	10,246	12,912			13,959
15	20,056	22,665	14,536	10,698	9,361		15,463
16	12,034	19,305	21,273	10,645	8,610		14,319
17	24,262	24,828	13,846	24,548	19,328		21,362
18		5,932	20,368	14,183	13,488	18,330	14,460
19			11,389	18,421	19,580	10,153	14,886
20				10,659	18,828	13,717	14,401
21					12,297	11,452	11,875
(22–24)						(9,913)	(9,913)

Age Effects

In Tables 4.2 and 4.3, age and period specific prevalence and general offending rates are presented for general delinquency and Index offending, respectively. Age 11 has been eliminated because data were available for only 1 year, and ages 22–24 have been aggregated because data were available for only 1 year for each of the three age groups, and we wished to base our age-specific means on at least two years of data to minimize the effect of random error on conclusions. In addition, by basing age-specific mean rates on more than one year, we average across at least two cohorts, so no mean can be attributed to the effect of a single cohort. This approach does not eliminate, but may reduce, the impact of cohort effects on trends across age. Since the data for ages 22–24 are aggregated across three age groups, they should be regarded as tentative estimates of age-specific patterns shortly following age 21.

In Table 4.2 it appears that both prevalence and general offending rates for general delinquency peak, as expected, in mid-adolescence. (This

TABLE 4.3.Index offenses.

Age	1976	1977	1978	1979	1980	1983	Age-specific mean
			Prevalence rate				
12	20	14					17
13	21	16	12				17
14	19	16	12	14			15
15	24	21	16	17	14		18
16	19	22	19	15	14		18
17	24	14	17	20	13		18
18		13	14	14	12	11	13
19			10	11	14	9	11
20				7	8	13	9
21					9	12	11
(22–24)						(6)	(6)
			General offending rate (per thousand)				
12	696	1,654					1,312
13	1,304	1,400	245				983
14	1,226	748	673	874			880
15	1,147	5,370	1,079	848	770		1,843
16	793	1,519	1,164	524	697		939
17	995	2,035	787	1,851	584		1,250
18		335	790	1,032	621	544	664
19			250	1,814	652	236	738
20				352	691	619	554
21					200	217	209
(22–24)						(228)	(228)

result is consistent with the analysis of the relationship between age and delinquency in Chapter 3). Prevalence is highest at age 16, but there is little difference among ages 11–17 in age-specific mean prevalence. It is clear from the period figures (columns) that those aged 12 and 13 have consistently (in every period) lower rates than those aged 16 and 17, and that those aged 19 and 20 also have consistently lower rates than those aged 16 and 17, for years in which comparable data are available. This indicates that the age differences are not merely artifacts of period or cohort trends. General delinquency offending rates peak sharply at age 17, and comparisons with rates for ages 12–14 and (with the possible exception of the year 1980) ages 19–21 again suggest the presence of a true age effect.

In Table 4.3 prevalence of Index offenses peaks at ages 15–17. Comparisons with younger and older ages in different years are not as conclusive in ruling out the possibility of a combined cohort-period effect as was the case for general delinquency, but averaging the prevalence figures for ages 11–13, 15–17, and 19–20 produce the same conclusion— that there is indeed a true age effect. General offending rates are highest for age 15 but fluctuate considerably across age in early adolescence.

From age 18 onward, however, mean age-specific general offending rates are consistently lower than rates for ages 12–17. General offending rates at age 15 are (with one exception in 1976) consistently higher than rates for ages 19–20. Overall, fluctuations in the rates over time and across ages are sufficient to raise the question of whether the apparent age differences are artifacts of cohort and period effects and to call into question the Maturational Reform hypothesis for serious crime.

Tables 4.4, 4.5, and 4.6 present age- and period-specific prevalence and general use rates for alcohol, marijuana, and polydrug use. Both prevalence and mean annual frequency of alcohol use increase with age from age 12 to age 20 (Table 4.4). After age 20, consistent with the Maturational Reform hypothesis and Kandel (1980), they appear to level off but not (yet) to decline. These age effects are consistent within each of the periods studied and across cohorts as well. The same pattern applies to prevalence and mean annual frequency of marijuana use (Table 4.5), which also increases until age 20. Unlike alcohol use, however, marijuana use shows some evidence of a decline in prevalence and frequency of use after age 21.

TABLE 4.4. Alcohol use.

Age	1976	1977	1978	1979	1980	1983	Age-specific mean
				Prevalence rate			
12	23	27					25
13	31	47	39				39
14	55	56	53	51			54
15	65	79	63	63	66		67
16	70	78	81	73	74		75
17	82	84	82	79	80		81
18		83	89	86	85	83	85
19			87	90	86	87	88
20				88	91	89	89
21					86	92	89
(22–24)						(89)	(89)
				General use rate (per person per year)			
12	1	1					1
13	2	5	2				3
14	8	6	5	7			7
15	11	9	12	12	11		11
16	16	19	25	19	23		20
17	18	21	34	30	28		26
18		26	46	59	40	43	43
19			47	71	71	50	60
20				69	86	53	69
21					68	56	62
(22–24)						(69)	(69)

TABLE 4.5. Marijuana use.

Age	1976	1977	1978	1979	1980	1983	Age-specific mean
			Prevalence rate				
12	2	4					3
13	9	9	12				10
14	18	19	20	22			20
15	28	32	30	31	30		30
16	31	38	45	35	35		37
17	39	43	49	46	42		44
18		49	52	50	53	41	49
19			49	52	51	44	49
20				56	49	46	50
21					52	47	50
(22–24)						(41)	(41)
			General use rate (per person per year)				
12	0	1					1
13	2	1	2				2
14	8	6	6	5			6
15	12	18	17	16	19		15
16	13	19	28	19	24		21
17	18	21	38	36	30		29
18		18	36	36	32	28	30
19			39	38	44	29	38
20				46	40	40	42
21					46	35	41
(22–24)						(32)	(32)

Prevalence of polydrug use (Table 4.6) increases until age 21, then appears to stabilize or to decline slightly. (Extended data for ages 22, 23, and 24 separately suggest the possibility that prevalence of polydrug use declines after age 21.) Age-specific prevalence rates within each year are (except for ages 18–19 in 1979) consistent with this pattern. Mean frequency of polydrug use is very low at all ages, but appears to be highest at age 20 and to stabilize or decline thereafter. Within individual years, however, there is no clear pattern. Rather than suggesting that the age effect is really an artifact of period and cohort trends, the data suggest that random variation or random measurement error are causing the fluctuations across age for specific years. Given this assumption, the data on polydrug prevalence and frequency of use are consistent with the Maturational Reform hypothesis, and all three substances (alcohol, marijuana, and multiple illicit drugs) appear to demonstrate true age effects.

Table 4.7 presents age- and period-specific prevalence rates and mean scale scores for mental health problems. Both prevalence and mean scale

TABLE 4.6. Polydrug use.

Age	1976	1977	1978	1979	1980	1983	Age-specific mean
				Prevalence rate			
12	1	0					1
13	1	1	2				1
14	5	5	5	8			6
15	8	8	7	11	9		9
16	10	11	14	11	13		12
17	16	10	14	18	12		12
18		16	15	21	19	19	16
19		17	18	21	21		19
20			25	21	21		22
21				24	23		24
(22–24)						(23)	(23)
				General use rate (per person per year)			
12	0	0					0
13	0	0	1				0
14	3	1	2	2			2
15	1	4	1	5	4		3
16	1	1	4	2	1		2
17	2	7	5	13	3	10	6
18		4	4	9	7	7	7
19			5	6	11	10	7
20				5	8	7	8
21					6	(7)	7
(22–24)							(7)

scores for mental health problems appear to decline with age. Examination of data for individual years, however, indicates that this apparent age effect is really an artifact of a secular negative trend in mental health problem prevalence and scale scores. Age-specific prevalence declines almost monotonically for each age group over time; other than this decline, there is no clear pattern to the prevalence of mental health problems. (By contrast, polydrug use demonstrated no such monotonic trend.) Mental health problem scale scores, in addition to showing a clear, monotonic, declining trend over time are nearly constant within each year. Therefore we may be able to rule out the existence of an age effect in the mental health problem data for the National Youth Survey.

With the exception of mental health, then, there appear to be genuine age effects in our data on delinquency and ADM problems. The data on general delinquency, alcohol use, marijuana use, and polydrug use all support the Maturational Reform hypothesis (the more so considering the apparent declines in marijuana and polydrug use, which are illegal, as opposed to the apparent stability in alcohol use, which is legal after age

TABLE 4.7. Mental health problems.

Age	1976	1977	1978	1979	1980	1983	Age-specific mean
				Prevalence rate			
12	15	7					11
13	10	7	5				7
14	13	9	7	6			9
15	9	9	6	8	6		8
16	13	7	8	5	6		8
17	14	10	5	4	5		8
18		8	6	8	4	7	7
19			8	7	8	6	7
20				6	5	5	5
21					5	5	5
(22–24)						(7)	(7)
				Mean scale score			
12	40	38					39
13	39	38	36				38
14	39	38	37	35			37
15	39	38	37	37	34		37
16	40	38	37	36	36		37
17	39	38	37	36	36		37
18		38	37	36	36	32	36
19			37	36	36	32	35
20				37	35	33	35
21					36	33	34
(22–24)						(32)	(32)

21). The data on Index offenses are more equivocal but are at least consistent with the Maturational Reform hypothesis and the existence of a true age effect. With regard to Index offenses, the issue may better be resolved after an examination of period and cohort effects.

Period Effects: Trends Over Time

Because there exist demonstrable age effects on delinquency, alcohol use, and drug use, we cannot use the National Youth Survey data to examine trends in these behaviors without first controlling for age. Absent such controls, we might compare 11–17-year-olds in 1976 with 18–24-year-olds in 1983. Any differences we found could not be attributed to period effects, because age effects would provide a very plausible alternative hypothesis. Controlling for age, however, limits the number of years we can use for any examination of trends. Data were collected annually for 1976 to 1980, then again for 1983.[1] (Data were also collected for 1986, but are not available at the time of writing.) For any given age, we have at most five data points, because by 1983 there were no more 11 to 17-year-olds, and before 1977 there were no 18-year-olds in the sample.

The inability to deal with long-term age-specific trends in behavior is an inherent weakness in any longitudinal panel study, and it points to the need for series of cross-sectional studies to supplement longitudinal panel studies. With the NYS data, it is still possible to examine trends for 15 to 17-year-olds for the 5-year period from 1976 to 1980. Mean age-specific rates, obtained by summing the age-specific rates from Tables 4.2–4.7 and dividing the total by three, are presented in Table 4.8 for general delinquency, Index offenses, alcohol use, marijuana use, polydrug use, and (despite the already evident absence of any age effect) mental health problems.

The age-specific prevalence of general delinquency declines monotonically over time from 1976 to 1980. Examination of the trends for each of the component ages (15–17), however, indicates that this monotonic decline is reflected only for age 15. For age 16, general delinquency prevalence is highest in 1977. For age 17, prevalence is highest in 1976, but prevalence in 1977 is lower than prevalence in 1978. Notice also that for age 18 (see Table 4.2), prevalence is highest in 1979, not in 1977. For ages 15, 16, and 18, prevalence is highest for the cohort born in 1961, the largest of the seven cohorts and the one with the second-highest average birth order. These results suggest that the period trend may be a result of cohort differences. (Note also the difference between the results for 15- to 17-year-olds on General Delinquency C, presented here, and those for 16- to 17-year-olds on General Delinquency B, presented in Menard, 1987.)

General delinquency offending rates for ages 15–17 are highest in 1977 and decline monotonically thereafter. Once again, this finding is inconsistent with the trends for two of the three age groups, but the cohort pattern is not as clear. Although random variation or random measurement error may play a role here, it is possible that the variations in age-specific general delinquency offending are a result of a combination of cohort effects and period effects. Age-specific Index offense prevalence and offending rates follow the same pattern as the corresponding rates for general delinquency. Again, inconsistencies between the average rates for

---

[1] Data were collected retrospectively for 1981 and 1982 for prevalence but not for offending rates. Aside from the problem of not having offending rates available at all for these years, the age-specific prevalence rates for 1981 and 1982 were substantially lower than those for 1980 or 1983, leading us to suspect that the retrospective data for 1981 and 1982 seriously underestimated the prevalence, especially of general and Index offending, for those years. Because of these problems in the data, data for 1981 and 1982 are not used in the analyses in this chapter.

TABLE 4.8. Age-specific trends over time.

	1976	1977	1978	1979	1980
	Mean prevalence rates (age 15–17)				
	1976	1977	1978	1979	1980
General delinquency	68	66	60	55	49
Index offenses	22	19	17	17	14
Alcohol use	72	80	75	72	73
Marijuana use	33	38	41	37	36
Polydrug use	11	10	12	13	11
Mental health problems	12	9	6	6	6
	Mean offending rates (age 15–17)				
General delinquency[a]	18,784	22,266	16,551	15,297	12,433
Index offenses[a]	978	2,974	1,010	1,074	684
Alcohol use[b]	15	16	24	20	21
Marijuana use[b]	14	19	28	24	18
Polydrug use[b]	1	4	3	6	3
Mental health problems[c]	39	38	37	36	35

[a] Offending rate per thousand.
[b] Mean annual frequency of use.
[c] Mean scale score.

ages 15–17 and the disaggregated rates for each separate age point to the possibility of a cohort effect as the explanation for the secular trend.

Alcohol use rates for ages 15–17 peak in 1978 and decline thereafter, but the lowest alcohol use rates for ages 15–17 are in 1976. Alcohol prevalence is highest in 1977; aside from this, there is little change in the prevalence of alcohol use for ages 15–17 over time. Marijuana use rates, like alcohol use rates, are highest in 1978 and lowest in 1976. Marijuana prevalence rates, however, peak in 1978, a year later than those for alcohol use (and at the same time as marijuana use rates). Prevalence of marijuana use is lowest for 1976. Both use rates and prevalence of polydrug use are highest for 1979, a year later than for marijuana use. The lowest polydrug use rate occurs in 1976, and the lowest prevalence in 1977. Taken together, these trends are consistent with those in Johnston et al. (1984), which indicated increasing alcohol, marijuana, and drug use from 1975 until 1979 (± 1 year), and declining rates of alcohol, marijuana, and drug use thereafter for high school seniors. The NYS data are also consistent with the suggestion (e.g., Kandel, 1982) that alcohol use is prerequisite to marijuana use, which in turn is prerequisite to polydrug use, since the sequence of peak years for use of these substances (particularly prevalence of use) goes from alcohol to marijuana to polydrug use.

Disaggregated trends for ages 15–17 taken separately are not consistent with trends for (aggregated) ages 15–17 taken together for alcohol prevalence. For the separate age groups alcohol prevalence is lowest in 1976 only for those 16 years old, and for this same age the highest prevalence of alcohol use occurs in 1979, not in 1978. For ages 15 and 16, cohort 5 has the highest prevalence; for ages 17 and 18, cohort 6 has the highest prevalence. There is no clear cohort pattern to the lowest age-specific prevalence rates for ages 15–18. These patterns would be compatible with the existence of a combined period and cohort effect on prevalence of alcohol use. Disaggregated trends for frequency of alcohol use, however, are generally consistent with the aggregate trends and suggest that frequency of alcohol use may be declining after 1978 independently of any cohort effects.

Disaggregated trends for frequency and prevalence of marijuana use are generally consistent with aggregate trends for ages 15–17. For ages 15, 16, and 18, however, cohort 4 has the highest age-specific prevalence of marijuana use, and there is some indication of a cohort effect for average frequency of marijuana use for ages 15–18. Both mean frequency and prevalence of polydrug use vary considerably within age groups and only weakly mirror the aggregated trends for ages 15–17. No cohort trends are obvious.

Taken together, the patterns of temporal variation in alcohol, marijuana, and drug use suggest that as we enter the 1980s, age-specific frequency of use of all three substances may be declining independently of cohort effects. Prevalence of alcohol and marijuana use, however, appears to be at least partially determined by cohort effects, although there is little evidence of such effects on polydrug use. Cohort effects will be examined in greater detail in the next section.

Both averaged and separate trends in mental health problem scale scores show a monotonic decline over time. Mental health problem prevalence also declines over time, monotonically when ages 15–17 are averaged, but not monotonically when ages 15–17 (and 18) are considered separately. There is little apparent evidence of any cohort effect, however, and the nonmonotonicity of the decline in prevalence scores may be a result of random variation or random error.

Cohort Effects: Preliminary Patterns

In the absence of a clear rationale which suggests some theoretical linkage between a cohort, as such, and the behavior in question, it would be substantively meaningless to attribute variations in offending rates, frequency of substance use, mental health problem scale scores, or prevalence of delinquency and ADM problems to age- and period-specific cohort effects. The Easterlin hypothesis provides us with just such a theoretical linkage.

The existence of a cohort effect will be inferred only if there appears to be a relationship between average parity or birth order and the behavior in question. To the extent that absolute cohort size is the variable of concern, we can measure it directly as the number of births in a given year. The measurement of relative cohort size is more problematic.

A common method of measuring relative cohort size is to use the ratio of persons under a certain age to persons over a certain age, or to use a ratio involving two age ranges, one of which may reasonably be interpreted as the "parental" generation with respect to the other. Steffensmeier, Steifel, & Harer, (1987) use the ratio of those aged 15–24 to those aged 24–64. Easterlin (1987) uses the ratio of those aged 15–29 to those aged 30–64. These ratios measure the number of adolescents and young adults relative to the number of older adults, but they do not really get at the relative size of parental and filial cohorts, because some of the older adults included in the comparison have no children or have children none of whom fall within the age range specified, and some of those in the younger cohort have parents older than 64 or brothers or sisters (same generation) a few years older who fall within the age boundaries of the older adults.

As an alternative measure of relative cohort size, we use *average parity*, or average birth order, of each cohort. The parents who have children in a particular year are thus defined as an *event cohort* (Graetz, 1987), the event being the birth of a child in any year from 1959 to 1965. For these seven event cohorts of parents, and the birth cohorts (children born between 1959 and 1965, where one's own birth is the "event" of concern) to which they correspond, average parity is the ratio of children, including siblings of those in the birth cohort, to parents in the event cohort, in the year of the event (the year in which the parent in the event cohort gives birth to the child in the birth cohort). The result is equivalent to the mean family size at birth of the child in the relevant birth cohort, for both the parent in the event cohort and the child in the birth cohort. It does not, however, correspond necessarily to subsequent family size. Whether it is thought of as a measure of relative cohort size or as a measure (at one particular point in time) of family size, average parity is an indicator of the relative availability of parental attention, the resource most relevant in early childhood.[2]

For the preliminary analysis of cohort effects, we focus on extreme (highest and lowest) age-specific rates of prevalence, rates of general

---

[2] This conclusion also may apply to the development of intelligence, according to Zajonc and Markus's (1975) confluence model of absolute intelligence. Zajonc's (1976) argument, that family configuration (birth order, family size, and child spacing) may have been responsible for declines in standardized test scores from 1965 to 1980, is one of the few that cannot be readily dismissed (Menard, 1981), especially since Zajonc correctly predicted the turnaround in SAT scores in the 1980s based on that model.

offending, frequency of substance use, and mental health problem scale scores. Although we use average parity or birth order as an indicator of relative cohort size, the present study should not be confused with previous studies (e.g., Biles, 1971; Lees & Newson, 1954; Nye, 1958; Rahav, 1980) of the relationship between *individual* birth order and *individual* levels of delinquent or problem behavior. Here, we are not concerned with the impact of birth order as such, or with whether middle-born children have higher or lower rates of illegal behavior than first-born or last-born children. Neither is the close relationship between *individual* birth order and *individual* family size (Menard, 1981, p. 197 and note 6) problematic. Our concern here is with *aggregate* cohort differences based on relative cohort size, for which average parity is one (macrosocial) indicator. Also, although results are discussed primarily in terms of *relative* cohort size (as indicated by average parity) we have also checked for effects of *absolute* cohort size. With the aid of Table 4.1 in conjunction with Tables 4.2–4.7, the reader may readily duplicate our analysis.

DELINQUENCY

Age-specific prevalence of general delinquency is consistently lowest for the cohort with the latest birthdate (see Table 4.1 for cohort numbers and years of birth). There is also a general tendency for the cohort with the earliest birth date to have the highest age-specific prevalence of general delinquency. These results indicate that there may be a slight cohort effect (one concentrated in those ages examined in the analysis of period trends), but the dominant effect appears to be a period trend toward declining prevalence.

Age-specific general offending rates are highest for cohorts 3, 4, 5, and 6 (the cohorts with highest average birth order) except once for cohort 2 (compared to cohort 1) and once for cohort 7. They are lowest for cohorts 1, 2, and 3 (the cohorts with lowest average birth order) except once for cohort 4 and once for cohort 5. Changes in offending rates of general delinquency appear to be a function of both cohort effects and period trends, with the former perhaps predominating.

The highest age-specific prevalence rates for Index offenses occur in cohorts 3, 4, 5, and 6, except once in cohort 7 and once (compared to cohort 1) in cohort 2. The lowest prevalence of Index offenses *always* occurs in cohort 1, 2, or 7 (and in 7 only if neither 1 nor 2 has data for the age in question). This finding strongly suggests that cohort effects may explain any apparent period trends in Index offense prevalence (particularly since, when neither 1 nor 2 are available, the fact that cohort 7 has the lowest prevalence effectively *reverses* the trend for those ages).

Age-specific general offending rates for Index offenses are highest for cohorts 4, 5, and 6, except once each for 1 (compared to 2) and 2. They are lowest for cohorts 1, 2, 7, and 3; observe that 3 has lower average birth order than 4, 5, or 6. These results again suggest the presence of a cohort effect, albeit not with the same division of cohorts (3, 4, 5, 6 vs. 1, 2, 7) as before. In 6 of 10 age-specific comparisons, the most recent cohort had the lowest offending rate, and in all of the remaining comparisons (two of which involve only two cohorts) the second-most recently born cohort had the lowest rate. This result suggests the presence of a period effect, a decline over time. Index offending rates, therefore, appear to have trends based on both period and cohort effects, with no clear evidence indicating which is stronger.

DRUG USE

For age-specific alcohol prevalence each cohort has the lowest prevalence rate in at least one comparison, and each except for cohort 5 also has the highest rate for at least one comparison. Except for age 16 (when it has the lowest prevalence rate), cohort 6 has the highest prevalence rate whenever age-specific data on cohort 6 are available. Except for age 16, age-specific prevalence rates prior to age 18 are highest for 1977, regardless of cohort. It seems most reasonable to conclude that for prevalence of alcohol use, period effects dominate adolescence but cohort effects begin to take over after age 17, with cohort 6 (the largest cohort) having the highest prevalence rates. Age-specific alcohol frequency rates are highest at least once for every cohort except cohort 5. If there is a cohort effect, it is not at all clear from the data. Trends in frequency of alcohol use thus appear to be independent of any cohort effects.

Age-specific prevalence of marijuana use is lowest at least once for each cohort, and highest at least once for every cohort except cohort 2 and cohort 3. The cohorts with the highest and the lowest average birth order (cohorts 1 and 4) rank highest on prevalence three times apiece. More important, lowest prevalence rates all occur in 1975 (for ages 12–17) or 1983 (ages 18–21), and highest prevalence scores occur in 1977–1980. These results suggest a curvilinear trend in prevalence of marijuana use, independent of cohort effects. There is no clear cohort effect on mean age-specific frequency of marijuana use either, suggesting that frequency, like prevalence, is subject to period but not cohort effects.

Each cohort has the lowest age-specific prevalence rate of polydrug use at least once, and all except 3 and 6 have the highest rate at least once. With the exception of age 12 (which has data only for 1976 and 1977), the highest prevalence of polydrug use occurs in 1979 or in a year immediately prior or subsequent to 1979. For all but ages 20 and 21 (for which there are no data prior to 1979), the lowest age-specific rate of polydrug use occurs 1 year before or after 1977. As with marijuana prevalence, there is an absence of any clear cohort effect on prevalence of polydrug use. There is also no clear cohort pattern for frequency of polydrug use.

There is some tendency for the lowest frequencies to occur in earlier years and for the highest frequencies to occur in later years. It appears once again that for polydrug use, period effects are independent of cohort effects.

MENTAL HEALTH PROBLEMS

As indicated earlier, variations in mental health problem scale scores and prevalence appear to be independent of both age and cohort effects. Only a secular declining trend is evident especially for scale scores. If cohort size is used instead of average birth order, there is no clear cohort effect for delinquency or alcohol and drug use, but an apparent cohort effect for mental health problems. For prevalence of mental health problems, highest age-specific prevalence occurs among the largest cohorts (4, 5, 6, and 7) except when they are not available for the age in question. When only cohorts 1, 2, or 3 are available, the largest of them has the highest prevalence. Lowest age-specific prevalence occurs in the smallest cohorts (1, 2, and 3) except twice for cohort 4 (the next smallest cohort). For mental health problem scale scores, the pattern of temporal decline coincides perfectly with the pattern of the smallest cohort at a given age having the lowest age-specific mean scale score, but not as perfectly with large cohorts having higher scores. Mental health problem scale scores, though consistent with absolute differences in absolute cohort size, can be explained completely in terms of period effects without reference to cohort effects. This does, nonetheless, raise the possibility that mental health problems (particularly prevalence) may be related to absolute rather than relative cohort size.

Age, Period, and Cohort Effects: Formal Analysis

Since the development of methods for parameterizing age, period, and cohort effects (Mason, Mason, Winsborough, & Poole, 1973) several attempts have been made to examine age, period, and cohort influences on crime, with a particular focus on juvenile delinquency (Greenberg & Larkin, 1985; Maxim, 1985; Pullum, 1977; Smith, 1986; Steffensmeier et al., 1987). The studies by Maxim, by Smith, and by Steffensmeier and co-workers purport to examine the hypothesis stated by Easterlin (1987, p. 101–104) that cohorts which are large relative to their parents' cohorts will experience greater frequency of crime among the young. These studies have all used age-and-period police or court data, which are relatively easy to obtain for criminal offenses but are much more difficult to obtain for alcohol use and drug use, especially if, with regard to the latter category, one wishes to separate relatively more serious and less frequent multiple illicit drug use (heroin, cocaine, hallucinogens, barbiturates, amphetamines) from the relatively less serious and more common offense of marijuana use. It is therefore not surprising that, to date, alcohol and illicit drug use has not been accorded the same attention as crime and delinquency with respect to age, period, and cohort effects (but with regard to alcohol, see Glenn, 1981). We are presently aware of no previous attempts at formal analysis of age, period, and cohort effects on mental health problems. In the present study, we extend the domain of concern from previous studies of age, period, and cohort effects to include patterns of licit (alcohol) and illicit (marijuana and polydrug) substance use and mental health problems.

In all five studies of crime and delinquency, some measure of official age-and-period-specific criminality is used as the dependent variable. Pullum (1977) uses odds of arrest for those aged 15–24 from 1964 to 1973. Maxim uses the prevalence of referral to juvenile court (subjected to a weighted arcsin transformation) for males and females (analyzed separately) aged 7–15 from 1952 to 1981. Smith (1986) uses age- and period-specific homicide arrest rates for those aged 15–49 (in 5-year intervals) during the years 1952–1976 (also in 5-year intervals). Steffensmeier et al. (1987) use the logarithm of age- and period-specific arrest rates for Index offenses (murder, robbery, aggravated assault, burglary, larceny, and motor vehicle theft, but not rape), separately and aggregated into a single measure, for ages 15–24 from 1953 to 1984. They also use a derivative measure, proportional age involvement in Index crimes.

The studies by Pullum (1977) and Greenberg and Larkin (1985) differ from the other three studies in two important ways. First, they are primarily methodological, and are not concerned with the Easterlin hypothesis or other explanations of the age, period, or cohort effects evident in the data. Second, Pullum used a multiplicative model, in contrast to the additive model used in the other three studies. Within this context, Pullum detected all three types of effects—age, period, and cohort—in his analysis. Greenberg and Larkin used a logistic regression model and also found all three types of effects.

Maxim (1985), Smith (1986), and Steffensmeier et al. (1987) all used the additive, dummy-variable model developed by Mason et al. (1973). For both males and females (between whom there appeared to be little substantive difference) Maxim found age, period, and cohort effects in the prevalence of juvenile court referral, and the cohort effect was correlated with cohort size, consistent with the Easterlin hypothesis. Smith found that cohort and age effects effectively explained period trends in homicide and that the correlation between cohort size and the cohort effect once again supported the Easterlin hypothesis. Steffensmeier and colleagues, in contrast to Smith, found only a weak cohort effect for Index offenses, including homicide considered separately from the other offenses, and they concluded, based on the weakness of the cohort effect and its insignificant correlation with their measure of relative cohort size, that the Easterlin hypothesis was not supported.

Data and Measurement

Data on age, period, and self-reported delinquency, substance use, and mental health problems are taken from the NYS. Data on cohort size (births and parity) are taken primarily from the U.S. Bureau of the Census (1975); see also Easterlin (1987) and Zajonc (1976). Included are data on absolute cohort size (total number of births in a year divided by 1,000) and relative cohort size (average parity in a year). For the formal analysis, the full range of ages (11–24) is used, for 1976–1980 and 1983, for which years data are available on both prevalence and offending rates, use rates, or scale scores (as appropriate).

The use of official arrest and court referral data as indicators of delinquency or crime is one reservation we have about prior studies of age, period, and cohort effects on crime and delinquency. The relative advantages and disadvantages of official and self-report data as indicators of criminal or delinquent behavior have been reviewed in detail elsewhere (for example, O'Brien, 1985) and we do not want to present yet another general discussion of official and self-report data here. Specific to the present analysis, however, we wish to suggest that official statistics may not be good indicators of period trends in illegal behavior, and period is one of three major variables in any analysis of age, period, and cohort effects. O'Brien (1985), after a review of the literature, comes to the conclusion that "it is not, in general, safe to consider changes in official crime rates over time as changes in rates of offending." Maxim (1985) found evidence in his data that official policies, perhaps in response to "saturation" of the juvenile justice system by large cohorts of youth, may have had an impact on trends in age-specific prevalence of juvenile court referral. Menard (1987) documented the existence of divergent period trends between official statistics (offenses known to the police and arrest rates) as compared to victimization and self-report (prevalence and mean frequency) data. Indeed, Menard found that trends in rates of arrest (the usual measure in age-period-cohort studies) and rates of offenses known to the police may diverge from one another, even for homicide, a finding that further calls into question the validity of arrest statistics as indicators of criminal behavior. For substance use, we have the additional problem that official sources do not disaggregate by type of substance. For mental health problems, we have no clear idea how official statistics on mental health problems are related to our mental health problem scale.

The measurement of the age effect would be straightforward only if the effect of age on substance use turned out to be linear. The Maturational Reform hypothesis, however, leads us to expect a nonlinear relationship between age and substance use, and does not specify at what age the prevalence and mean frequency of substance use should reach its maximum. In the present analysis, we shall consider chronological age (age at last birthday) as one variable that may influence substance use, but we shall also examine the results of replacing chronological age with the *absolute deviation* from the age of maximum prevalence or mean frequency of use. The absolute deviation from the age of maximum prevalence or mean frequency of use refers to the absolute value of the difference between chronological age and age of maximum offending, or | (chronological age) − (age of maximum offending) |. Consistent with the Maturational Reform hypothesis, the absolute deviation from age of maximum substance is, by definition a U- or J-shaped function of age. If substance use has a similar (or inverted) nonlinear relationship with age, then substance use should have an approximately linear relationship with absolute deviation from age of maximum substance use.

The measurement of time period as calendar year is straightforward. We have also considered the possibility of a curvilinear period relationship. The appropriate measures for cohort size are a little more problematic. Maxim (1985) and Smith (1986) used measures of absolute cohort size, and we will consider this measure here, but Easterlin's hypothesis deals generally with the *relative* sizes of cohorts of parents and children. For the reasons detailed above, we use average parity as our measure of relative cohort size.

METHODS

In addition to concerns about the use of arrest or court referral statistics and the measurement of relative cohort size in past studies, we question the use of the additive dummy-variable model developed by Mason et al. (1973) in the studies by Maxim (1985), Smith (1986), and Steffensmeier et al. (1987). We are not echoing Glenn's (1976) reservations about the additive model for parameterizing age, period, and cohort effects, nor do we question Pullum's (1977) use of a similar but multiplicative model, given the atheoretical context within which it was presented. Indeed, the Mason et al. model is extremely valuable in the analysis of age, period, and cohort effects when there is no *a priori* specification of the form (linear, logarithmic, polynomial) that those effects may take or of the relevant variables (absolute or relative cohort size) for which those effects act as proxies. Instead, we wish to reiterate a crucial point stated by Mason, Mason, and Winsborough (1976, p. 905):

What deserves special emphasis here is that in models of the sort considered in our article, age, period, and cohort are proxies for unmeasured mechanisms or variables. If these mechanisms or variables were measured and available for analysis, the estimability problem dealt with in our paper either would not occur or would be different. For example, if cohort size is held to be the variable which causes cohort differentiation in the context of a specific substantive problem, then, if size measurements can be constructed, it is unnecessary to include cohorts as such in the specification because the preferred variable is available. Under circumstances like this the results of cohort analysis become less tentative, since the estimability problem as we described it is eliminated. The replacement of proxies by the variables they index is a universal goal of research.

Mason et al. (1973) were concerned with the estimation of cohort effects when cohort itself, operationalized as year of birth, had to be entered into an analysis as an independent variable along with chronological age and period (year). As they indicate, for these measures, cohort=year−age. By contrast, relative or absolute cohort *size* bears no such fixed, linear relationship to year and age. For that matter, the absolute deviation of age from some specified age also bears no such fixed, linear relationship to cohort and year. Use of either cohort size or absolute deviation of age eliminates the problem of estimability that the Mason et al. method was designed to solve. Instead of estimating 39 (Pullum), 54 (Smith), 77 (Maxim), or 79 (Steffensmeier et al.) dummy-variable parameters, and losing some information when we impose constraints on the model to make it estimable, we really need estimate only three parameters per dependent variable (12 if we consider all possible combinations of age, period, and cohort size effects) if we want to test the Easterlin or Maturational Reform hypotheses.

We shall proceed by assuming a linear, additive relationship between the dependent and independent variables. The assumption of additivity is no different from that made by the Mason et al. dummy-variable model. The assumption of linearity is tested to some extent by examining (a) the explanatory power of the model—that is, how well a linear model explains each of the dependent variables; (b) the effect of taking the natural logarithm of the dependent variables; (c) the effect of substituting the absolute deviation from the age of maximum offending for chronological age, consistent with the Maturational Reform hypothesis; and (d) the effect of substituting the absolute deviation from the calendar year of the year of maximum offending, $|$ (calendar year)−(year of maximum offending) $|$. The use of the natural logarithm in (b) has some precedent (Steffensmeier et al., 1987) and seems appropriate, given the skewness of some of the data, especially with regard to mean frequency of offending. We use ordinary least-squares regression to calculate the magnitude and statistical significance of age, period, and cohort size effects, and consider reduced models that include only statistically significant regression coefficients. Principal components tests for collinearity and the Durbin-Watson test for autocorrelated error are also considered.

For each dependent variable, regression equations were calculated for several combinations of age, period, and cohort size indicators. The *best-fitting equations* were defined as those equations that satisfied two criteria: (a) the explained variance was maximized subject to the requirement that (b) all regression coefficients in the equation were statistically significant with probability less than or equal to .050. Greater detail on the relative explanatory power of different combinations of indicators for delinquency, alcohol use, marijuana use, and polydrug use may be found in Menard and Elliott (1988a) and Menard and Huizinga (1988).

DELINQUENCY

For general delinquency and Index offenses, the best-fitting equations are presented in Table 4.9. For each variable in Table 4.9, GDC refers to general delinquency or crime, IND refers to Index offenses, a P-suffix (as in GDCP) refers to prevalence, and an F-suffix (as in INDF) refers to a general offending rate. An L-prefix (as in LGDCP) refers to the natural logarithm of the variable (in this example, the natural logarithm of the prevalence of general delinquency). Durbin-Watson tests for each equation in Table 4.9 indicate that we may accept the hypothesis of no autocorrelated error.

For prevalence of general delinquency, we find both the curvilinear age effect suggested by the Maturational Reform hypothesis and the cohort size effect predicted by the Easterlin hypothesis. In addition, there is a statistically significant period effect. For each year of age younger than 15 or older than 16, prevalence of general delinquency is reduced by 1.6%, and for each year after 1976, it declines by 2.5%–3%, according to the equations in Table 4.9. For each reduction of .026 (one-half standard deviation) in average parity, prevalence of general delinquency is reduced by 0.07%–1.0%. For the logarithmic transformation of prevalence of general delinquency, the level of explanation is the same ($R^2 = .86$), and the best-fitting equations include a curvilinear age effect (absolute deviation from age 15), a period effect, and either absolute or relative cohort size effects. In all of the best-fitting equations, with or without logarithmic transformation, period has the strongest influence, and cohort size the weakest, on prevalence of general delinquency. The period trend is not, as suggested in connection with Table 4.8 above, merely a combination of age and cohort effects.

The offending rate for general delinquency, with or without logarithmic transformation, appears to reach its peak at age 16, a year later than for prevalence. Again, there is both a curvilinear age effect and a cohort size effect, as predicted by the Maturational Reform and Easterlin hypotheses, but for the offending rate of general delinquency there is no statistically significant period effect. The weak negative period trend indicated in connection with Table 4.8 is apparently a result of combined age and cohort effects for the general delinquency offending rate. For each year of age younger or older than 16, the offending rate for general delinquency decreases by 906 offenses per 1,000 people, or almost one offense per person. A reduction of .026 in average parity produces a reduction of more than 1,300 offenses per thousand people. In the

TABLE 4.9. Best-fitting equations for self-reported delinquency.

Dependent variable	R^2 (explained variance)	Independent variable	β (standardized regression coefficient)	B (unstandardized regression coefficient)	Significance of B	Intercept
GDCP	.86	|Age − 15| Year Parity	−.379 −.620 .216	−1.63 −2.56 39.7	.000 .000 .001	143.
GDCP	.86	|Age − 16| Year Parity	−.322 −.701 .141	−1.64 −2.89 25.9	.000 .000 .027	209.
LGDCP	.86	|Age − 15| Year Parity	−.421 −.594 .171	−.036 −.049 .625	.000 .000 .007	6.06
LGDCP	.86	|Age − 15| Year Parity	−.465 −.565 .149	−.040 −.046 .00016	.000 .000 .030	7.05
GDCF	.37	|Age − 16| Parity	−.314 .479	−906. 51417.	.019 .000	−134.919.
LGDCF	.41	|Age − 16| Parity	−.297 .532	−.066 4.43	.021 .000	−3.40
INDP	.67	Age Parity	−.886 .510	−1.38 47.2	.000 .000	−101.
LINDP	.72	Age Parity	−.929 .467	−.112 3.34	.000 .000	−5.36
LINDP	.72	|Age − 15| Year	−.550 −.385	−.092 −.062	.000 .001	7.74
INDF	.27	Age Parity	−.508 .446	−142. 7386.	.002 .005	−18.564.
LINDF	.53	Age Parity	−.772 .520	−.193 7.71	.000 .000	−12.9

best-fitting equations for offending rate of general delinquency, the effect of cohort size is greater than the effect of age.

For prevalence of Index offenses, there appears to be no curvilinear age effect, but instead a fairly strong negative trend with increasing age. Inspection of the age- and period-specific data confirms that there is no clear unimodal, curvilinear pattern, but there is a general decline from age 11 to age 24. The effect of relative cohort size is once again evident, and there is no statistically significant period trend. This agrees with the conclusion suggested in connection with Table 4.8 above. An increase of 1 year in age is associated with a decrease of 1.4%, and a decrease of .026 in average parity is associated with a decrease of 1.2% in the prevalence of Index offenses.

When a logarithmic transformation of Index prevalence is used, the results are equivocal. There appears to be either a cohort size effect or a combined period plus maturation effect, but not both. For the logarithmic transformation, even a period effect coupled with an effect of chronological age (not curvilinear) is plausible. The combination of chronological age and parity is the combination of variables that appears in the best-fitting equation for the prevalence of Index offenses whether or not the dependent variable is subjected to a logarithmic transformation (and also, as noted below, in the best-fitting equations for frequency of Index offending) and as such seems the more plausible of the two possibilities, but it is necessary to acknowledge that there is some ambiguity here. For all of the best-fitting equations, age has the stronger effect of the two variables in the equation.

The Index offending rate, whether the logarithmic transformation is applied or not, is best explained by chronological age and average parity. Each additional year of age after age 11 is associated with a decrease of 142 Index offenses per 1,000 people, and each reduction of .026 in average parity is associated with a decrease of 192 Index offenses per 1,000 people. The apparent period decline in Index offending rates may thus be explained as a combination of age and cohort effects, again consistent with the analysis of Table 4.8. Unlike previous dependent variables, the Index offending rate is substantially affected by the logarithmic transformation in another way. Using the logarithmic transformation approximately doubles the explained variance in mean frequency of Index offending. Otherwise, however, the structure of the model remains the same, with age having the larger and parity the smaller effect on the dependent variable.

ALCOHOL, MARIJUANA, AND POLYDRUG USE

Table 4.10 presents the best-fitting equations for alcohol, marijuana, and polydrug use. The prefixes and suffixes used are the same as in Table 4.9, with the F-suffix standing for use rate or mean frequency of use and ALC,

TABLE 4.10. Best-fitting equations for self-reported substance use.

Dependent variable	R^2 (explained variance)	Independent variable	β (standardized regression coefficient)	B (unstandardized regression coefficient)	Significance of B	Intercept
ALCP[a]	.88	|Age − 20|	−.631	−5.60	.000	−203.
		Year	.202	1.87	.015	
		Births	.288	.036	.007	
LALCP[b]	.72	|Age − 20|	−.725	−.139	.000	−1.10
		Parity	.222	1.98	.024	
ALCF	.86	Age	.872	7.31	.000	−84.9
		|Year−1980|	−.164	−3.10	.012	
LALCF[c]	.95	|Age − 20|	−.589	−.285	.000	−16.6
		Year	.318	.160	.000	
		Births	.290	.002	.000	
MRJP	.92	|Age − 20|	−.811	−5.32	.000	−81.8
		|Year−1980|	−.150	−1.72	.006	
		Parity	.157	47.7	.005	
MRJP	.92	|Age − 20|	−.763	−5.00	.000	−15.1
		|Year−1980|	−.170	−1.95	.002	
		Births	.193	.018	.002	
LMRJP[d]	.76	|Age − 20|	−.662	−.234	.000	−6.67
		|Year−1980|	−.181	−.112	.049	
		Parity	.232	3.79	.016	
MRJF	.89	|Age − 20|	−.798	−4.82	.000	−66.1
		|Year−1980|	−.166	−1.76	.010	
		Parity	.134	37.5	.041	

Model	R²	Variable				
MRJF	.89	|Age − 20|	−.767	−4.64	.000	−8.21
		|Year−1980|	−.178	−1.89	.007	
		Births	.149	.013	.043	
LMRJF[c]	.88	|Age − 20|	−.746	−.335	.000	−9.38
		|Year−1980|	−.156	−.123	.019	
		Parity	.224	4.65	.001	
DRGP	.92	|Age − 20|	−.573	−1.83	.000	−121.
		Year	.394	1.31	.000	
		Births	.204	.009	.003	
LDRGP	.85	|Age − 20|	−.704	−.260	.000	−11.5
		Year	.211	−.081	.016	
		Parity	.167	2.86	.034	
LDRGP	.85	|Age − 20|	−.617	−.228	.000	−9.56
		Year	−.261	.100	.005	
		Births	.229	.001	.014	
DRGF	.60	|Age − 20|	−.538	−.800	.000	−32.6
		Year	.328	.507	.012	
LDRGF	.72	|Age − 20|	−.683	−.224	.000	−4.29
		Year	.244	.083	.024	

[a] In a similar equation with parity in place of births, the regression coefficient for year was not quite statistically significant ($p = .053$); the substantive results were otherwise the same.

[b] In a similar equation with births in place of parity, the regression coefficient for births was not quite statistically significant ($p = .059$); the substantive results were otherwise the same.

[c] In a similar equation with parity in place of births, the explained variance was .93; the substantive results were otherwise the same.

[d] In a similar equation with births in place of parity, the explained variance was .75, and births had a slightly greater influence on the dependent variable than year.

[e] In a similar equation with births in place of parity, the explained variance was .87; the substantive results were otherwise the same.

MRJ, and DRG referring to alcohol, marijuana, and polydrug use, respectively. Durbin-Watson tests for autocorrelated error (Kelejian & Oates, 1974, pp. 200–203) indicate the presence of autocorrelated error in some of the equations: the equations for the natural logarithm of alcohol prevalence, the (untransformed) alcohol use rate, the natural logarithm of marijuana prevalence, and the (untransformed) prevalence of polydrug use. There is no autocorrelated error in the equations for the natural logarithms of alcohol, marijuana, or polydrug use rates or in the equation for marijuana use rate (untransformed) when absolute cohort size is in the equation. For the other equations, the test is inconclusive about the presence of autocorrelated error. The presence of autocorrelated error suggests that caution is necessary in interpreting some of the results in Table 4.10.

For alcohol prevalence, both the Maturational Reform hypothesis and the Easterlin hypothesis are supported. Prevalence of alcohol use is better explained by absolute deviation from age 20, which is also the strongest predictor of alcohol prevalence in the best-fitting equation. The negative regression coefficient indicates that, as expected, alcohol prevalence increases up to age 20, and for each year of age over or under 20, prevalence of alcohol use is lower by 5.6%,

For alcohol prevalence it appears to make little difference whether absolute or relative cohort size is used to test the Easterlin hypothesis. In either case, the hypothesis is supported and cohort size has the second strongest effect on alcohol prevalence, although its statistical significance (see note a to Table 4.10) when measured by average parity is somewhat marginal. Recalling that births are measured in thousands, a reduction in absolute cohort size of 100,000 births is associated with a reduction in alcohol prevalence of 3.6%. Alternatively, a reduction in average parity of .026 (one-half standard deviation) is associated with a 2.4% decrease in alcohol prevalence.

Of the three independent variables, period has the weakest effect on the prevalence of alcohol use. In the first (unlogged) equation, there is an increase in alcohol prevalence of about 1.9% per year from 1976 to 1983, and the exclusion of period from the equation would reduce explained variance alcohol prevalence by only 2% (see Table 4.10). In the best-fitting equation for the natural logarithm of alcohol prevalence, there is no period effect.

Results for alcohol use rates are consistent with neither maturational reform nor the Easterlin hypothesis when the logarithmic transformation is not used. Instead, frequency of alcohol use appears to have increased with age from ages 11 to 24 and to have increased over time from 1976 to 1980, and then to have declined from 1980 to 1983. Each year of age is associated with an average increase in use of 7 times per person per year. For each year's difference from 1980, an average decrease in frequency of 3 times per person per year is indicated.

By contrast, the equation for the natural logarithm of alcohol use rate supports both the Maturational Reform and Easterlin hypotheses. The logarithmic equation, moreover, has higher explained variance and no autocorrelated error, a problem that does affect the first equation. For the logarithmic equation, absolute deviation from age 20 has the strongest effect, followed in order by period and cohort size.

Whether the logarithmic transformation is used or not, the prevalence of marijuana use is best explained by a combination of the Maturational Reform hypothesis, the Easterlin hypothesis (with either absolute or relative cohort size; it makes little difference which is used), and a curvilinear period trend with a peak in 1980. The age effect is the strongest of the three, and each year of age over or under age 20 is associated with a 5% reduction in prevalence of marijuana use. Cohort size has the next strongest effect, and a reduction in average parity of .026 (one-half standard deviation) or a reduction of 100,000 in the number of births is associated with a decrease of a little over 1% in the prevalence of marijuana use. Finally, for each year earlier or later than 1980, there is nearly a 2% reduction in marijuana prevalence. As with alcohol prevalence, the equation without the logarithmic transformation has the higher explained variance for marijuana prevalence.

The use of the logarithmic transformation for the marijuana use rate affects only whether period (in the logarithmic equations) or cohort size (in the unlogged equations) has the smallest effect on the marijuana use rate. Otherwise, the explained variance is about the same, and both the Maturational Reform and Easterlin hypotheses are supported. The age effect is strongest, with each year younger or older than age 20 being associated with a decrease of about 5 occasions of use per person, or 4,600 to 4,800 occasions of use per 1,000 people. For each year before or after 1980, a reduction of nearly 2 occasions of use per person is indicated, and for each reduction of nearly .026 in average parity or each reduction of 100,000 births, a reduction of 1 occasion of use per person occurs.

Prevalence of polydrug use also produces results consistent with both the Maturational Reform and Easterlin hypotheses. Age has the strongest influence on polydrug use prevalence, followed in turn by period and cohort size. For each year of age older or younger than age 20, polydrug use prevalence is reduced by about 2%. Each year after 1976 is associated with an increase in polydrug use prevalence of a little over 1%, and a reduction of 100,000 births is associated with a reduction of about 1% in polydrug use prevalence.

For mean frequency of polydrug use, there appears to be a maturational effect but not a cohort size effect. For each year of age older or younger than age 20, polydrug use declines by 800 occasions of use per 1,000 people, or a little under one occasion of use per person. In addition, for each year after 1976, polydrug use mean frequency increases at a rate of 507 occasions per person, or about 1 occasion of use for every 2 people.

MENTAL HEALTH PROBLEMS

Table 4.11 presents the best-fitting equations for prevalence and mean scale scores of mental health problems. As expected from the preliminary analysis, mental health problem scale score shows a pure, linear, period effect, and this period effect accounts for 94% of the variance in the mental health problem scale scores. A change of 1 year produces nearly a 1-point change in the mental health problem scale.

For prevalence, however, there appear to be age and cohort size effects, as well as a curvilinear period trend with a *low* point in 1980. The formal analysis clarifies the difficulties in interpreting the earlier tables. The period effect is still strongest, and a change of 1 year, moving closer to 1980, produces a decrease of 1% in mental health problem prevalence. Mental health problems decline with age, and an increase of 3 years of age is associated with a reduction in prevalence of a little more than 1%. Absolute cohort size is weakest in its effect, and a reduction of 20,000 births is associated with 1% reduction in the prevalence of mental health problems.

For mental health problems, then, there is clear evidence of a period trend, but for prevalence that trend is curvilinear with a nadir in 1980, whereas for mean scale score the trend is linear and declining over time. There is no evidence of a maturational reform effect. For prevalence, the relationship with age is linear and declining. For mean scale score there is no statistically significant relationship with age. Finally, the Easterlin hypothesis is confirmed with respect to prevalence but not with respect to mean scale score for mental health problems. Those born into larger cohorts (in absolute size) are more likely to be classified as having mental health problems than those born into smaller cohorts.

Conclusions

For prevalence of general delinquency, we find, in descending order of magnitude, period, age (absolute deviation from age 16), and cohort size effects, and confirmation of both the Easterlin and Maturational Reform hypothesis. For offending rates of general delinquency, the effect of cohort size dominates, with a secondary effect of age (absolute deviation from age 15), again confirming both the Maturational Reform and Easterlin hypotheses. For prevalence of Index offenses, there is clearly an age effect and probably a cohort size effect, but we can neither accept nor reject either the Maturational Reform or the Easterlin hypothesis. Finally, the mean frequency of Index offending appears to be influenced

TABLE 4.11. Best-fitting equations for mental health problem prevalence and mean scale scores.

Dependent variable	R^2 (explained variance)	Independent variable	β (standardized regression coefficient)	B (unstandardized regression coefficient)	Significance of B	Intercept
MHPP	.53	Age	−.434	−.387	.004	−8.64
		|Year−1980|	.542	1.090	.000	
		Births	.306	.005	.034	
LMHPP	.51	Age	−.432	−.048	.005	.030
		|Year−1980|	.530	.133	.000	
		Births	.297	.001	.043	
MHPF	.94	Year	−.968	−.968	.000	113.
LMHPF	.94	Year	−.969	−.027	.000	5.73

by chronological age and cohort size, contrary to the Maturational Reform hypothesis but consistent with the Easterlin hypothesis.[3]

Our substantive conclusions regarding age, period, and cohort size effects are generally consistent with those of Smith (1986), who found that trends in homicide rates may be explained by age and cohort effects, just as we find that trends in the mean frequency of Index offenses can be explained in terms of age and cohort effects. Our results with regard to prevalence of general delinquency are also consistent with Maxim's (1985) findings concerning prevalence of juvenile court referral, particularly insofar as confirmation of the Easterlin hypothesis is concerned. Our findings regarding mean frequency of Index offending, however, contradict those of Steffensmeier et al. (1987). The agreement of our results with those of Smith (1986) and Maxim (1985) suggests that the disparity of findings may be attributable not to differences between official arrest and self-report data, but to the choice of cohort indicators for testing the Easterlin hypothesis.

Substance use, like other forms of criminal or delinquent behavior, appears to be subject to a Maturational Reform effect. Unlike other forms of criminal or delinquent behavior, which tend to peak at mid-adolescence (Farrington, 1986; Gold, 1970; Hirschi, 1969), substance use appears to peak at the end of adolescence and the beginning of adulthood, around age 20. Again, like other forms of criminal or delinquent behavior (Maxim, 1985; Pullum, 1977; Smith, 1986), substance use appears to be affected by cohort size, as predicted by Easterlin (1987). In contrast, however, to other forms of criminal or delinquent behavior (Menard, 1987) there is a consistent, *increasing* period trend in substance use from 1976 to 1980, and a continuing positive trend after 1980 in alcohol and polydrug use.

The overall image that emerges from this analysis is that substance use does differ in some respects (age of maximum prevalence and mean frequency, presence of an increasing period trend) from other forms of criminal and delinquent behavior. In future research it would be worth determining whether such patterns are unique to substance use or also characteristic of other consensual or "victimless" offenses. As more data become available, it would also be worthwhile to extend this analysis to include a wider range of ages and time periods. Finally, introduction of other theoretical variables to help explain the period effects (and also, perhaps, the age and cohort size effects) would be an appropriate focus for future research.

---

[3] If the relationship between average birth order and academic aptitude and intelligence also holds, relative cohort size may be the one explanation for the allegedly spurious relationship between intelligence and delinquency (Menard & Morse, 1984, 1986).

Mental health problem prevalence, but not mean scale score, yields results consistent with the Easterlin cohort size hypothesis. In addition, prevalence of mental health problems, like prevalence and offending rates of Index offenses, has a linear negative relationship to age. Both prevalence and mean scale score for mental health problems show period effects but for prevalence the effect is curvilinear and for mean scale score it is linear.

The presence of a period effect for the prevalence of general delinquency, for all of the substance use measures, and for mental health problems, is problematic, not from an analytical perspective but from a theoretical viewpoint. As Hobcroft, Menken, and Preston (1982, p. 5) explained:

Age is a surrogate—probably a very good one in most applications—for aging or more generally for physiological states, amount of exposure to certain social influences, or exposure to social norms. . . . indicators of period and cohort are much further removed from variables that presumably influence social processes. "Period" is a poor proxy for influences in the past. Measured "effects" of periods and cohorts are thus measures of our ignorance: in particular, of whether the factors about which we are ignorant are more or less randomly distributed along chronologically measurable dimensions.

Hobcroft et al. (1982), like Mason et al. (1976), emphasized the importance of substituting, when possible, the variables for which period or cohort act as proxies (for example, the use of cohort size rather than year of birth). With regard to the effect of period, however, it would be correct to infer that further explanation or elaboration is necessary. Although the Maturational Reform and Easterlin hypotheses help us to understand the presence of age effects and cohort size effects, we have no such basis for understanding period effects. Elaboration of period effects is beyond the scope of the present chapter but would be an appropriate topic for future research. At the individual level, this problem is addressed to some extent in Chapter 6.

5
Developmental Patterns

Age, period, and cohort effects, as described in Chapter 4, constitute one three-dimensional aspect of variation in delinquency and ADM problem behaviors over time. In this chapter, we consider three other aspects of temporal variation in delinquency and ADM problem behaviors. We begin by examining patterns of initiation (or onset) and suspension (or termination) of problem behavior. After that, we look at patterns of transition (escalation and de-escalation) *within* delinquency, drug use, and mental health problem types. Finally, we consider patterns of transition *among* the three types of problem behavior, with a special concern for the temporal order in which the problem behaviors occur.

Initiation and Suspension

Table 5.1 presents annual data on initiation, suspension, prevalence, and mean number of years of activity for general delinquency, Index offenses, alcohol use, marijuana use, polydrug use, and mental health problems. *Initiation* refers to the first instance of active involvement in one of the problem behaviors (i.e., active involvement in the absence of any prior active involvement). Data on initiation are not presented for 1976 because that was the first year in which data were collected and we do not know whether participation in delinquency, drug use, or mental health problems in 1976 was preceded by participation in earlier years or not. Judging from initiation rates in 1977, it seems likely that for all offenses, except perhaps for marijuana and polydrug use, the prevalence rates for 1976 include both initiation and continuation of behavior previously initiated. Data for 1983 include initiation that occurred in 1981 and 1982.

Suspension refers to the temporary or permanent cessation of active participation in any of the problem behaviors. Initiation can occur only once, the first time an individual becomes an active participant in the behavior in question. Suspension, by contrast, may occur several times, interspersed with periods of active participation. A negative rate of

TABLE 5.1. Initiation, suspension, and participation in delinquency and ADM problems.

Problem behavior	1976	1977	1978	1979	1980	1983	Total sample	Active only
			Percent				Years	
General delinquency								
Annual initiation	NA	12	4	3	1	1		
Annual suspension	NA	17	9	6	6	8		
Annual prevalence	67	62	58	55	49	43		
Mean years active participation							3.7	4.1
Index offenses								
Annual initiation	NA	8	4	4	1	2		
Annual suspension	NA	12	7	3	4	6		
Annual prevalence	24	19	16	16	13	10		
Mean years active participation							1.1	2.2
Alcohol use								
Annual initiation	NA	22	9	6	5	5		
Annual suspension	NA	4	3	2	−1	−2		
Annual prevalence	48	65	71	76	82	89		
Mean years active participation							5.3	5.6
Marijuana use								
Annual initiation	NA	19	10	6	7	7		
Annual suspension	NA	11	1	1	3	9		
Annual prevalence	19	27	36	41	44	43		
Mean years active participation							2.8	4.0
Polydrug use								
Annual initiation	NA	5	6	6	4	12		
Annual suspension	NA	2	3	1	3	7		
Annual prevalence	6	8	12	17	18	23		
Mean years active participation							1.2	2.9
Mental health problems								
Annual initiation	NA	4	2	2	1	2		
Annual suspension	NA	9	4	3	1	1		
Annual prevalence	15	10	8	7	6	7		
Mean years active participation							0.5	1.8

initiation is impossible, but a negative rate of suspension may occur if fewer individuals enter a state of suspension (by ceasing to participate in delinquency, substance use, or mental health problems) than leave that state of suspension (by renewing their participation in a previously initiated behavior after a temporary period of suspension). Annual suspension rates are therefore *net* rates reflecting both entry into and exit from a state of suspension of delinquency, substance use, or mental health problems. Technically, initiation rates are also net rates, but by definition the number who exit from a state of initiation (that is, who go from having *ever* committed at least one offense to having *never* committed an offense) is zero. Data for 1983 include the net of suspension rates for 1981 and 1982.

Annual prevalence is used here in the same way that prevalence has been used in previous chapters. It refers to the percentage of the sample that, in a given year, actively participates in delinquency, substance use, or mental health problems. Because of problems in data that involve a recall period of more than 1 year (Elliott et al., 1985), data for 1981 and 1982 are considered questionable with respect to validity and are not presented here. Annual prevalence in any year is the sum of annual prevalence in the prior year plus initiation in the current year minus suspension in the current year. (In some cases, results will be off by 1% because of rounding error.) Cumulative initiation rates may be calculated by adding prevalence in 1976 to initiation in subsequent years. The data in Table 5.1 indicate that about two-thirds of the sample have initiated general delinquency by 1976. Indeed, if we consider only those aged 11 in 1976, 60% already participate in general delinquency. For each year from 1977 to 1983, net suspension rates were higher than initiation rates (a pattern generally characteristic of the seven cohorts taken separately); as a result, prevalence rates of general delinquency declined from 1976 to 1983. A similar pattern occurred for Index offense prevalence. Nearly one-fourth of the sample initiated Index offending by 1976 (20% of the 11-year-olds), and prevalence rates show a general decline over time. As suggested by the data presented in Chapter 4, this decline appears to reflect the combined effects of maturation and either a period effect (for general delinquency) or a chort effect (for Index offenses). For the period 1979–1983, it appears that fewer than 10% of the sample changed from active to inactive or vice versa in any given year. For both general and Index offenses, rates of initiation declined over time, while rates of suspension were fairly stable or (after 1978) increased slightly.

Alcohol use, marijuana use, and polydrug use show the opposite pattern. With the exception of marijuana use in 1983, initiation exceeds net suspension for all three substances in each year. For alcohol use alone, more people resumed use (after having suspended it) than suspended use in 1980 and 1983, as indicated by the negative percentages in the table. Prevalence increases over time for all three, reflecting a combination of age and period effects. By 1976, nearly half of the sample, 48% (but only 9% of the 11-year-olds) had initiated alcohol use, 19% (0.4% for 11-year-olds) had initiated marijuana use, and 6% percent (and none of the 11-year-olds) had initiated polydrug use. Rates of initiation and suspension of polydrug use tend to be small compared to those for general and Index delinquency; rates of initiation and suspension (combined) of alcohol and marijuana use are more comparable in magnitude to those for delinquency. Rates of initiation for alcohol and marijuana use declined over time, but rates of initiation of polydrug use (bearing in mind that the 1983 data incorporate 1981 and 1982 as well) appear to be stable. Rates of suspension also declined for alcohol use, but increased for marijuana and polydrug use after 1979.

Rates of initiation (onset) and suspension of mental health problems are small, and the difference between initiation and suspension rates decreases over time. By 1976, 15% have experienced the onset of mental health problems, and prevalence tends to stabilize at about 40% to 50% of that level after 1978. From 1977 to 1979, initiation rates were lower than suspension rates, but suspension rates declined more rapidly over time than initiation rates. From 1979 to 1983, initiation and suspension rates were nearly equal.

Table 5.1 also presents the mean number of years of active participation in delinquency, substance use, and mental health problems, using both the total sample (some of whom have zero years active participation) and only those with one or more years of active participation as the denominator. For general delinquency and alcohol use, the two most widespread behaviors, the choice of denominators makes little difference. For Index offenses, marijuana use, polydrug use, and mental health problems, the difference is considerable. Focusing on the last column, those who ever use alcohol tend to do so for an average of 5.6 of the 8 years for which we have data. Those who ever commit general delinquency or use marijuana are active an average of 4 years, polydrug users for 3 years, and Index offenders and those with mental health problems average 2 years of active participation.

All of these are underestimates. First, we lack data prior to 1976 and subsequent to 1983. Second, data for 1981 and 1982 underestimate prevalence in those years (Elliott et al., 1985) or, in the case of mental health problems, are simply unavailable. The estimates of mean years of active participation should therefore be regarded as minimum estimates of participation limited to the 8-year period from 1976 to 1983.

Termination Prior to the End of Adolescence

Juvenile delinquency is conceptually and legally distinct from adult crime, even though the specific behaviors involved may be indistinguishable for minors and adults. Conceptually, much juvenile delinquency is regarded as a transient response to the particular conditions of adolescence, which the juvenile will outgrow in time (Briar & Piliavin, 1965; Greenberg, 1977; Hirschi & Gottfredson, 1983; Matza, 1964). This view of delinquency underlies the Maturational Reform hypothesis, which received support from the data analyzed in Chapter 4. Legally, juvenile delinquency encompasses a wider range of behaviors (notably status offenses) than adult crime. Even for actions that would be considered criminal for an adult, minors do not have the same rights and are not subject to the same penalties as adults unless the juvenile court waives its jurisdiction and remands them to adult court. In effect, waiver of jurisdiction and transfer to adult court denies the minor "juvenile" status and defines the act as (adult) criminal rather than (juvenile) delinquent.

Implicit within the Maturational Reform hypothesis is the suggestion that most adolescents who initiate delinquency will discontinue it when they leave adolescence, and few who have not initiated delinquent behavior will do so after leaving adolescence. Insofar as marijuana and polydrug use are illegal for both minors and adults, they may be expected to follow a similar pattern (although results of the age period-cohort analysis in Chapter 4 suggest that this decline in substance use may not occur until the early 20s). No clear expectations exist for patterns of suspension of mental health problems, but their short average duration, as indicated in Table 5.1, suggests a high rate of suspension prior to the end of adolescence.

Table 5.2 presents data on noninitiation (the absence of initiation) and suspension prior to age 17, and on initiation subsequent to age 17, for three birth cohorts, aged 11, 12, and 13 in 1976. Age 17 is chosen as the last year of adolescence (and correspondingly, age 18 as the first year of adulthood) because at age 17, most individuals are still in school, and in most states are still initially under the jurisdiction of the juvenile court, but at age 18 most either graduate or have left high school and all are under the jurisdiction of the adult criminal court (Gibbons & Krohn, 1986, p. 21). The transition from age 17 to age 18 is thus critical in defining the adolescent period. Only the first three birth cohorts are examined because a substantial amount of suspension takes place prior to normal entry into high school at age 14. Of the 1965 cohort (age 11 in 1976), 5.0% have initiated and suspended general delinquency by age 12, and another 5.9% have done so by age 13. By age 14, a total of 17.6% have initiated general delinquency and then suspended it with no further delinquent activity through age 18. For Index offenses, figures are comparable, with 17.1% suspending their involvement in Index offending by age 14. Noninitiation rates in Table 5.2 may therefore be slightly inflated, and suspension rates slightly deflated, for the older cohorts. The problem would be even more severe were we to include those cohorts aged 14–17 in 1976.

For present purposes, we will regard individuals as having *terminated* a behavior prior to the end of adolescence if they meet all of three conditions. First, they must have *initiated* the behavior (i.e., actively participated in it at least once) by age 17. Second, they must have suspended that same behavior for at least 1 year prior to age 17. Third, their last known year of active participation in the activity must occur at or prior to their 17th year of age (i.e., there must be no active participation *after* age 17). Clearly, it is possible that *termination*, as we have defined it here, may represent a permanent suspension of the behavior in question or, for some, a temporary hiatus between juvenile delinquency and adult crime. Until we have more extensive data (indeed until everyone in the panel dies!) we cannot be certain that criminal behavior will not be resumed (or initiated) at a later date, but at the very least, termination here represents a break between juvenile and adult offending, rather than a continuous progression from juvenile delinquency to adult crime.

TABLE 5.2. Termination of adolescent problem behavior at or prior to age 17.

Problem behavior	Cohort	Noninitiation prior to age 17 (percent)	Initiation followed by suspension prior to age 17 (percent)	Total of noninitiation and suspension prior to age 17 (percent)	Initiation subsequent to age 17 (percent)	Suspension prior to age 17 as percent of ever-active participants prior to age 17
General delinquency	1965	14	42	56	0	49
	1964	12	47	59	1	53
	1963	13	44	57	1	51
Index offenses	1965	60	35	95	3	88
	1964	58	36	94	1	86
	1963	59	32	91	4	78
Alcohol use	1965	20	9	29	8	11
	1964	11	11	22	4	12
	1963	11	13	24	6	15
Marijuana use	1965	51	14	65	2	29
	1964	47	14	61	2	26
	1963	49	19	68	9	37
Polydrug use	1965	79	10	89	8	48
	1964	77	11	88	12	48
	1963	80	8	88	12	40
Mental health problems	1965	76	20	96	2	83
	1964	74	24	98	3	92
	1963	80	19	99	2	95

As Table 5.2 indicates, most of the sample (86%–88%) have initiated general delinquency by age 17, and very few (0%–1%) initiate at age 18 or older. Of those who initiated general delinquency during adolescence, half discontinued for one or more years while still under 18 years of age and did not resume general delinquency by 1983 (age 18, 19, or 20). These are the individuals whom we regard as having terminated their juvenile delinquency prior to the end of adolescence. If we include those who did not initiate delinquency at or prior to age 17, more than half of the sample were not involved in general delinquency by age 18.

Fewer than half of the individuals in the sample (40%–42%) initiated Index offenses by age 17, and the vast majority of these (78%–88%) suspended their involvement in Index offending by age 17 and did not resume it by 1983. Initiation after age 17 is slightly higher for Index offending than for general delinquency, but it is still very small (1%–4%). Over 90% of the sample either terminated or did not initiate Index offending by age 17.

Alcohol use initiation rates by age 17 are comparable to those for general delinquency (80%–89%) but suspension rates are much lower (11%–15%). Initiation continued after age 17 (4%–8%), and the vast majority of the sample (71%–78%) used alcohol by age 18. Alcohol use is also the behavior for which the greatest differences occur among cohorts, with the youngest cohort having the highest percentage not initiating alcohol use by age 17, but the lowest percentage (whether of the active users or the total sample) suspending use by age 17.

About half of the sample initiated marijuana use by age 17, and initiation continued (2%–9%) after age 18. Of those who started using marijuana during adolescence, 26%–37% percent stop, and by age 18 nearly two-thirds of the sample are no longer or never have been marijuana users. Only 20%–23% of the sample initiated polydrug use by age 17, and of those who did, 40%–48% discontinued use by age 17. Rates of initiation after age 18 are relatively high (8%–12%), about half the adolescent initiation rate, but by age 18 more than 80% of the subsample no longer use or never did use multiple illicit drugs.

The pattern of mental health problems is somewhat similar to that for polydrug use. The rate of initiation by age 17 is about the same (20%–26%), but the percentage who terminate by age 17 is much higher (83%–95%) and the rate of initiation after age 17 is lower (2%–3%). By age 18, more than 95% no longer have or never had mental health problems.

On the whole, the results for delinquency and especially for Index offenses are consistent with the Maturational Reform hypothesis, but a substantial percentage continue directly from juvenile delinquency to adult crime. Alcohol use, which may be legal for some respondents by age 18, shows the lowest rates of termination, and termination rates are lower for marijuana and polydrug use than for general or Index offenses. Mental health problems have the highest termination rates of all, and it appears to be this result, coupled with low initiation rates, that accounts for the secular decline in mental health problem prevalence observed in Chapter 4.

Demographic Correlates of Termination Prior to the End of Adolescence

Demographic correlates of adolescent termination of problem behavior are similar to those for prevalence of the same behavior. The principal difference is that termination of problem behavior is less likely than prevalence to be statistically significantly related to sex, race, social class, or urban/rural residence. Age is not examined here because we used only three cohorts (aged 11, 12, and 13) in 1976. Table 5.3 presents the percent terminating prior to adolescence by sex, race, social class, and place of residence, along with a Chi-square test of the significance of the difference in proportions terminating each behavior by each demographic variable, and a measure of the strength and significance of the correlation (Kendall's tau-b) between termination prior to adolescence and each of the demographic variables for each problem behavior. Given our definition of termination, the data in Table 5.3 refer only to those in the selected cohorts who initiated each behavior prior to age 17.

As seen in Table 5.3, females are more likely than males to have terminated both general and Index offenses prior to the end of adolescence. Both the differences in proportions terminating and the correlations between sex and termination are statistically significant. For alcohol use and mental health problems, by contrast, neither the difference in the proportion of males and females terminating nor the correlation is statistically significant. Marijuana and polydrug use represent marginal cases, in which the difference in proportions is not quite statistically significant but the correlation is (barely) statistically significant. In every instance, statistically significant or not, females are more likely than males to terminate delinquent and ADM behavior prior to the end of adolescence, but the difference is unequivocally statistically significant only for general and Index offenses.

According to the data in Table 5.3, neither race nor social class is statistically significantly related to termination of alcohol use, marijuana use, polydrug use or mental health problems. Race bears an interesting relationship to termination of delinquency. Blacks are more likely to terminate general delinquency prior to the end of adolescence than whites, but whites are more likely than blacks to terminate Index delinquency prior to the end of adolescence. There is no difference by social class in the termination of general delinquency prior to the end of

TABLE 5.3. Demographic correlates of termination prior to the end of adolescence: 1963, 1964, and 1965 cohorts.

	General delinquency	Index offenses	Alcohol use	Marijuana use	Polydrug use	Mental health problems
			Problem behavior			
Sex						
Male[a]	31.9%	56.1%	7.5%	13.3%	17.5%	68.7%
Female	49.4%	79.5%	7.6%	19.6%	27.6%	72.9%
Sig. of χ^2	.000	.000	1.000	.120	.123	.724
tau[b]	.177	.228	.002	.085	.121	.045
Sig. of tau	.000	.000	.478	.046	.044	.296
Race						
White	36.8%	67.9%	7.1%	15.3%	22.4%	69.5%
Black	52.9%	46.5%	9.6%	11.3%	27.3%	73.1%
Sig. of χ^2	.008	.014	.528	.580	.995	.909
tau	.123	−.171	.034	−.040	.028	.032
Sig. of tau	.003	.004	.200	.224	.354	.362
Social class						
Middle	34.9%	78.3%	8.0%	20.8%	22.2%	65.0%
Working	40.0%	64.9%	5.9%	15.9%	20.6%	69.0%
Lower	40.9%	56.2%	8.2%	15.6%	23.4%	73.1%
Sig. of χ^2	.509	.028	.615	.570	.914	.753
tau	.046	−.170	.010	−.046	.018	.067
Sig. of tau	.143	.004	.400	.185	.401	.227
Residence[c]						
Urban	38.2%	56.3%	10.1%	20.3%	23.4%	71.7%
Suburban	38.5%	64.0%	7.1%	15.3%	22.3%	61.1%
Rural	42.1%	72.6%	5.7%	12.0%	20.9%	83.8%
Sig. of χ^2	.735	.133	.272	.260	.954	.064
tau	.029	.126	−.061	−.082	−.021	.091
Sig. of tau	.250	.022	.058	.052	.381	.147

[a] Percent of those active prior to the end of adolescence who terminate prior to the end of adolescence
[b] Kendall's tau-b; for sex and race, this will be equal to Pearson's r and also to phi.
[c] 1976.

adolescence, but for Index offenses the middle class is the most likely and the lower class the least likely to terminate.

None of the differences in proportion terminating by place of residence is statistically significant, although there is some suggestion that termination of mental health problems has a curvilinear, marginally significant ($P = .064$) relationship with place of residence. Suburban residents appear least likely, and rural residents most likely, to terminate mental health problems prior to the end of adolescence. Although the differences in proportions terminating Index offenses by residence is not statistically significant, the correlation between residence and termination of Index offending is significant, with urban residents least likely and rural residents most likely to terminate Index offending. Correlations between residence and termination of alcohol and marijuana use are weak and do not quite reach statistical significance.

With the exception that prevalence of general delinquency tends to be higher in urban than rural areas, the demographic correlates of termination of general delinquency and Index offenses are the same as the demographic correlates of the prevalence of general and Index offenses, respectively. That females are marginally significantly more likely to terminate marijuana and polydrug use but not alcohol use by age 17 is consistent with correlations between sex and the prevalence of alcohol, marijuana, and polydrug use in Chapter 3. Although prevalence rates (in Chapter 3) of alcohol, marijuana, and polydrug use show some differences by race, social class, and residence, termination of the three substances by age 17 is not statistically significantly related to any of the demographic variables other than sex. Mental health problems tend to be more prevalent among blacks and among the lower class (Chapter 3), but termination of mental health problems (once initiated) is unrelated to sex, race, social class, or place of residence. In short, with the possible exception of the absence of some (weak) relationships expected on the basis of differential prevalence of problem behavior from Chapter 3, the relationships of termination of problem behavior prior to age 17 with sex, race, social class and urban/rural residence produce no surprises.

Risk of Progression to States of Greater Involvement in Delinquency and Drug Use

In examining patterns of temporal ordering for delinquency and drug use, it is interesting to examine the probability that youth engaging in these behaviors at one level will progress to states of greater involvement at a later time and to examine the intervening levels of involvement. A major question is whether individuals become serious offenders or heavy users of drugs in a short period of time or whether there is a slower progression through intermediate levels of involvement. In the following section, this issue is considered separately for delinquency, drug use, and mental health problems.

Table 5.4 presents mean transition matrices for the three problem behavior typologies described in Chapter 1. Each entry in each matrix represents the proportion of individuals in the category defined by the row who, in the next year, move into the category defined by the column. For example, 31% (.31) of those who are exploratory offenders in one year remain exploratory offenders in the next year, and 16% (.16) of exploratory offenders in one year become nonserious offenders in the next year.

The transition probabilities in the matrices of Table 5.4 are computed by averaging the transition probabilities for 1976–1977, 1977–1978, 1978–

TABLE 5.4. Mean transition matrices for problem behavior types, 1976–1980[a].

Self-reported delinquency type	Nonoffender	Exploratory	Nonserious	Serious
(1) Nonoffender	.84	.10	.05	.01
(2) Exploratory	.47	.31	.16	.06
(3) Nonserious	.33	.27	.32	.09
(4) Serious	.21	.14	.26	.40

Drug user type	Nonuser	Alcohol	Marijuana	Polydrug
(1) Nonuser	.72	.20	.07	.02
(2) Alcohol	.15	.62	.20	.03
(3) Marijuana	.08	.15	.59	.18
(4) Polydrug	.04	.07	.22	.68

Mental health problem type	Nonproblem	Problem		
(1) Nonproblem	.96	.04		
(2) Problem	.61	.39		

[a] Rows may not sum to exactly 1.00 because of rounding error.

1979, and 1979–1980. Since we lack data on offending rates, frequency of substance use, and mental health problem scale scores for 1981 and 1982, we cannot create the same topologies for those years, and it would be inappropriate to average a 3-year (1980–1983) transition matrix with the 1 year (annual) transition matrices, because the 3-year transition matrix contains the *cumulative* effect of 3 years of transitions and typically will not have the same transition probabilities as an annual matrix.

Before computing the mean transition matrices in Table 5.4, a Chi-square test of homogeneity of the annual transition matrices (Markus, 1978) was performed. For the offender typology, a statistically significant difference was obtained only when comparing the 1976–1977 and 1979–1980 transition matrices. All of the other five comparisons failed to achieve a statistically significant difference at the .05 level of probability. It is possible that the transition matrix for the offender typology changes gradually over time, or that the one statistically significant difference out of six trials is attributable to random error. Annual transition matrices for the offender typology are presented along with 1980–1983 and 1976–1983 transition matrices in Table D.1 (Appendix D). On the whole, the mean transition matrix in Table 5.4 appears to represent the annual transition matrices well.

For the substance use typology, all six comparisons of annual transition matrices resulted in statistically significant (probability ≤ .05) differences. Annual, 1980–1983, and 1976–1983 transition matrices are presented in Table D.2. There appears to be little that is systematic about the change except perhaps for an increase in the overall likelihood of remaining within a given category (as indicated by the sum or average of the diagonal elements of the matrix) from one year to the next. For the mental health typology, there is no statistically significant difference (probability ≤ .05) between any pair of annual transition matrices. Annual, 1980–1983, and 1976–1983 transition matrices are presented in Table D.3. It appears that the transition probabilities between the two mental health types are quite stable from one pair of years to the next. For the drug user typology, then, the mean transition matrix does not accurately reflect any given annual transition matrix. For the offender and mental health problem typologies, the mean transition matrices do reflect annual transition matrices from 1976 to 1980.

In all three problem typologies, the most likely transition is from the nonoffender, nonuser, or nonproblem type to that same nonoffender, nonuser, or nonproblem type, respectively. For exploratory and nonserious offenders, the most probable transition is to nonoffender status, followed in turn by remaining in the current status (exploratory or nonoffender, respectively). Least likely for each is escalation to serious offender status. Serious offenders are most likely to remain in that status, with de-escalation to nonserious offender status the next most likely transition.

The majority within each drug user type remains within that type from one time to the next. For each type except polydrug users (than which there is no more serious category) the second most likely transition is to the next most serious type, that is, from nonuse to alcohol, alcohol to marijuana, and marijuana to polydrug use. Polydrug users, having nowhere to go but down, are likely to de-escalate to marijuana use if they do not remain polydrug users. Least likely for all four types is movement to a nonadjacent type. For the mental health problem typology, there are only two types (perforce adjacent), and the most likely transition for both problem and nonproblem types is to nonproblem status.

As can be seen in Table 5.4, among those increasing their delinquent involvement there is an indication of a progression from nonoffender to exploratory to nonserious to serious offending. While the bulk of nonoffenders remain nonoffenders, for those who increase their involvement the most common movement from one year to the next is to an exploratory state. Similarly, although the bulk of exploratory offenders remain exploratory or return to a nondelinquent status, those whose delinquency increases are more likely to become nonserious than serious offenders. Finally, those nonserious delinquents who increase their delinquency level become serious delinquents. It is interesting to note that serious offenders have a relatively high probability of remaining in that status (40%) from year to year. While there are exceptions, a general rule controlling movement between delinquency states is that the bulk of individuals in a given state will either remain in that state or return to a state of lesser involvement; among those increasing their delinquent involvement, the most common movement is to an adjacent, more delinquent, status.

Although the exact magnitudes of the probabilities change from year to year, the same general pattern of movement between drug use types can be seen in the transition matrices. Nonusers (i.e., no use of any drug more than three times) are most likely to remain nonusers; if they begin to use drugs, they most commonly become alcohol users. Alcohol users are most likely to remain alcohol users and those who expand their drug use most commonly begin to use marijuana. Similarly, users of both alcohol and marijuana are most likely to remain in this status, although some begin to use other illicit drugs. Users of alcohol, marijuana, and other illicit drugs tend to remain in this status, although, as with all user types, there is some regression to earlier types with decreased drug involvement.

Although these patterns are insufficient to draw firm conclusions, they suggest a progression of no use to alcohol use, alcohol use to marijuana use, and marijuana use to use of other illicit drugs, with many youth remaining at each step of the progression. This progression is similar to the developmental stages of drug use described by Kandel (1975, 1978), Kandel and Faust (1975), and Jessor et al. (1980). It should be noted that this progression is simply descriptive and provides no conclusive evidence for the "stepping-stone" theory that the use of one drug necessarily or inevitably leads to the use of another. Although the use of one drug is associated with a higher probability of subsequent use of other drugs, there is no evidence of a causal relationship, and the probabilities of progression are not very high.

The Temporal Priority of Delinquency, Substance Use, and Mental Health Problems

To examine the temporal order of delinquency, substance use, and mental health problems, we use two approaches. The first approach is to examine the entire NYS sample and determine in what percentage of cases one behavior is initiated *prior to or in the absence of* another. The second is to determine in what percentage of cases one behavior is initiated prior to another for *only* those cases in which *both* types of behavior are initiated.

In some cases, two behaviors (for example, marijuana use and Index offending) may be initiated in the same year, thereby making it impossible to ascertain from our data which behavior was initiated first. In other cases, an individual may initiate one behavior in one year and the other behavior the following year or later, thus allowing us to conclude that initiation of the one precedes initiation of the other. What about those cases in which the individual initiates one behavior but does not, during the period for which we have data, initiate the other? In the first approach, we allow for the possibility that the "other" behavior may be initiated at a later date and say, for example, that those who initiate marijuana use but not Index offending (during the period for which we have data) have initiated marijuana use prior to the initiation of Index offending.

This first approach has the advantage of being applicable to a large number of cases, and it seems reasonable to conclude that if an individual has initiated one behavior (at time *t*) but not another, the initiation of the first has clearly not occurred subsequent to or contemporaneously with the second, leaving priority as the only logically possible time ordering. It may be the case, however, that a large percentage of the sample *rarely* initiates a particular behavior, but *when they do,* it precedes another behavior that is, nonetheless, more frequently initiated by the individuals in the sample. The low relative frequency of the first behavior might then lead us to conclude, in this case incorrectly, that the second behavior usually preceded the first. This concern leads us to the second of our two approaches to studying the temporal priority of delinquency, substance use, and mental health problems. In this second approach, we examine only those who have engaged in some delinquency, some substance use, and who have had some mental health problems on at least one occasion. Although this technique substantially reduces the size of the sample under study, it allows us to determine if and when a low-prevalence behavior precedes a high-prevalence behavior.

For purposes of this temporal comparison, we consider the prevalence of Index offenses, alcohol use, marijuana use, polydrug use, and mental health problems. In addition, because general delinquency includes Index offenses, we use minor or non-Index delinquency (general delinquency except for Index offenses) in place of general delinquency. This allows us to examine the extent to which minor and Index offending occur prior to each other, and the results for minor offending with respect to alcohol use, marijuana use, polydrug use, and mental health problems are practically identical to those for general delinquency.

Table 5.5 presents the results of the first approach, using the total NYS sample, for studying the temporal priority of problem behavior. Minor delinquency occurs before any other type of problem behavior. It is almost never preceded by Index offenses, polydrug use, or mental health problems, and rarely by marijuana use. In most cases, it is not possible to ascertain whether minor delinquency or alcohol use occurs first; therefore it is suggested (since both have high prevalence rates) that they tend to be initiated at about the same time, but for those cases in which temporal order can be ascertained, minor delinquency is about twice as likely to precede alcohol use as alcohol use is to precede minor delinquency.

Alcohol use comes next, preceding Index offenses, marijuana use, polydrug use, and mental health problems in a clear majority of cases. Reversal of this order is rare. Marijuana use comes next, but in a substantial number of cases it may be preceded by Index offenses or mental health problems. Index offenses follow, but again there exist a substantial number of cases that counter the dominant trend, and most of

TABLE 5.5. Temporal priority of problem behaviors: Total sample.

Usual order of initiation	Consistent with usual order of initiation			Inconsistent with usual order of initiation			Missing or unascertainable	
	N	Total percent[a]	Ascertainable percent[b]	N	Total percent	Ascertainable percent	N	Total percent
Minor to Index offending	727	42	99.5	4	0.2	0.5	994	58
Minor offending to alcohol use	259	15	64	145	8	36	1321	77
Minor offending to marijuana use	711	41	93	51	3	7	963	56
Minor offending to polydrug use	987	57	99	13	1	1	725	42
Minor offending to mental health problems	889	52	97	25	1	3	811	47
Alcohol use to Index offending	971	56	86	159	9	14	595	35
Alcohol use to marijuana use	1017	59	95	52	3	5	656	38
Alcohol use to polydrug use	1218	71	99	9	0.5	0.7	498	29
Alcohol use to mental health problems	1086	63	90	126	7	10	513	30
Marijuana use to Index offending	560	33	63	331	19	37	834	48
Marijuana use to polydrug use	763	44	95	42	2	5	920	53
Marijuana use to mental health problems	724	42	78	206	12	22	795	46
Index offending to polydrug use	465	27	67	225	13	33	1035	60
Index offending to mental health problems	427	25	68	201	12	32	1097	64
Polydrug use to mental health problems	370	21	59	260	15	41	1095	64

[a] Percent of total sample.
[b] Percent of cases for which temporal order of initiation was clearly ascertainable, i.e., for which initiation occurred in separate years for the two behaviors being compared.

the cases have a temporal order that is unascertainable. This uncertainty also holds for the priority of polydrug use over mental health problems. For these last three, the temporal order is not as clear as we might like, but the dominant pattern is Index offenses, then polydrug use, then mental health problems.

Bear in mind that in Table 5.5 a behavior in many cases is initiated *in the absence of*, rather than (strictly speaking) prior to the initiation of a behavior placed later in the temporal ordering. Somewhat different results are obtained when we restrict our analysis to those individuals who have initiated all three types of problem behavior (delinquency, substance use, and mental health problems). Table 5.6 presents the temporal ordering of problem behaviors for those who have initiated at least one type of delinquency (minor or Index), at least one type of substance use (alcohol, marijuana, or polydrug), and mental health problems.

Note that in Table 5.6, an individual need not have initiated all six behaviors (minor delinquency, Index offending, alcohol use, marijuana use, polydrug use, mental health problems) to be included in the table as a multiproblem youth. This means that in some cases the comparisons will still involve the "prior to or in the absence of" criterion. To overcome this problem, separate examination was made for each pair of the six behaviors, looking only at those who had initiated both behaviors. This, in conjunction with Table 5.6, allows us to ascertain which behavior is more likely to be initiated first according to a strict "prior to only" criterion.[1]

In Table 5.6 the priority of minor delinquency over the other types of behavior is even more evident than in Table 5.5. For those experiencing all three types of problem behavior, *no one* initiates marijuana or polydrug use before minor delinquency, and practically no one initiates Index offenses, alcohol use, or mental health problems before minor delinquency. Alcohol use clearly comes second, with little change in its relationship to polydrug or marijuana use, but with substantial percentages for which Index offenses and mental health problems precede alcohol use. Separate analysis of those who have ever initiated each

---

[1] The alternative, examination of only those who had initiated all six behaviors, would reduce the number of cases in question to only 120. For this group of 120, the temporal priority of problem behavior runs from minor delinquency to alcohol use, then Index offenses, then marijuana use, then mental health problems, and finally polydrug use. The only difference between these results and those discussed in the main text of this chapter involve the relative priority of mental health problems and marijuana use. In Table 5.8, and for those who initiate both marijuana use and mental health problems between 1976 and 1983 ($N = 282$), mental health problems are more often initiated prior to marijuana use (41.1% of all cases, 58.3% of ascertainable cases) than is marijuana use prior to mental health problems (29.4% of all cases, 41.7% of ascertainable cases).

TABLE 5.6. Temporal priority of problem behaviors: Multiple problem youth.

Usual order of initiation	Consistent with usual order of initiation			Inconsistent with usual order of initiation			Missing or unascertainable	
	N	Total percent	Ascertainable percent	N	Total percent	Ascertainable percent	N	Total percent
Minor to Index offending	148	43	99	1	0.3	0.7	198	57
Minor offending to alcohol use	60	17	98	1	0.3	2	286	82
Minor offending to marijuana use	142	42	100	0	0	0	201	58
Minor offending to polydrug use	218	63	100	0	0	0	129	37
Minor offending to mental health problems	89	26	99	1	0.3	1	257	74
Alcohol use to Index offending	179	52	75	59	17	25	109	31
Alcohol use to marijuana use	196	57	97	7	2	3	144	42
Alcohol use to polydrug use	252	73	99	2	0.6	0.8	93	27
Alcohol use to mental health problems	130	38	57	97	28	43	120	35
Mental health problems to Index offending	168	48	73	62	18	27	117	34
Mental health problems to marijuana use	170	49	67	85	25	33	92	27
Mental health problems to polydrug use	224	65	86	36	10	14	87	25
Marijuana use to Index offending	122	35	56	98	28	45	127	37
Marijuana use to polydrug use	178	51	93	14	4	7	155	45
Index offending to polydrug use	135	39	70	57	16	30	155	45

behavior or pair of behaviors confirms that minor delinquency is characteristically initiated first and alcohol use second.

The biggest change between Tables 5.5 and 5.6 is that mental health problems move from last (sixth) to third in temporal priority. Although there are substantial percentages for whom Index offenses, marijuana use, and polydrug use precede mental health problems, the dominant pattern for multiple problem youth generally is for mental health problems to precede Index offenses, marijuana use, and polydrug use. In part, however, this reflects the initiation of mental health problems in the absence of the other three behaviors. Examination of those who have initiated both mental health problems and Index offenses indicates that, for those cases in which temporal order is ascertainable, Index offenses more often precede mental health problems (54% of the cases) than vice versa (46%). Examination of those with both mental health problems and either marijuana or polydrug use, however, confirms that mental health problems are more likely to precede marijuana use (57%) and polydrug use (72%). In all three comparisons, the percentage for which the dominant temporal ordering is reversed is substantial.

For multiple problem youth generally, marijuana use comes next, followed by Index offenses and finally polydrug use. Comparing those who have initiated both Index offenses and marijuana use, however, suggests that the apparent temporal priority of marijuana use results from its higher rate of prevalence. Among those who have initiated both Index offenses and marijuana use, and for whom temporal priority is ascertainable, Index offenses are more likely to precede marijuana use (64%) than marijuana use is to precede Index offenses. Similar comparisons confirm that both marijuana use (95%) and Index offenses (87%) precede polydrug use. With the exception of alcohol use, then, delinquency occurs first, followed by mental health problems, and drug use occurs last among multiple problem youth.

We cannot use the patterns of temporal ordering to infer the validity of any causal ordering among the behaviors listed here. We can, however, infer that if one behavior causes another, since the cause must temporally (as well as logically) precede the effect, certain causal orderings are probably *not* valid. In particular, neither alcohol, marijuana, nor polydrug use causes minor delinquency, and neither marijuana nor polydrug use leads to Index offenses, because the most common pattern is for delinquent offending to precede substance use. Mental health problems also do not appear plausible as causes of delinquent behavior, but our sampling of mental health problems in this analysis is much less inclusive than our sampling of delinquent behaviors. Although it is logically possible that drug use leads to mental health problems, particularly problems other than those considered in this analysis, it appears that mental health problems as defined here are more likely to precede than to be a consequence of the use of psychoactive drugs.

The most important conclusion to be drawn from the analysis of temporal order and the transitions within the delinquency, drug use, and mental health types is that there is support for the idea that there is a developmental progression of delinquent and ADM behaviors. Relatively minor involvement in problem behavior (minor delinquency, alcohol use) consistently tends to precede more serious involvement. Within delinquency and drug use types, progression seems to occur in small, gradual steps. There are exceptions, of course, but gradual progression—with many individuals stopping permanently at each stage—seems to be the dominant pattern. Finally, most youth either do not initiate or else suspend their involvement in problem behavior prior to leaving adolescence, a pattern consistent with the developmental progression implied by the Maturational Reform hypothesis.

6
The Etiology of Delinquency and ADM Problems

An integrated social psychological model that incorporated elements of traditional strain theory, social control (bonding) theory, and social learning theory was tested and presented by Elliott et al. (1985). A satisfactory integration required some modification of the "pure" forms of these theoretical perspectives, and a detailed logical and empirical justification of the modifications was also presented. Here, we present a brief overview of the theoretical model, a discussion of the methods used to test that model for the present chapter, and a test of that model for adolescent delinquency and alcohol, drug, and mental health (ADM) problems.

The Theoretical Model

The terminology and concepts utilized in the integrated model are those of social control theory, since it is our belief that the integrated model best fits this historical tradition and that this theory best captures the intended balance and interaction between the ecological environment, the perceived environment, and individual personality variables. The basic modification to classical control theory required by the integration concerns the natural motivation assumption—that is, the assumption that motivation for deviance is a constant and that the *only* source of variation related to delinquency or illicit drug use is variation in social controls or *restraints* on these behaviors. Kornhauser (1978) notes that the natural motivation assumption is unreasonable and not critical to a social control argument and Hirschi (1969) rejected this assumption on empirical grounds. In our own review of the empirical evidence, we found little or no support for a natural motivation for delinquency or illicit drug use (Elliott et al., 1985). The integrated model thus assumes variation in motivation for deviance as well as in restraints against deviance; it assumes that involvement and commitment (i.e., social bonding) to deviant persons and groups provides positive social rewards (motivation) for deviant behavior in the same way that bonding to conventional persons and groups provides positive rewards (motivation) for prosocial behavior; it assumes variation in the normative content of socialization experiences as well as in the effectiveness of socialization processes.

Four direct causal paths to delinquent behavior are identified in the integrated model presented in Figure 6.1. Path (1) represents a pure strain theory hypothesis that limited or blocked opportunities to achieve personal success goals lead directly to delinquent behavior, independently of conventional or delinquent bonding. Path (2) is a pure control theory hypothesis, that weak internal and external controls against delinquent behavior lead directly to delinquent behavior, independently of delinquent bonding. The dashed lines for paths (1) and (2) indicate that we expect these paths to be weak or insignificant in predicting and explaining delinquent behavior. Path (3) is primarily a social learning theory hypothesis, that exposure to and invovlement with delinquent others leads directly to delinquent behavior, independently of conventional bonding. Path (4) is a new causal path postulated in the integrated theoretical model, asserting that the joint occurrence of weak conventional controls and reinforcements for deviant acts predicts delinquent behavior and illicit drug use. Paths (3) and (4) are viewed as the primary causal paths to delinquency and drug use. Path (4) reflects our belief that although bonding to deviant peers is the most proximate cause of delinquency and drug use, this relationship is specified by levels of

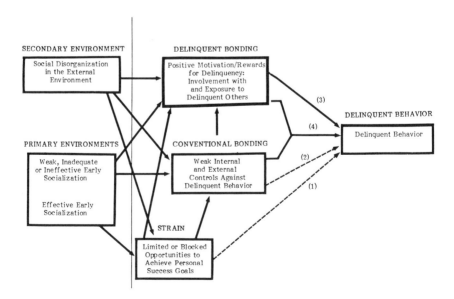

FIGURE 6.1. Integrated social psychological model.

bonding to conventional persons, norms, and institutions. We have shown this conditional relationship as an interaction effect in Figure 6.1. Path (4) combines weak bonding to conventional persons, institutions, and norms with strong bonds to persons and groups who provide some modeling and reinforcement for delinquency and drug use. (We will refer to such groups as "deviant groups" but are not asserting that such groups are homogeneous with respect to attitudes, values, or behavior.) Involvement and commitment to deviant groups are thus viewed as a necessary, but not as sufficient, causal explanations for a sustained involvement in deviant behavior.

Individuals with strong bonding to the family and school are not likely to develop bonds to delinquent or drug-using peers; even if they did, their conventional bonds should limit their involvement in these behaviors. Likewise, weak conventional bonding without bonding to deviant others should not result in any sustained involvement in deviant behavior; that is, we expect the effect of weak conventional bonding to be mediated by bonding to deviant peers. Whereas paths (1) and (2) may account for some temporary, trivial, and/or exploratory involvements in deviant behavior, we postulate that these paths do not account for a sustained involvement in either delinquency or drug use, since there is no social reinforcement for this behavior to offset the general societal proscriptions and formal controls against such behavior. Social control, therefore, influences delinquency primarily by inhibiting or facilitating the development of social bonds to deviant peers. Correspondingly, strain influences delinquency primarily by attenuating the conventional bonds of those who enter adolescence with strong conventional bonds, thereby opening the door to delinquent bonding. The major effects of both strain and weak conventional controls are thus postulated to operate primarily through an attachment to deviant peers or in interaction with deviant peers. This position is clearly at odds with a "pure" social control perspective, which views youth who have weak bonds to peers and parents as the most vulnerable to delinquency and drug use. In the pure control model, deviant youth are unbonded youth, marginal to all groups and institutions. In the integrated model, deviant youth are bonded youth. However, they are bonded to deviant rather than conforming peers, or to deviant rather than conforming adults. Paths (3) and (4) are postulated to be the major causal paths to delinquency and drug use.

General Structure of the Analysis

Prior to the analysis presented in this chapter, we performed a series of analyses leading up to, and including, a general test of the integrated model (Elliott et al., 1985). As a means of reducing the number of predictor measures to be included in the causal modeling analysis, we completed several preliminary analyses. First, we examined the psychometric properties and intercorrelations of all predictor measures over the first three data waves (ages 11–19). Second, we did a series of lagged stepwise multiple regression analyses with each set of predictors representing a given theoretical construct (e.g., strain, internal conventional bonding, external conventional bonding, internal deviant bonding, and external deviant bonding), using our measures of delinquent behavior and drug use as dependent variables. On the basis of these analyses, one or two variables representing each theoretical construct was selected for inclusion in the causal modeling analysis. In nearly all instances, the "best" variable(s) captured the bulk of the explained variance attributable to the complete set. Third, we completed a series of Lazarsfeld 16-fold table analyses to examine the temporal ordering of the predictor variables. The theoretical model specifies that bonding to deviant peers mediates the impact of conventional bonding and strain on delinquent behavior, and we attempted to verify this temporal ordering. We also varied the location of the deviant bonding variable in a series of path analyses (from an intervening to endogenous predictor, and to a position temporally following delinquent behavior as suggested by Hirschi, 1969) so as to establish the correct temporal ordering of the variables in the theoretical model. These analyses verified the order as postulated theoretically, although in some instances the evidence was not particularly strong.

We then tested the full model controlling for the temporal ordering of the variables, predicting delinquent behavior and drug use. We next replicated the analysis, predicting delinquent behavior and drug use at wave 3. Finally, we examined the postulated interaction effect between conventional and deviant bonding on delinquent behavior and drug use. The results of these analyses may be found in Elliott et al. (1985, chap. 6).

Our analysis here differs from previous analyses in several important respects. First, although the theoretical model was not formulated with the intention of explaining mental health problems, we consider in this chapter the possibility that the thereotical model, or elements thereof, may predict mental health problems as well as delinquency and drug use. Our mental health problem scale is therefore included as a dependent variable. Second, given the results presented in Chapters 3 and 4, we include demographic variables (age, sex, race, social class, urban-rural residence, cohort size) as well as theoretical variables in the model. We should note, however, that the present analysis is at the individual rather than the aggregate (age and period-specific group means) level considered in Chapter 4, and that the range of ages considered is (necessarily for the type of analysis presented here) more limited than that considered in Chapter 4. Also, although average parity or number of births were appropriate measures for the aggregate analysis in Chapter 4, individual birth order would perhaps have been preferable (but was unavailable) for the individual level analysis presented in this chapter.

A third difference between this analysis and previously published analyses is the absence from the present regression equations of a lagged endogenous variable—that is, an equation for current delinquency (or ADM problem behavior) that includes a previous level of delinquency (or ADM problem behavior) as a predictor. The use of lagged endogenous variables is appropriate for models of *change* (Kessler & Greenberg, 1981: pp 9–12; Liker, Augustyniak, & Duncan, 1985) as an alternative for example, to first-difference models. Here, we focus on the explanation of *levels* of the dependent variable, without recourse to the use of previous levels of that same variable. Although this method generally reduces the level of explained variance by comparison to the use of lagged endogenous variables, it permits us to assess the impact on delinquency of such variables as sex (i.e., gender) and race. These variables do not change over time, and if their impacts on delinquency or ADM problems is fairly constant over age and time, the use of lagged endogenous variables or other change models may mask their effects by including those effects as part of the stability coefficient (the influence of previous level on current level of the dependent variable). The present analysis avoids that potential problem.

A fourth major change in the present analysis is a reconceptualization of our measures of strain. One measure of strain, employment expectations, asks respondents how good they think their chances are of getting the kind of job they would like after finishing school. This single-item measure replaces the home strain measure used in previous analyses. The second measure of strain is a composite of a previously used school strain scale, self-reported grade point average, and how good the respondents think their chances are of completing college. Measures of normlessness, involvement, attitudes toward delinquency, and combined exposure to and involvement with delinquent peers are measured as in previous studies, and are described in detail elsewhere (Elliott et al., 1983, 1985). For offending rates, instead of raw frequency scores we here use the categorical scores described in Chapter 1 because their psychometric properties are preferable for use in a regression analysis.

All of these differences should be borne in mind when comparing the results of the present study to those presented in previous analyses (for example, Elliott et al., 1985). In addition, when comparing the results presented in this chapter to those presented in Chapter 4 with regard to age and cohort effects, it is important to remember that the anlysis in Chapter 4 was an *aggregate* analysis involving 42 data points (age and period-specific means), but the results in this chapter are for an *individual* analysis of over 1,200 respondents, and in which the range of ages is seriously truncated by comparison with the range available in Chapter 4. The principal effect of both of these changes is to reduce the explained variance (R^2) in the dependent variables, relative to previously published results and the results in Chapter 4. This does not imply that one analysis is more or less valid than another; it only indicates that there are important differences which should be recognized in the types of analysis we have performed.

Methods

VARIABLES

The dependent variables in this chapter are the categorical general offending rates (described in Chapter 1) for general delinquency and Index offenses, categorical rates of alcohol, marijuana, and polydrug use, and the mental health problem scale score. As exogenous variables, we use sex (1 = male, 2 = female); race (1 = white, 2 = nonwhite); urban-rural residence (1 = urban, 2 = suburban, 3 = rural); parents' social status as measured by the Hollingshead two-factor index, recoded so that a high score indicates high social status; absolute (births) and relative (parity) cohort size; and three measures of age (chronological age, absolute deviation from age 15, and absolute deviation from age 20). The cohort and age measures are described in more detail in Chapter 4. With the restriction placed on age in this analysis, chronological age and absolute deviation from age 20 are equivalent measures. The latter measure is used for the analyses involving alcohol and drug use because of its apparent importance in the results in Chapter 4. Use of absolute deviation from age 20 does not affect the correlation or the standardized regression coefficient (β), but it does affect the values of the unstandardized regression coefficient (B) and the intercept (A).

Strain, as noted above, is measured by two indicators. One, future job strain or occupational strain, asks respondents how good they think their chances are of getting the kind of job they would like after they finish school. For the present analysis this has been reverse-coded so that a high score on future job strain indicates the presence, not absence of strain. The second measure, school strain, combines an objective measure of school success (grade point average), subjective perceptions of school success ("how well are you doing . . . ?"), and the subjective likelihood of obtaining a college education. The school success scale and the single-item indicators of grade point average and college expectations were standardized (*z*-scores), then added to form a single scale (Cronbach's alpha = .67 to .72 for 1976–1980). School strain was also coded so that a high score on the school strain scale indicates the presence of strain, and a low score indicates the absence of strain.

Internal bonding is measured by three indicators. Two, family normlessness and school normlessness, are context-specific. Normlessness in both contexts indicates the extent to which a respondent in a particular context believes it is necessary or acceptable to engage in societally disapproved behavior (lying, cheating, breaking rules) to achieve desired goals within that context. The third indicator, belief, measures the extent to which an individual believes it is morally wrong for someone the same age as the respondent to commit a variety of illegal (assault, theft, drug use) or rule-violating (cheating on tests) acts. Belief is a measure of internal bonding to society in general rather than to a specific context. All three measures tap the dimension of internalized norms or beliefs. All three measures are described in more detail, with psychometric scale properties, elsewhere (Elliott et al., 1985).

External bonding is also measured by three indicators, of which two are context-specific. Family involvement and school involvement measure the amount of time devoted to family and school (excluding athletic or extracurricular) activities, respectively. Both measure bonding to conventional institutions or social contexts. By contrast, the third measure of external bonding measures the extent to which an individual is bonded to deviant or delinquent friends. A measure of peer group delinquency (how many of the respondent's friends have engaged in a variety of illegal acts or encouraged the respondent to break the law) was recalculated by subtracting the mean (that is, a mean deviation score was obtained) and multiplied by a measure of peer group involvement (how much time a respondent spends with friends) to obtain a measure of delinquent peer group involvement times exposure, or delinquent peer group bonding (DPGB). Although we describe this as an external bonding measure, implicitly invoking control theory, it is more directly derived from learning theory.

METHODS OF ANALYSIS

The general path model we analyze is diagrammed in Figure 6.2, in which the demographic variables are self-evidently exogenous. Age for a given year (or deviations from some age for a given year), sex, race, and cohort size are all determined in the year of birth. Parental social class and urban/rural residence may vary over the lifetime of the child, but they are not influenced by any of the child's characteristics; instead, they are determined by characteristics of the parents themselves.

For purposes of the present model, strain is placed causally prior to conventional and deviant bonding. Briefly, strain is the element of the model that provides the motivation for deviant, delinquent, or problem behavior. More extensive justification for this aspect of the causal ordering is detailed in Elliott et al. (1985). For adolescents, we hypothesize that internal bonding comes next, followed by external bonding. In terms of strict temporal priority (onset of internal bonding vs. onset of external bonding), external bonding in the form of time spent with family, in school, and with friends probably precedes internal bonding in the form of beliefs regarding right and wrong in the context of family, school, and

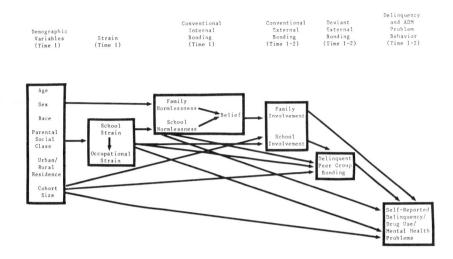

FIGURE 6.2. Complete path model.

society in general. However, we assume that for adolescents, early socialization by family, school, and friends is already reflected in the belief structure of the respondents. The extent of their involvement with family, school, and friends then is influenced by their beliefs or attitudes, whether general or context-specific. We assume that the general context-independent bond comes after the context-specific bond, and that conventional bonding precedes deviant bonding. We also assume that school strain precedes and influences occupational strain.

Path models were calculated using 1976 as time 1 and 1977 as time 2, then replicated using 1977 as time 1 and 1978 as time 2. Note that the demographic, strain, and conventional internal bonding measures are all point measures, taken at the end of time 1. By point measures, we mean that they are attitudes or attributes of an individual on a particular day at the end of time 1. By contrast, conventional external bonding, deviant external bonding, and delinquency and ADM problem behavior are all interval measures—that is, measures of time spent on certain activities or behavior performed during a certain time interval (from the beginning of time 1 to the beginning of time 2). The external bonding measures are thus contemporaneous with the delinquency and ADM measures (in effect assuming a zero or very short time lag), while the strain, and internal bonding measures are taken for a time immediately prior to the period in which the delinquent or ADM problem behavior occurs (in effect assuming a time lag of zero to 12 months). The demographic measures are all obtained for 1976; most (age, sex, race, cohort size) are invariant or completely predetermined for any time after birth, and the others (residence, social class) tend to be stable over short periods of time.

Path coefficients were calculated using ordinary least-squares regression. This was done for the demographic and the theoretical variables separately, then for the demographic and theoretical variables combined. For 1977 and 1978, the demographic variables alone could account for 8% to 10% of the variance in general delinquency offending, 4% to 6% in Index offending, 18% to 26% in alcohol use, 10% to 11% in marijuana use, 3% to 4% in polydrug use, and 3% to 5% in mental health problems. The theoretical variables alone explained 30% to 31% of the variance in general delinquency offending, 14% in Index offending, 30% to 40% in alcohol use, 40% to 41% in marijuana use, 14% to 16% in polydrug use, and 17% to 23% in mental health problems. Combining the demographic and theoretical predictors in the same equation results in an explained variance of 34% for general delinquency offending, 16% to 17% for Index offending, 36% to 49% for alcohol use, 42% for marijuana use, 15% to 16% for polydrug use, and 21% to 25% for mental health problems. The theoretical variables consistently provide higher levels of explained variance than the demographic variables when the two sets of variables are considered separately, but the two sets of variables taken together explain more of the variance in the dependent variables than either set taken separately. The increase in explained variance obtained by combining the theoretical and demographic variables, compared to using the theoretical variables alone, is small (0%–2%) for marijuana and polydrug use, larger (2%–4%) for general delinquency offending, Index offending, and mental health problems and substantial (6%–7%) for alcohol use.

Reduced models were calculated by eliminating variables from the equation if they failed to meet criteria of statistical significance here defined as probability of .010 (1.0%) of obtaining a nonzero regression coefficient when the true value of the regression coefficient is zero; and substantive significance, here defined as a standardized regression coefficient (β) of .100, meaning that a change of one standard deviation in the independent variable is associated with at least a one-tenth standard deviation change in the dependent variable. Statistically or substantively insignificant variables were deleted from the model, least statistically significant first, using stepwise regression with backward elimination. For more detailed discussion of statistical significance, substantive (or practical) significance, and the use of regression analysis with backward elimination, see Agresti and Finlay (1986, pp. 152–153, 211–213), Bohrnstedt and Knoke (1982, pp. 101, 1976), and Weisberg (1980, pp. 190–196). Once reduced models were calculated for 1976–1977, we attempted to replicate our findings by testing the same reduced models for 1977–1978.

Whenever we seek to eliminate meaningless paths or causal influences from a regression or path analysis equation using the above methods and criteria or any other set of criteria, we run the risk of eliminating or retaining variables arbitrarily. Accordingly, although we concentrate on the results using the above criteria, we also give some attention to what happens when we "bend" the above rules a little. Thus we pay special attention to the replicability of the findings with the orientation that findings replicated for 1977–1978 as well as 1976–1977 may be viewed with greater confidence than findings that appear for one but not the other time period.

To maintain some consistency in the type of samples being analyzed, it was necessary to choose between maintaining a constant distribution of cohort sizes or a constant distribution of ages. If we use all seven cohorts, the age range would be 12–18 in 1977 and 13–19 in 1978. Alternatively, if we do the analysis only for those aged 13–18 in 1977 and those aged 13–18 in 1978, we lose the third smallest cohort in 1977 and the smallest cohort in 1978. Either way, inconsistencies in age distribution or cohort size would raise some question about the validity of our results with respect to those variables. Given the relatively weaker impact of cohort size on most of the dependent variables (as indicated in Chapter 4) and the ubiquity of age effects for all except mental health problems, we chose the latter option, constancy of age distribution.

In the presentation which follows, we focus primarily on path models that (a) are restricted to ages 13–18 for both 1977 and 1978, (b) include only statistically (probability $\leq$ .010) and substantively ($\beta \geq$ .100) significant causal paths, and (c) include both demographic and theoretical variables. Although we focus on models sharing all three of the above criteria, other models, not presented in detail, were also considered as explanations for delinquency and ADM problems among adolescents. In general, models with only demographic variables achieved less explanatory power (R^2) than models with only theoretical variables. For marijuana and polydrug use the addition of the demographic variables to the equation, which already included the theoretical variables, produced little or no increase in the explanatory power of the model, but for the other dependent variables the addition of the demographic variables increased the explained variance in both the full (all variables included) and reduced models.

Results

DEPENDENT VARIABLES

Table 6.1 presents the regression equations for each of the dependent variables, measured in 1977 and 1978. The last column, directly attributable variance (DAV), is the product of the two preceding columns (β and r), and is the variance in the dependent variable that is directly attributable to the independent variable in that row. The sum of the DAVs is equal to R^2. All of the regression coefficients in Table 6.1 are statistically significant (probability < .0005).

Delinquency

Given the *a priori* criteria of substantive and statistical significance, two variables, delinquent peer group bonding and sex, significantly influence levels of both general delinquency and Index offending in 1977. The 1977 results were successfully replicated for 1978. DPGB has the strongest influence on delinquency, and the other theoretical variables influence delinquency only (if at all) through DPGB. The influence of sex is weaker, but statistically and substantively significant. As expected, males and those who are frequently involved with delinquent friends have the highest levels of delinquency.

Alcohol and Drug Use

As it was for general delinquency and Index offenses, DPGB is the principal influence on alcohol, marijuana, and drug use. Those who have frequent contact with delinquent peer groups show higher rates of alcohol, marijuana, and polydrug use. Unlike general delinquency and Index offending, none of the three forms of substance use appears to be directly influenced by sex. This result is not surprising for marijuana or polydrug use. The results in Chapter 3 indicated no significant correlation between sex and either type of illegal drug use in adolescence (1976). The relationship between sex and alcohol was statistically significant, but weak. Instead of sex, however, belief is a significant influence on all three types of substance use, with those having stronger internal bonds to society having lower rates of all three substance types in adolescence. No other variable emerges as a predictor of polydrug use. For marijuana use, family involvement has a weak, negative influence, indicating that those who spend more time in family activities have lower rates of marijuana use. Age, here represented by absolute deviation from age 20, has an influence on alcohol use. As indicated in Chapter 4, alcohol use increases as age increases, at least up to age 20. All of the results for 1977 were successfully replicated for 1978.

Mental Health Problems

Unlike delinquency and drug use, mental health problems appear to be largely unrelated to delinquent peer group bonding, sex, belief, or age. The strongest influences on mental health problem scale scores are school strain and family normlessness, both of which are associated with higher scores (more problems) on the mental health problem scale. Family involvement is third in influence, with those more involved in family activities having lower mental health problem scale scores. Finally, nonwhites have higher mental health problem scale scores than whites; the relationship is weak, but statistically and substantively significant. All of these results were successfully replicated for 1978.

TABLE 6.1. Regression equations for delinquency and ADM problems.

Dependent variable	Year	R^2 (explained variance)	Independent variable	A (intercept)	B (unstandardized regression coefficient)	β (standardized regression coefficient)	r (zero-order correlation)	DAV (directly attributable variance)
General delinquency offending rate	1977	.31	DPGB	26.1	.046	.505	.530	.268
			Sex (1 = male, 2 = female)		−1.67	−.164	−.239	.039
	1978	.31	DPGB	25.5	.042	.515	.533	.274
			Sex		−1.45	−.153	−.213	.033
Index offending rate	1977	.15	DPGB	9.63	.0078	.344	.362	.125
			Sex		−.309	−.123	−.174	.021
	1978	.14	DPGB	9.54	.0065	.334	.349	.117
			Sex		−.285	−.127	−.166	.021
Alcohol use rate	1977	.35	DPGB	6.54	.012	.353	.482	.170
			Belief		−.081	−.174	−.410	.071
			|Age − 20| (absolute deviation from age 20)		−.322	−.275	−.393	.108
	1978	.47	DPGB	7.78	.012	.355	.531	.189
			Belief		−.112	−.236	−.517	.122
			|Age − 20|		−.384	−.324	−.481	.156

Marijuana use rate	1977	.41	DPGB	5.53	.017	.468	.590	.276
			Belief		−.108	−.224	−.457	.102
			Family involvement		−.060	−.106	−.266	.028
	1978	.40	DPGB	6.87	.014	.394	.557	.219
			Belief		−.143	−.291	−.504	.147
			Family involvement		−.063	−.107	−.291	.031
Polydrug use rate	1977	.13	DPGB	6.90	.0061	.249	.326	.081
			Belief		.057	−.175	−.285	.050
	1978	.15	DPGB	6.63	.0075	.302	.368	.111
			Belief		−.048	−.142	−.283	.040
Mental health problems scale score	1977	.17	Family involvement	31.4	−.362	−.161	−.209	.034
			Family normlessness		.656	.204	.284	.058
			School strain		.774	.227	.271	.062
			Race (1 = white, 2 = other)		3.28	.140	.145	.020
	1978	.22	Family involvement	27.3	−.261	−.113	−.180	.020
			Family normlessness		.979	.297	.390	.116
			School strain		.771	.224	.322	.072
			Race		2.80	.115	.121	.014

Depression and Mental Health Service Use

Data on depression and mental health service use were not collected until 1983, when the respondents in the NYS were 18–24 years old. This poses a problem for etiological analysis of depression and mental health service use with NYS data, because (a) we are no longer analyzing the data for respondents who are all adolescents, and (b) we have no data collected in 1982 on the exogenous and intervening variables, so we cannot preserve strict temporal ordering. With regard to the mental health problem scale, data on social isolation were not collected in 1983, so we have data only on emotional problems (self-perceived "sick" labeling). In addition, data were collected on family involvement, as measured in previous waves of data collection, only for those who indicated that they were not in a heterosexual (boyfriend/girlfriend/spouse) living arrangement in 1983. School normlessness and school strain are available in 1983 only for those enrolled in school in 1983.

This shortage of data makes it difficult to replicate our analysis of the mental health problem scale for 1983 and thus increases the difficulty in comparing the etiology of other mental health measures (depression, mental health service use) with that of the mental health problem scale. As an exploratory attempt at replication, however, we restricted our sample to those for whom the family involvement measure was available in 1983 (those not living with spouse, boyfriend, or girlfriend) and for whom normlessness could be measured either at school, at work, or both. From the school and work normlessness measures (standardized), we constructed a single measure of work/school normlessness. For school strain, we substituted highest grade completed, and for occupational strain a new measure was introduced indicating how much strain the respondent experienced at work instead of whether the respondent felt it likely that he or she would get the kind of job he or she wanted.

We began by using the emotional problems measure as a dependent variable in place of the mental health problem scale, and attempted to replicate the reduced equation for the mental health problem scale from Table 6.1. The attempt at replication was fairly successful. Family normlessness ($\beta = .390$), family involvement ($\beta = -.109$), and highest grade completed ($\beta = -.220$) explained 22% of the variance in emotional problems. Race, however, dropped out of the equation because of substantive insignificance ($\beta < .100$). Because the equations for mental health/emotional problems were reasonably consistent over time (suggesting stability in the etiological pattern), we attempted to replicate the same equations for depression and mental health service use. In both cases, all four variables from the reduced equation for mental health problems dropped out of the models because of statistical or substantive insignificance.

We next performed a stepwise regression using all of the variables in the model. As in the replication, family normlessness ($\beta = .287$), family involvement ($\beta = -.105$), and highest grade completed ($\beta = -.178$) were retained in the model for emotional problems, and together with work/ school normlessness ($\beta = .135$) and the new occupational strain measure ($\beta = .138$), which were also retained, they explained 25% of the variance in emotional problems. These results suggest that for those aged 18–24, the work context becomes important as an influence on mental health problems. Using the same set of variables, however, only sex ($\beta = .118$) emerged as an influence on depression with females being more likely to suffer depressive symptoms than males, but with only 1% of the variance in depression explained. Mental health service use was unexplained by the demographic and theoretical variables in the model. Even with all variables in the equation, less than 0.5% of the variance in mental health service use was explained.

These results raise some question about the adequacy of all three of our mental health measures. Clearly, the etiological patterns for the three measures differ, and it may well be that with respect to etiology, there is more difference among measures of mental health than among measures of delinquency or substance use. As we indicated earlier (Chapter 1) our mental health measures are much less exhaustive of the range of mental health problems than are our measures of delinquency and substance use for their respective domains. For the present, we may conclude that the variables in our model do a fair job of explaining the mental health problems scale (emotional problems and social isolation), that they do a poor job of explaining depression, and that they completely fail to explain mental health service use. In the remainder of this chapter, insofar as we discuss explanations of mental health problems, we will be referring only to emotional problems and social isolation.

EXOGENOUS AND INTERVENING VARIABLES

In Table 6.2, three variables directly influence DPGB: belief, school normlessness, and school involvement.[1] Belief and school normlessness are both elements of the belief structure of individuals, and the results in Table 6.2 suggest that those people with conventional beliefs tend not to

---

[1] Family involvement may be substituted for school involvement with no loss in statistical or substantive significance and little change in explained variance. Using standardized regression coefficients, the alternate equations are

$$\text{DPGB (1977)} = -.366(\text{belief}) + .169(\text{school normlessness}) - .109(\text{family involvement})$$
$$\text{DPGB (1978)} = -.345(\text{belief}) + .164(\text{school normlessness}) - .143(\text{family involvement}),$$

with R^2 of .23 and .26, respectively. When both school and family involvement are used in the same equation, however, one of the two has a standardized regression coefficient less than .100. These results suggest that it may be general involvement in conventional social contexts, rather than specific involvement in a particular conventional social context, that reduces the level of DPGB.

TABLE 6.2. Regression equations for independent and intervening variables.

Dependent variable	Year	R^2 (explained variance)	Independent variable	A (intercept)	B (unstandardized regression coefficient)	β (standardized regression coefficient)	r (zero-order correlation)	DAV (directly attributable variance)
Delinquent peer group bonding	1977	.24	Belief	143.	−4.46	−.337	−.442	.149
			School involvement		−2.36	−.140	−.244	.034
			School normlessness		3.13	.159	.344	.055
	1978	.25	Belief	161.	−4.97	−.363	−.466	.169
			School involvement		−2.10	−.126	−.245	.031
			School normlessness		2.92	.147	.355	.052
Family involvement	1977	.10	Belief	86.8	.122	.143	.250	.036
			Family normlessness		−.179	−.126	−.219	.028
			|Age − 15| (absolute deviation from age 15)		−.757	−.194	−.058	.011
			Parity (relative cohort size)		−26.4	−.211	−.109	.023
	1978	.10	Belief	29.3	.184	.219	.276	.060
			|Age − 15|		−.456	−.121	−.142	.017
			Parity		−8.29	−.129	−.058	.011
	1977 (alt.)	.09	Belief	84.4	.173	.203	.250	.051
			|Age − 15|		−.770	−.197	−.191	.025
			Parity	−26.6	−26.6	−.213	−.109	.023
School involvement	1977	.14	Belief	.495	.116	.147	.216	.032
			School strain		−.359	−.256	−.295	.076
			Sex (1 = male, 2 = female)		.884	.134	.176	.024
			Race (1 = white, 2 = other)		1.15	.120	.113	.014
	1978	.18	Belief	.985	.106	.129	.234	.030
			School strain		−.458	−.315	−.362	.114
			Sex		.864	.124	.186	.023
			Race		1.04	.102	.101	.010

	Year	R²	Predictor					
Belief	1977	.14	School strain	81.9	−.277	−.156	−.190	.030
			Urban-rural residence		.634	.112	.097	.011
			Sex		.962	.115	.141	.016
			Births (absolute cohort size)		−.013	−.283	−.300	.085
	1978	.19	School strain	59.3	−.359	−.203	−.248	.050
			Urban-rural residence		.594	.104	.101	.011
			Sex		1.16	.138	.173	.024
			Births		−.0077	−.312	−.338	.105
Family normlessness	1977	.06	School strain	−38.8	.137	.129	.153	.020
			Sex		−.644	−.129	−.147	.019
			$\lvert Age - 15 \rvert$		.481	.175	.042	.007
			Parity		16.2	.185	.077	.014
	1978	.09	School strain	−6.88	.282	.270	.282	.076
			Parity		5.24	.116	.144	.017
School normlessness	1977	.10	School strain	13.2	.311	.259	.265	.069
			Urban-rural residence		−.455	−.119	−.106	.013
			Sex		−.666	−.118	−.143	.017
	1978	.16	School strain	13.2	.415	.342	.351	.120
			Urban-rural residence		−.567	−.144	−.129	.019
			Sex		−.707	−.122	−.169	.021
Occupational strain	1977	.10	School strain	2.65	.066	.312	.312	.097
	1978	.13	School strain	2.69	.073	.365	.365	.133
School strain	1977	.09	Parents' social status	12.8	−.040	−.280	−.278	.078
			Births		.0027	.104	.097	.010
	1978	.08	Parents' social status	7.50	−.038	−.259	−.259	.067
			Births		.0014	.102	.102	.010

become involved in delinquent peer groups, but those who believe it is necessary or acceptable to lie, cheat, or break the rules (particularly in the school context), or are more tolerant of these behaviors, do become involved in such groups. Those who invest more time in conventional social contexts (family or school) are less likely to invest time in delinquent peer groups. These results are successfully replicated for 1978.

For 1977, *family involvement* appears to be positively influenced by belief and negatively influenced by family normlessness, absolute deviation from age 15, and relative cohort size (parity). In attempting to replicate these results for 1978, we found that in 1978 the influence of family normlessness on family involvement was not substantively significant. If we drop family normlessness from the equation for 1977, the variance explained in family involvement decreases by 1% and the influence of belief on family involvement increases. Otherwise, there is no substantial change in the model. Based on these results, we may regard the influences of belief, absolute deviation from age 15, and parity as confirmed, and that of family normlessness as questionable. The fact that family involvement decreases with average parity is consistent with Easterlin's (1987) analysis, as described in Chapter 4. That absolute deviation from age 15, instead of chronological age, is retained in the equation indicates the presence of an unexpected curvilinear relationship between age and time spent in family activities, with the lowest level of family involvement occurring in mid-adolescence, around age 15, and increasing involvement thereafter. This relationship may bear further investigation in future analyses. Whether family normlessness is included in the equation or not, belief structure has an influence on family involvement.

School involvement is influenced by belief,[2] school strain, sex, and race. The strongest influence is school strain, presence of which decreases school involvement, followed by belief, which increases school involvement. Females are more likely than males, and nonwhites more likely than whites, to report higher levels of involvement in school. The male-female difference is probably not surprising, but the white-nonwhite difference may run counter to expectations based on the relative levels of school achievement (grade point average, test scores) and attainment

---

[2] School normlessness, the context-specific measure of internal bonding, may be substituted for belief, the more general measure, with no loss of statistical or substantive significance and little or no loss of explained variance:

$$\text{School involvement (1977)} = -.124(\text{school normlessness})$$
$$- .251(\text{school strain}) + .138(\text{sex}) + .137(\text{race})$$
$$\text{School involvement (1978)} = -.113(\text{school normlessness})$$
$$- .307(\text{school strain}) + .129(\text{sex}) + .123(\text{race})$$

with $R^2 = .14$ and .17, respectively. This result suggests that belief structure, whether general or specific, influences involvement in school.

(years of school completed, highest degree received) of whites and nonwhites. It is consistent, however, with previous findings that nonwhites (including both blacks and orientals) spend more time on homework than whites, are less likely to miss school because of truancy, and are more likely to read outside the school than whites (Coleman et al., 1966, chap. 3).

It appears in Table 6.2 that the primary influence on *belief* in the conventional normative order is absolute cohort size (births), followed by school strain, sex, and urban-rural residence. Those from the larger birth cohorts are less likely to accept conventional definitions of the wrongness of certain actions, and we may speculate that this effect, consistent with the Easterlin hypothesis, is a result of less adequate socialization when parental resources are more thinly spread among larger numbers of children. Conventional beliefs are stronger among those without school strain, perhaps indicating that those who are succeeding in the system are less likely to question its legitimacy. Females have more strongly held conventional beliefs than males, and rural residents, consistent with past analyses (Abrahamson, 1980, chap. 9), have more strongly held conventional beliefs than urban residents.

From Table 6.2 it appears that in 1977 *family normlessness* was influenced by school strain, sex, absolute deviation from age 15, and relative cohort size (parity). Given our criteria of statistical and substantive significance, however, we fail to replicate these results for 1977: Sex and absolute deviation from age 15 drop out of the equation, leaving school strain and parity. If we attempt to use only school strain and parity for 1977, the standardized regression coefficient for parity is less than .100, and the explained variance decreases to 3%. Further attempts at reconciling the two equations for family normlessness suggested that school strain and chronological age might be used, with an explained variance of 4% in 1977 and 10% in 1978, but overall the results indicate poor agreement between the models for family normlessness in 1977 and 1978. The lack of agreement and the low levels of explained variance suggest that further work is needed to explain family normlessness, but school strain probably forms part of that explanation, and either age or relative cohort size (parity) may also be useful.

With *school normlessness* we encountered no problems in replicating the 1977 results for 1978. School strain has the strongest influence, and sex and urban-rural residence also influence school normlessness. All three variables had similar patterns of influence on belief (with opposite signs because belief and normlessness refer, respectively, to strength and weakness in internal bonding), and the discussion of their influences on belief also applies here. For *occupational strain,* only school strain has any influence, and this result is replicated for 1978. This finding suggests that respondents who have or expect to have problems with regard to academic achievement or attainment also anticipate problems in getting the kind of job they want after completing school. *School strain* is influenced by parents' social status, as we would expect from Merton (1938), and by absolute cohort size, as Easterlin (1987) would lead us to expect.

THEORETICAL IMPLICATIONS

Elements of three theoretical perspectives are included in this analysis. Delinquent peer group bonding was derived most directly from learning theory. Relative and absolute cohort size are derived from a macrostructural variant of anomie or strain theory (Easterlin, 1987) and school strain and occupational strain from a microsocial variant of strain theory (Cloward & Ohlin, 1960). Strain theory also implies the inclusion of race and parental social status as relevant variables. Family and school normlessness may also be germane to strain or anomie theory (anomie is defined as a state of normlessness), but they are more directly derived from control theory, in which, along with belief, they are operational measures of internal bonding. Also, from control theory, we include school and family involvement as measures of external bonding. Delinquent peer group bonding may also be considered a measure of (deviant) external bonding, but as noted above, this measure is more directly derived from learning theory. In the way they have been operationalized here, school and occupational strain resemble measures of commitment used by Hirschi (1969), although they are more directly pertinent to strain theory.

If we view these variables as components of a single, integrated theory, the general conclusion to which we come is that the integrated theory works moderately well at explaining delinquency and ADM problem behavior in adolescence. If, however, we consider the three theoretical perspectives separately, some important distinctions emerge in their utility for explaining delinquency and ADM problem behavior. Strain theory variables influence delinquency and substance use only indirectly, but (at the microsocial level) strain has a direct impact on mental health problems. Control theory variables, particularly belief, directly influence substance use, and family-related control theory variables directly influence mental health problems. Control theory has no direct impact, however, on delinquent behavior. Learning theory provides the principal explanation for both delinquency and substance use but does not help explain mental health problems. One might reasonably argue that volitional deviance (delinquency, substance use) is learned, but involuntary deviance (mental health problems) is spontaneous and not learned. Learning theory is the only one of the three theories to be completely excluded from the explanation of any of the mental health dependent variables. Strain and control theory have at least indirect influences on all of the dependent variables in our models.

Summary

Figure 6.3 presents a visual summary of the results discussed above. Solid lines represent those paths found to be statistically and substantively significant in both the original test with 1976–1977 data and in the replication with 1977–1978 data. Dashed lines represent either paths which were significant in 1977 but not 1978 (sex to family normlessness, absolute deviation from age 15 to family normlessness, family normlessness to family involvement) or paths that, though not selected in the model for 1977, are plausible alternatives (statistically and substantively significant) to other paths in the model (school normlessness—as an alternative for belief—to school involvement; family involvement—as an alternative for school involvement—to delinquent peer group involvement times exposure). Path coefficients are excluded from the model because of its complexity, but they may be found in Tables 6.1 and 6.2. Also, occupational strain is excluded from the model because it has no influence, direct or indirect, on delinquency or ADM problem behavior for the 13- to 18-year-olds in our sample.

Sex indirectly influences both delinquency and substance use through its influences on belief, school involvement, and delinquent peer group bonding. It also has a direct influence on both general delinquency and Index offending. In each case, being female is associated, as we would expect, with a lower risk of delinquency or substance use. There is also some weak indication that being female indirectly reduces the risk of

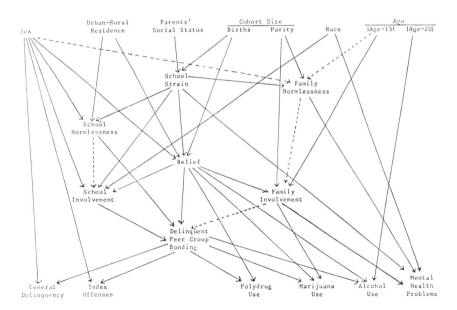

FIGURE 6.3. Verified path model.

mental health problems, through its influence on family normlessness. Race has an indirect effect on delinquency and substance use through school involvement, which places nonwhites at *lower* risk of delinquency than whites. Insofar as race is correlated with parents' social status ($r = -.281$ for 1977 and $-.282$ for 1978), it is associated with higher rates of delinquency and substance use because social status has an indirect influence (with lower-class respondents at greater risk of delinquency or substance use) through school strain. One might reasonably argue that parental race is the same as respondents' race (although this assumption need not always be valid in mixed-race marriages or adoptions), and that race could be placed causally prior to parental social status, but both race and parental social status are regarded as exogenous variables here, relative to respondent characteristics.

Age appears to have a direct influence on alcohol use and an indirect influence (through family involvement and maybe through family normlessness) on marijuana use and mental health problems. For all practical purposes, the age effect on alcohol use for ages 13–18 is positive, with alcohol use increasing with age. The influence of age on family involvement (and family normlessness), however, appears to be curvilinear, with a nadir in mid-adolescence, around age 15. Despite the restricted range imposed by eliminating one cohort in each model (to keep the ages constant), cohort size indirectly affects all of the dependent variables. Through school strain and belief, larger absolute cohort size (births) brings an increased rate of both types of delinquency and all three types of substance use. Greater relative cohort size (parity) appears to increase the rate of mental health problems (through family normlessness and family involvement), marijuana use (through family involvement), and perhaps (through family involvement) alcohol and polydrug use and general and Index offending.

The influence of school strain is pervasive. It influences mental health problems directly and (through family normlessness) indirectly, with greater school strain increasing the risk of mental health problems. It also influences delinquency and substance use indirectly, through school normlessness, school involvement, and belief. Occupational strain has no apparent effect on any of the other measures. School normlessness and school involvement also have indirect influences on delinquency and substance use (through delinquent peer group involvement times exposure), but no apparent impact on mental health problems. Family normlessness and involvement, by contrast, both have direct effects on mental health problems. Except for the direct influence of family involvement on marijuana use, the evidence for an influence of family normlessness or involvement on delinquency and substance use is equivocal. Such an influence may exist, but it was not initially found and then replicated in the present analysis. Notice that of the five equivocal relationships (dashed lines) in Figure 6.3, all but one involves either family normlessness or family involvement, or both. All three of the unreplicated paths are either to or from family normlessness.

Belief and delinquent peer group bonding have direct influences on alcohol, marijuana, and polydrug use. DPGB also directly influences general delinquency and Index offending. Belief indirectly influences delinquency (through school involvement and DPGB) and mental health problems (through family involvement). As expected, DPGB increases and belief decreases the rate of delinquency and ADM problem behavior.

The four variables with the most pervasive influence on the fully elaborated model in Figure 6.3, as indicated by the number of paths that originate at those variables are sex, school strain, belief, and DPGB. The last of the variables directly influences all of the dependent variables except mental health problems; sex, school strain, and belief directly or indirectly influence all of the dependent variables without exception. School strain influences all three of the internal bonding measures (belief, school normlessness, family normlessness). Belief influences all three of the external bonding measures (DPGB, school involvement, family involvement), in contrast to the context-specific internal bonding measures (school and family normlessness), which influence either delinquency and substance use or mental health problems but (ignoring the questionable relationships indicated by the dashed lines) not both. The influence of sex appears to be more evident in the school context than in the family. With regard to the dependent variables, sex has its strongest influence on delinquency, and its weakest on mental health problems.

If we disregard the dashed lines in Figure 6.3, an interesting pattern emerges. One measure of cohort size, parity, has an indirect influence only on mental health problems, and both family normlessness and family involvement (which are influenced by parity) affect mental health problems but not delinquency, alcohol, or polydrug use. School normlessness, school involvement, and DPGB influence delinquency and substance use, but not mental health problems. Age does not influence delinquency or polydrug use but does influence alcohol use (directly), marijuana use, and mental health problems (through family involvement). School strain and belief directly or indirectly influence all of the dependent variables, as does race (directly for mental health, indirectly through school involvement for everything else). Sex, urban-rural residence, parents' social status, and absolute cohort size (births) indirectly (through either or both of school strain and belief, as well as through other variables) influence all of the dependent variables.

The overall picture that emerges is one of three distinct etiological paths for delinquency, substance use, and mental health problems. The path for both general delinquency and Index offending involves sex and delinquent peer group bonding. The path for substance use involves belief and DPGB, with some additional, unique influence for marijuana use (family involvement) and alcohol use (age). The presence of DPGB as the principal influence on both delinquency and substance use makes the etiological paths for delinquency and substance use more similar to each other than either path is to that for mental health problems. For mental health problems, the etiological path involves the two family context variables (family involvement and normlessness), neither of which is strongly related to delinquency (and only one of which, family involvement, has anything to do with substance use), along with race and school strain, both of which have indirect influences on delinquency and substance use. Our measure of mental health problems, then, appears to tap a very different etiological domain than that tapped by our measures of delinquency or substance use. Nonetheless, once we move back past the direct influences on each variable, there does appear to be some etiological linkage among all three types of behavior.

The Interaction Between Conventional and Delinquent Bonding

The foregoing analysis does not take into account the conditional relationship (Path 4 in Figure 6.1) postulated in our theoretical model, namely, that the relationship between delinquent peer group bonding and delinquent behavior is conditioned by weak conventional bonding. To probe for the existence of this interaction effect, we constructed a typology with six categories:

1. Low conventional bonding, low DPGB.
2. High conventional bonding, low DPGB.
3. Low conventional bonding, medium DPGB.
4. High conventional bonding, medium DPGB.
5. Low conventional bonding, high DPGB.
6. High conventional bonding, high DPGB.

High, low, and medium levels of DPGB are here defined, respectively, as one-half standard deviation or more above the DPGB mean, one-half standard deviation or more below the mean, and within one-half standard deviation of the mean. High and low levels of conventional bonding were obtained from an O-type cluster analysis of the NYS sample with respect to the five bonding measures (belief, family and school involvement, family and school normlessness) in the theoretical model. The cluster analysis produced a satisfactory two-group solution for both 1977 and 1978, in which cluster centroids were more than 2.5 standard deviations apart, and a distance of approximately one standard deviation was obtained between the group centroids on each of the five bonding variables.

BIVARIATE RESULTS AND THE
CONVENTIONAL-DELINQUENT BONDING INTERACTION

As a first step in examining the interaction between conventional bonding and DPGB, we compared mean levels of categorical scores (general offending and use rates, the same as used in the regression equations) for general delinquency, Index offenses, alcohol use, marijuana use, and polydrug use. The mental health problem scale score is excluded from this analysis because DPGB had no impact on mental health problems in the regression equations (Table 6.2 and Figure 6.3). Means for each group are presented in Table 6.3 and the statistical significance of the differences between the means for each group, based on an unequal-variances t-test (Bulmer, 1979, p. 151), are presented in Table 6.4. Of particular interest in Table 6.4 are the contrasts between types 1 and 2 (both with low delinquent bonding; 1 with low conventional bonding and 2 with high conventional bonding), 3 and 4 (both medium delinquent bonding; 3 low and 4 high conventional bonding), and 5 and 6 (both high delinquent bonding; 5 low and 6 high conventional bonding) for the effect of conventional bonding, with deviant bonding held constant; and between groups 1 and 3 (low conventional bonding, low to medium deviant bonding), 3 and 5 (low conventional bonding, medium to high deviant

TABLE 6.3. Mean categorical scores for delinquent offending rates and substance use rates by conventional/delinquent bonding type

	Conventional bonding	Delinquent bonding		
		Low (Type)	Medium (Type)	High (Type)
General delinquency, 1977	Low	23.08 (1)	25.07 (3)	29.81 (5)
	High	22.76 (2)	23.82 (4)	26.68 (6)
General delinquency, 1978	Low	22.25 (1)	26.33 (3)	30.23 (5)
	High	22.57 (2)	23.69 (4)	26.82 (6)
Index offenses 1977	Low	9.11 (1)	9.37 (3)	10.18 (5)
	High	9.07 (2)	9.20 (4)	9.69 (6)
Index offenses, 1978	Low	9.00 (1)	9.67 (3)	10.23 (5)
	High	9.05 (2)	9.18 (4)	9.58 (6)
Alcohol use, 1977	Low	2.14 (1)	3.25 (3)	4.56 (5)
	High	1.68 (2)	2.50 (4)	3.71 (6)
Alcohol use, 1978	Low	1.88 (1)	3.78 (3)	5.18 (5)
	High	1.59 (2)	2.66 (4)	4.25 (6)
Marijuana use, 1977	Low	1.11 (1)	2.38 (3)	4.52 (5)
	High	1.04 (2)	1.37 (4)	3.02 (6)
Marijuana use, 1978	Low	1.00 (1)	3.05 (3)	4.98 (5)
	High	1.13 (2)	1.73 (4)	3.63 (6)
Polydrug use, 1977	Low	5.00 (1)	5.37 (3)	6.19 (5)
	High	5.03 (2)	5.07 (4)	5.29 (6)
Polydrug use, 1978	Low	5.00 (1)	5.71 (3)	6.62 (5)
	High	5.05 (2)	5.08 (4)	5.58 (6)

TABLE 6.4. Significance of unequal-variance t-tests for conventional and delinquent bonding types

Types	General delinquency	Index offenses	Alcohol use	Marijuana use	Polydrug use
	1977 t-test results (significance level)				
1–2	.292	.476	.060	.433	.259
1–3	.000	.004	.000	.000	.001
1–4	.028	.148	.088	.008	.009
1–5	.000	.000	.000	.000	.000
1–6	.000	.001	.000	.000	.003
2–3	.000	.000	.000	.000	.002
2–4	.000	.001	.000	.000	.222
2–5	.000	.000	.000	.000	.000
2–6	.000	.000	.000	.000	.009
3–4	.000	.036	.000	.000	.008
3–5	.000	.000	.000	.000	.000
3–6	.015	.075	.027	.017	.513
4–5	.000	.000	.000	.000	.000
4–6	.000	.005	.000	.000	.031
5–6	.000	.019	.000	.000	.000
	1978 t-test results (significance level)				
1–2	.101	.000	.579	.000	.102
1–3	.000	.001	.000	.000	.001
1–4	.000	.000	.027	.000	.000
1–5	.000	.000	.000	.000	.000
1–6	.000	.000	.000	.000	.000
2–3	.000	.002	.000	.000	.003
2–4	.000	.000	.000	.000	.281
2–5	.000	.000	.000	.000	.000
2–6	.000	.000	.000	.000	.001
3–4	.001	.016	.000	.000	.005
3–5	.001	.062	.000	.000	.005
3–6	.594	.669	.062	.070	.602
4–5	.000	.000	.000	.000	.000
4–6	.000	.000	.000	.000	.001
5–6	.001	.009	.000	.000	.000

bonding), 2 and 4 (high conventional bonding, low to medium deviant bonding), and 4 and 6 (high conventional bonding, medium to high deviant bonding) for the effect of deviant bonding with conventional bonding held constant.

As Tables 6.3 and 6.4 indicate, the level of conventional bonding generally makes little difference in delinquent offending and drug use rates for those who belong to primarily prosocial peer groups, that is, those with low DPGB (types 1 and 2). Of ten comparisons only two, Index offending and marijuana use, both in 1978, indicate a statistically significant (probability $\leq$ .05) difference between types 1 and 2. Of the two, moreover, one (marijuana use) is in the opposite direction to what we would expect: those with stronger conventional bonds have higher marijuana use rates than those with weaker conventional bonds, when DPGB is low. Further examination of Table 6.3 indicates that there is no consistency in the direction of the relationships between delinquency or drug use and conventional bonding for those with low DPGB.

For those with medium and high DPGB (comparisons of type 3 to type 4, and type 5 to type 6), the differences in delinquent offending and substance use are all statistically significant, and those with higher levels of conventional bonding consistently have lower levels of delinquent offending and drug use than those with lower levels of conventional bonding. These results indicate that the effects of conventional bonding are influenced by the level of DPGB. In peer groups with moderate to high levels of delinquency, conventional bonding reduces the rate of delinquent offending or substance use; when delinquency in the peer group is low, conventional bonding makes little difference.

Comparisons between types 1 and 3, 3 and 5, 2 and 4, and 4 and 6 suggest that DPGB, by contrast, affects delinquent offending and substance use largely independently of levels of conventional bonding. The difference between medium and low levels of DPGB for those with high levels of conventional bonding (types 2 and 4) is statistically significant for all of the problem behavior except polydrug use. For Index offending in 1978, the difference between medium and high DPGB is not quite statistically significant for those with low levels of conventional bonding, but the difference is statistically significant in 1977. All of the other 37 comparisons between adjacent levels of DPGB with conventional bonding controlled, are statistically significant. Overall, these results indicate that the effects of DPGB do not depend on the level of conventional bonding. The one clear exception, as noted above, is the absence of a difference in polydrug use between those with low and those with medium DPGB when conventional bonding is strong. Individuals with higher levels of DPGB have consistently higher levels of delinquent behavior and substance use. It is also the case that the type with the highest rates of delinquent offending and drug use is always type 5, those with low levels of conventional bonding and high levels of bonding to delinquent peers. Those with the lowest offending and use rates are always types 1 or 2, i.e., with low levels of bonding to delinquent peers, but not necessarily with high levels of conventional bonding. This finding suggests the possibility of an interaction effect with conventional bonding having an effect only among those with high levels of bonding to delinquent peers.

REGRESSION RESULTS AND THE CONVENTIONAL-DELINQUENT BONDING INTERACTION

As a second test of whether the impact of DPGB on delinquent offending and substance use is conditional upon the level of conventional bonding, we recalculated the regression results separately for those with low conventional bonding and those with high conventional bonding, for both 1977 and 1978. The results are presented in Table 6.5. For 1977, for both types of delinquency and all three types of substance use, the explained variance is higher for those with low levels of conventional bonding. We are thus better able to predict delinquent offending and substance use rates for those with weak conventional bonds. For 1978, however, the explained variance is higher for those with weak conventional bonds only for Index offending and polydrug use. For general delinquency, alcohol use, and marijuana use, the explained variance is the same or slightly higher for those with high levels of conventional bonding. In both years, family involvement in the equation for alcohol use and belief in the equation for polydrug use become substantively insignificant ($\beta < .100$), a result that is not altogether surprising in view of the fact that controlling for levels of conventional bonding is, in part, controlling for levels on these variables.

Comparison of the results regarding explained variance in Table 6.5 to the results in Table 6.1 indicates that the equations calculated without controls for conventional bonding (Table 6.1) produce explained variances that are nearly as high (general delinquency offending in 1977, Index offending in 1977 and 1978, polydrug use in 1977) or, in most cases, higher than the explained variance for either the weakly or strongly conventionally bonded types. For alcohol, marijuana, and polydrug use, this finding is reflected also in smaller zero-order correlations not only for DPGB but also for belief and family involvement, two of the variables upon which the high/low conventional bonding dichotomy was based. It is also worth remarking that DPGB is influenced by three of the five bonding measures used in constructing the conventional bonding dichotomy. Based on this result, we would expect attenuated correlations associated with restrictions in the range of the bonding measures, including DPGB, when we split the sample into high and low conventional bonding types.

ANOVA RESULTS AND THE CONVENTIONAL-DELINQUENT BONDING INTERACTION

As a final, more formal test for the presence of an interaction effect between conventional and delinquent bonding, we examined the effect of using the conventional-delinquent bonding typology as an explanatory variable in an analysis of variance (ANOVA) and covariance. The results are presented in Table 6.6. Although unequal variances and unequal cell sizes render the inferential statistics for an ANOVA (for example, probability levels associated with independent variables and covariates) invalid, there should be little impact on the overall explanatory power of the model. The first part of Table 6.6 presents the variance explained in

Dependent variable	R^2 Low bonding	R^2 High bonding	Independent variable	β, low bonding	β, high bonding	r, low bonding	r, high bonding	n, low bonding	n, high bonding
1977									
General delinquency offending rate	.32	.19	DPGB	.516	.381	.537	.403	489	1148
			Sex	-.188	-.166	-.243	-.216		
Index offending rate	.18	.08	DPGB	.377	.255	.394	.269		
			Sex	-.159	-.102	-.200	-.136		
Alcohol use rate	.30	.24	DPGB	.373	.284	.411	.372		
			Belief	-.121	-.144	-.258	-.295		
			|Age − 20|	-.323	-.262	-.350	-.342		
Marijuana use rate	.36	.28	DPGB	.476	.469	.540	.509		
			Belief	-.237	-.114	-.334	-.262		
			Family involvement	-.148	-.075	-.141	-.104		
Polydrug use rate	.15	.03	DPGB	.276	.190	.328	.184		
			Belief	-.215	.018	-.282	-.042		
1978									
General delinquency offending rate	.26	.28	DPGB	.475	.483	.488	.493	289	1280
			Sex	-.133	-.186	-.179	-.213		
Index offending rate	.15	.11	DPGB	.349	.289	.363	.297		
			Sex	-.147	-.135	-.181	-.151		
Alcohol use rate	.34	.40	DPGB	.321	.375	.341	.487		
			Belief	-.187	-.198	-.315	-.406		
			|Age − 20|	-.413	-.322	-.422	-.435		
Marijuana use rate	.27	.29	DPGB	.360	.419	.424	.497		
			Belief	-.256	-.202	-.321	-.342		
			Family involvement	-.186	-.069	-.181	-.177		
Polydrug use rate	.11	.07	DPGB	.245	.254	.285	.260		
			Belief	-.180	-.021	-.234	-.101		

TABLE 6.6. Variance explained with and without conventional-delinquent bonding interaction.

| | Explained variance (R^2) | | | | | | | | | |
| Independent variable | General delinquency | | Index offenses | | Alcohol use | | Marijuana use | | Polydrug use | |
	1977	1978	1977	1978	1977	1978	1977	1978	1977	1978
DPGB (delinquent peer group bonding)	.28	.29	.14	.14	.21	.27	.36	.31	.11	.11
Interaction (conventional bonding by DPGB)	.19	.20	.08	.08	.23	.32	.33	.33	.08	.11
Sex (general delinquency and index offending only)	.06	.05	.03	.03						
|Age − 20| (alcohol use only)					.15	.24				
Family involvement (marijuana use only)							.08	.08		
Belief (alcohol, marijuana, and polydrug use only)					.16	.27	.21	.24	.08	.08
DPGB plus sex	.31	.31	.16	.15						
DPGB plus sex plus interaction	.36	.35	.23	.19						
DPGB plus belief plus |age − 20|					.33	.47				
DPGB plus belief plus |age − 20| plus interaction					.34	.48				
DPGB plus belief plus family involvement							.42	.39		
DPGB plus belief plus family involvement plus interaction							.43	.41		
DPGB plus belief									.13	.14
DPGB plus belief plus interaction									.15	.16

each of the five problem behavior variables by each of the independent variables, considered separately. The second half of the table compares the variance explained by the original reduced regression analysis model with that explained by the same model plus the interaction of conventional and delinquent bonding.[3]

For alcohol and marijuana use, the addition of the interaction effect increases the explained variance by only 1% in both 1977 and 1978. For polydrug use, the increase is 2%. For general and Index offending, however, the increases are more substantial: 4% to 5% for general delinquency and 4% to 7% for Index offending. From Tables 6.5 and 6.6 we have fairly consistent evidence that the interaction between conventional bonding and DPGB contributes substantially to the explanation of Index offending. The results also suggest that the interaction effect is not a particularly important variable in the explanation of alcohol or marijuana use. Finally, from both Table 6.5 and 6.6, it appears that the interaction between conventional and delinquent bonding may add somewhat to the explanation of delinquency and polydrug use.

CONCLUSION

The model diagrammed in Figure 6.1 receives qualified support from this analysis. For delinquent behavior, but not for substance use, there is moderate to strong evidence for an interaction effect between conventional and delinquent bonding. The direct effect of delinquent peer group bonding is the strongest effect on each of the delinquent behavior and substance use dependent variables. As expected, the conventional bonding measures, particularly belief and school-related bonding, influence DPGB. Also as expected, strain, particularly school strain, affects bonding. Both bonding and strain, then, affect delinquency and substance use indirectly, and bonding affects substance use directly.

The demographic variables also play a part in the etiology of delinquent and ADM problem behaviors. Sex has a pervasive influence on bonding, especially in the school context, and a direct influence on delinquent behavior. Urban-rural residence also influences the belief structure, particularly in the context of the school. Cohort size, as measured by births in a given year, affects school strain (consistent with the Easterlin hypothesis) and belief, while parity (family size at birth) influences the family bonding measures. Parents' social status has an indirect influence on delinquency through school strain, a relationship consistent with the

---

[3] The explained variances for the reduced models in Table 6.6 are not identical to those in Table 6.1 because valid data were necessary only for those variables actually included in the models, rather than the full set of variables from which the equations in Table 6.1 were calculated. The R^2 data in Table 6.6 is therefore based on slightly more cases than in Table 6.1; the differences are small.

strain theories of Merton (1938) and Cohen (1955). Age affects alcohol use directly, and also affects bonding in the family context. Race affects school involvement, with nonwhites being more involved than whites; and mental health problems, with nonwhites having more problems than whites.

The results presented here do not support the conclusion that there is a common etiological structure underlying delinquent and ADM problem behaviors. Delinquency is influenced by DPGB, sex, and the interaction between conventional and delinquent bonding. Alcohol, marijuana, and polydrug use are influenced by DPGB, but this is the only independent variable substance use has in common with delinquency. In place of sex, we find belief as a direct influence on all three types of substance use, along with age (for alcohol) or family involvement (for marijuana use), and there is little support for the presence of a nonlinear interaction effect of conventional and delinquent bonding for alcohol or marijuana use. Mental health problems have only family involvement in common with marijuana use, and no variables in common with delinquency, alcohol use, or polydrug use, as direct influences. Mental health problems are influenced by (weak) bonding in the family context, by school strain, and by race. Although the independent variables are interrelated, the results do not support a common etiology. Instead, they suggest separate but related etiological paths, with no *direct* influences common to all three types of problems (delinquency, substance use, mental health), but some *indirect* influences (sex, school strain, belief in conventional norms) common to all.

7
Prediction of Delinquent and ADM Behavior from Other Delinquent and ADM Behavior

In previous chapters we examined the common correlates of delinquent and ADM behavior, and (in Chapter 3) the direct correlation between different types of delinquent and ADM behavior. In Chapter 6 in particular, we found that although delinquency, substance use, and mental health problems share no direct causal influence common to all three types of behavior, all three had some indirect influences in common. In the present chapter we turn to the prediction of the different types of delinquent and ADM behaviors directly from one another. We do not suggest here that one type of behavior *causes* another, as, for example, we suggested in Chapter 6 that delinquent peer group bonding (DPGB) causes or leads to delinquent behavior. Instead, we are simply asking to what extent our knowledge of one type of behavior better enables us to predict another.

Prediction of Ever-prevalence of Delinquent and ADM Behaviors from Ever-Prevalence of Other Delinquent and ADM Behaviors

Annual prevalence of delinquent behavior, substance use, or mental health problems refers to the percentage or proportion of individuals who have committed an offense, used a substance, or had a mental health problem in a particular year; or, at the individual level, to whether an individual has committed an offense, used a substance, or had a mental health problem in a particular year. It is in this sense that we have used prevalence throughout most of this book. *Ever-prevalence* refers to the percentage or proportion of individuals who have committed an offense, etc., or on the individual level, to whether an individual has committed an offense, etc., in any one or more of the years under study; for the National Youth Survey, this period would refer to the years 1976–1983.

Table 7.1 presents the correlations among ever-prevalence of minor

TABLE 7.1. Correlations[a] among ever-prevalence measures.

Problem behavior	Minor delinquency	Index offenses	Alcohol use	Marijuana use	Polydrug use	Mental health problems
Minor offenses	1.00/1.00	.32./33	.15/.17	.30/.31	.25/.22	.11/.08[b]
Index offenses		1.00/1.00	.16/.20	.33/.29	.35/.32	.21/.17
Alcohol use			1.00/1.00	.33/.38	.19/.23	.03[b]/.06[b]
Marijuana use				1.00/1.00	.50/.53	.12/.15
Polydrug use					1.00/1.00	.16/.14
Mental health problems						1.00/1.00

[a] For total NYS sample/those aged 11–12 in 1976.
[b] *Not* statistically significant with probability ≤ .050.

offenses, Index offenses, alcohol use, marijuana use, polydrug use, and mental health problems for the years 1976–1980 and 1983. The minor (non-Index) offense measure is used in place of general delinquency here, as in the temporal-development analysis of Chapter 5, to avoid the problem of overlap between general delinquency and Index offenses. The correlations in Table 7.1 are weak to moderate (.03–.53). In each cell, the first correlation refers to the total NYS sample, aged 11–17 in 1976. The second correlation refers to the subsample consisting of those aged 11–12 in 1976, those who enter adolescence at the beginning (1976) and exit adolescence, at ages 18–19, at the end (1983) of the time period in question. As is evident in Table 7.1, the differences in the correlations between the total NYS sample and the 11- or 12-year-old (in 1976) subsample are small.

In Table 7.2 the conditional probability of ever-prevalence on one offense or ADM behavior, given each other offense or ADM behavior, is presented. Table 7.2 gives a more detailed picture of the predictability of one behavior from another. Although the correlation between minor offenses and Index offenses is only a little over .3, table 7.2 indicates that knowing someone has never committed a minor delinquent act allows us to predict with greater confidence (95%–98% probability) that that person has also never committed an Index offense, despite the fact that nearly half of those in the total sample (or of those aged 11–12 in 1976) have done so. Conversely, knowing that someone has committed at least one Index offense allows us to predict with virtual certainty (99% probability) that the same person has also committed at least one minor offense as well. This result is not as impressive, because such a high percentage (88%–90%) of the sample have committed minor offenses. Alcohol use, marijuana use, polydrug use, and mental health problems are similarly but less strongly related to both minor offenses and Index offenses.

Knowledge that a respondent has used marijuana or other illegal drugs allows us to predict with virtual certainty that the individual also used

TABLE 7.2. Conditional probability[a] of ever-prevalence of one delinquent or ADM behavior given ever-prevalence of another delinquent or ADM behavior.

Problem behavior	Conditional probability of . . .					
	Minor offenses	Index offenses	Alcohol use	Marijuana use	Polydrug use	Mental health problems
Given . . .						
No minor offenses	—	.02/.05	.86/.78	.30/.19	.08/.07	.15/.19
Minor offenses	—	.53/.53	.97/.93	.95/.65	.45/.37	.29/.30
No index offenses	.79/.77	—	.92/.85	.54/.46	.24/.19	.19/.21
Index offenses	.99/.99	—	.99/.97	.85/.74	.59/.50	.37/.37
No alcohol use	.69/.70	.12/.16	—	.03/.02	.01/.00	.21/.21
Alcohol use	.91/.89	.48/.50	—	.73/.65	.43/.36	.28/.30
No marijuana use	.75/.75	.22/.28	.84/.77	—	.05/.04	.19/.21
Marijuana use	.95/.96	.57/.57	1.00[b]/1.00[c]	—	.58/.54	.31/.34
No polydrug use	.82/.81	.29/.33	.91/.85	.48/.39	—	.20/.23
Polydrug use	.98/.97	.65/.67	1.00[d]/1.00[e]	.96/.95	—	.35/.37
No mental health problems	.86/.85	.36/.38	.94/.89	.63/.53	.33/.28	—
Mental health problems	.94/.91	.60/.58	.96/.93	.76/.69	.51/.42	—
Total sample	.90/.88	.47/.47	.96/.91	.70/.59	.41/.33	.28/.29

[a] For total NYS sample/those aged 11–12 in 1976.
[b] 1,082 out of 1,084.
[c] 270 out of 271.
[d] 580 out of 581.
[e] 142 out of 142.

alcohol. More powerfully, if an individual has never used alcohol, there is a 97% to 98% probability that he or she has never used marijuana, despite the fact that well over half of those in the sample have done so, and a near-certainty (99%–100%) that he or she has never used harder drugs (cocaine, heroin, hallucinogens, amphetamines, barbiturates), despite the fact that one-third or more of the sample have done so. Prediction of polydrug use based on minor delinquency is also fairly good; of those who have never committed minor delinquency, fewer than 10% ever initiate polydrug use (again compared with 33%–41% of the total sample). Polydrug use predicts marijuana use with very high (95%–96%) probability, and never having used marijuana reduces the probability of polydrug use to 4% to 5%, compared with 33% to 41% of the total sample.

Mental health problems are neither strongly predictive of nor particularly well predicted by delinquency, alcohol use, marijuana use, or polydrug use. The correlations of mental health problems with alcohol use and, for those aged 11–12 in 1976, minor offenses, are not statistically significant. It is clear that the delinquency measures are fairly predictive of one another, that the drug use measures are fairly predictive of one another, and that delinquency and drug use are more closely related to one another than either is to mental health problems. These findings only further confirm results obtained in previous chapters.

Substance Use Immediately Prior to Index Offenses

In 1979 and 1983, a series of follow-up questions were asked about selected offenses. The follow-up questions in 1979 asked about the most recent offenses committed by the respondent, and in 1983 questions were asked about the three most recent offenses committed by the respondent, specific to each separate offense. Included among the follow-up questions were items asking whether the respondent had used alcohol, drugs, or both immediately prior to committing the offense. Table 7.3 presents the percentages of the total sample and each drug use type who used alcohol, drugs, or both, immediately prior to the most recent commission of each of five offenses in 1979 and immediately prior to the three most recent commissions of six offenses in 1983.[1] The offenses in Table 7.3 are those that comprise the Index Offenses subscale of the NYS. Although there appears to be more alcohol and drug use immediately prior to delinquent or criminal offenses for polydrug users than for alcohol or marijuana users, the differences are generally small.

Follow-up data on sexual assault are not available for 1979. For 1983, however, it is clear that the vast majority of sexual assaults involved the use of alcohol immediately prior to the offense, and none involved the use of drugs. It may be important to note in this context that, *from the perspective of the offenders* who reported having sexually assaulted someone, none of the sexual assault incidents for which follow-up data were obtained involved attacking the victim with a weapon, hitting, beating, or choking the victim. The most serious behavior admitted by the offenders was mild roughness or verbal threats. More often, nothing more than verbal persuasion was attempted, according to the respondent. Unfortunately, data on the same incidents as viewed from the victim's perspective are not available. Still, the overwhelming presence of alcohol

---

[1] A substantial proportion (typically 10% to 20%) of persons classified as alcohol user types reported use of drugs prior to committing offenses. This report is not necessarily inconsistent with the alcohol user classification, which was based upon reported use of substances in a later section of the interview. Recall that alcohol user types could have used marijuana or the set of other illicit drugs used in the classification up to three times during the year and still be classified as alcohol users. Further, the offense follow-up questions did not ask about the specific type of drug used and could logically have involved drugs not included in the drug typology. Still, it is possible that the respondents report drug use in this section of the interview that they did not report in the later drug use section. There is no way to obtain a complete reconciliation of the two separate reports of substance use.

TABLE 7.3. Percent of most recent offenses involving alcohol or drug use immediately prior to the commission of the offense.

Offense	Subsample	Substance use immediately prior to commission of most recent offense (percent): 1979			Substance use immediately prior to commission of three most recent offenses (percent): 1983		
		Alcohol only	Drugs only	Both	Alcohol only	Drugs only	Both
Sexual assault	Total	NA	NA	NA	82	0	0
	Alcohol users	NA	NA	NA	82	0	0
	Marijuana users	NA	NA	NA	79	0	0
	Polydrug users	NA	NA	NA	100	0	0
Aggravated assault (including gang fights)	Total	23	1	9	19	1	13
	Alcohol users	24	2	10	24	0	10
	Marijuana users	25	2	13	33	1	16
	Polydrug users	23	2	20	28	1	24
Robbery	Total	10	10	6	0	0	0
	Alcohol users	10	10	6	0	0	0
	Marijuana users	13	13	8	0	0	0
	Polydrug users	10	16	10	0	0	0
Burglary	Total	14	2	12	22	4	8
	Alcohol users	15	2	13	22	4	8
	Marijuana users	18	3	16	26	5	10
	Polydrug users	20	4	20	24	5	10
Larceny over $50	Total	16	7	5	10	2	16
	Alcohol users	16	7	5	10	2	16
	Marijuana users	15	8	5	11	2	18
	Polydrug users	12	8	8	10	2	19
Motor vehicle theft	Total	20	5	15	0	38	13
	Alcohol users	21	5	16	0	33	11
	Marijuana users	22	6	17	0	38	13
	Polydrug users	20	7	20	0	43	14

in connection with sexual assault suggests (a) that the sexual assaults occurred in connection with social settings or occasions in which alcohol was used, or (b) that alcohol was a contributing factor (as a cause or an excuse) in the sexual assault itself. Alcohol use was also fairly common in connection with aggravated assault or gang fighting. Use of drugs alone was rare in this context, only 1% to 2%.

The only offense for which drug use (alone) immediately preceded the offense in 10% or more of the incidents was robbery in 1979. Alcohol use (alone) occurred with about the same frequency, and in more than 5% of the incidents both alcohol and drugs were used. In 1983, however, the few robberies reported (five) involved neither alcohol nor drug use. The use of alcohol or drugs immediately prior to robbery, then, was very low in 1979 and nonexistent in 1983, after the respondents were 18–24 years old.

By contrast with robbery, the use of both alcohol and drugs immediately prior to burglary increases from 1979 to 1983. The pattern for burglary in 1983 is very similar to that for aggravated assault in 1979. For larceny, the pattern shifts from one of alcohol use alone in 16% of the incidents to alcohol plus drug use in 16% of the cases, with no change in the total percent of incidents (28%) that involve alcohol, drugs, or both. Motor vehicle theft goes from a crime in which alcohol use, alone or in combination with drugs, immediately precedes the offense, to one in which drug use, alone or in combination with alcohol, precedes the offense. In 1983, half of the auto thefts for which we have follow-up data involve drug use immediately prior to the offense.

For sexual assault and motor vehicle theft, both in 1983, more than half of all offenses for which we have follow-up data involve alcohol and/or drug use immediately prior to the commission of the offense. For sexual assault, alcohol alone precedes the offense. For motor vehicle theft, drug use, alone or in combination with alcohol, precedes the offense. One-fifth to one-third of the aggravated assaults, burglaries, and larcenies over $50 involve either alcohol or drug use immediately prior to the offense. For aggravated assaults and burglaries, alcohol is the principal substance used, but for larcenies the pattern is not as clear and appears to change over time.

None of these findings can be taken to imply that alcohol or drug use "caused" the offenses to which they were immediately prior. In particular, we do not know the extent to which alcohol and/or drugs were used immediately prior to other noncriminal activities (sexual intercourse with one's spouse, going to sleep, watching television, etc.), so we do not know whether the rate of alcohol or drug use prior to delinquent or criminal activity exceeded or was less than normal for the individuals involved. It might also be argued that the anticipation of committing a criminal act stimulated the use of alcohol or drugs. It is clear, however, that alcohol and drug use do not immediately precede most cases of robbery, burglary, larceny over $50, or aggravated assault, but they do precede about half of all auto thefts and the vast majority (80%) of all sexual assaults.

Prediction of Classification as Serious Delinquent, Polydrug User, and Mental Health Problem Types

In Chapter 1 we described three typologies, one each for delinquency, drug use, and mental health problems. In Table 7.4, we examine the extent to which knowledge of an individual's classification on any one of those three typologies allows us to predict whether that individual will subsequently be classified as a serious delinquent, a polydrug user, or as having mental health problems, according to the classification rules detailed in Chapter 1. Two sets of results are presented in Table 7.4. In each cell of the table, the first figure refers to the total NYS sample, aged 11–17 in 1976. The second figure refers to a subsample just entering adolescence in 1976, aged 11–12 in 1976. Both correlations (Pearson's r) and the probabilities of ever being classified as a serious delinquent, a polydrug user, or a person with mental health problems from 1977 to 1983 are presented.

TABLE 7.4. Conditional probability[a] of serious delinquent, polydrug user, and mental health problem type classification given prior (1976) delinquency type, drug use type, and mental health problem type.

		Subsequent classification, 1977–1983		
Typologies in 1976		Serious delinquent	Polydrug user	Mental health problem
Correlations	Delinquency Typology	.35/.31	.25/.17	.14/.11
	Drug Use Typology	.12/.07	.26/.06	.07/.03
	Mental Health Typology	.06/.07	.01/−.03	.33/.29
Transition probabilities	Delinquency typology			
	Nondelinquent	.05/.08	.16/.16	.14/.17
	Exploratory	.16/.10	.30/.18	.16/.14
	Nonserious	.22/.23	.39/.36	.24/.19
	Serious	.47/.49	.47/.34	.32/.37
	Drug use typology			
	Nonuser	.11/.12	.17/.19	.16/.18
	Alcohol	.14/.14	.29/.14	.19/.14
	Marijuana	.21/.00[b]	.59/1.00[b]	.20/.00[b]
	Polydrug	.28/.100[b]	.79/1.00[b]	.29/1.00[b]
	Mental health typology			
	Nonproblem	.12/.11	.24/.20	.12/.13
	Problem	.18/.18	.26/.16	.51/.46
	Total sample			
	Ever-prevalence	.13/.12	.24/.19	.17/.18

[a] For total NYS sample/those aged 11–12 in 1976.
[b] $N = 1$ for marijuana users and $N = 1$ for polydrug users at ages 11–12 in 1976.

The correlations at the top of Table 7.4 indicate that the 1976 types are only weak to moderate predictors of subsequent classification as a serious delinquent, polydrug user, or mental health problem type. Whether one becomes a serious delinquent in 1977–1983 is best predicted by the delinquency typology, followed by the drug use typology and, lastly, the mental health typology, but there is no difference in the predictive accuracy of the drug use and mental health typologies for the youngest cohorts, aged 11–12 in 1976. For the full NYS sample, subsequent classification as a polydrug user is best predicted by the drug use typology, followed by the delinquency typology and then the mental health problem typology. For the 11- to 12-year-olds in 1976, however, subsequent classification as a polydrug user is best predicted by the delinquency typology, followed by the drug use typology and, weakly and negatively, the mental health problem typology. Classification as having mental health problems is best predicted by the 1976 mental health problem typology, followed by the delinquency typology and, finally, the drug use typology.

As the transition probabilities indicate, individuals initially classified as nondelinquents have less than a 10% chance of becoming serious delinquents between 1977 and 1983. Those who are serious delinquents in 1976, by contrast, have almost a 50% chance of being serious delinquents in subsequent years, and there is a clear ordinal progression in the probability of being a serious delinquent from 1977 to 1983, from nondelinquents with the lowest probability to delinquents with the highest, based on the 1976 types. There is a similar but much weaker ordinal progression for the total sample by drug use type, from 11% for nonusers to 28% for users. Because there are so few 11- to 12-year-old marijuana and polydrug users, prediction of classification as a serious delinquent from marijuana user or polydrug user type in 1976, at those ages, is pointless. Individuals classified as having mental health problems in 1976 are slightly more likely than those not so classified to become serious delinquents in subsequent years.

Prediction of classification as a polydrug user from the delinquency typology is stronger than prediction of classification as a serious delinquent from the drug use typology, probably because (as we saw in Chapter 5) delinquency characteristically precedes drug use. Again, there is a clear ordinal progression in the transition probabilities for the total sample, with nondelinquents least likely and serious delinquents most likely to become polydrug users. For those aged 11–12 in 1976, however, nondelinquents and exploratory delinquents are almost equally likely (16%–18%) to become polydrug users, and nonserious and serious delinquents are almost equal to each other (34%–36%) and are twice as likely as nondelinquents and exploratory delinquents to become polydrug users.

A clear, moderately strong ordinal progression exists for the total sample across the drug use typology in the probability of subsequently being a polydrug user, from nonusers (17%) to polydrug users (79%). Once initiated, polydrug use tends to be fairly stable in prevalence. Among 11- to 12-year-olds, however, the 1976 drug use typology is practically useless in predicting future polydrug user classification, both because of the low number of marijuana and polydrug users at ages 11–12 and because the difference between nonusers and alcohol users is small (and, incidentally, in the opposite direction of what would have been expected). As a predictor of future polydrug use, the mental health problem typology is also practically useless, even weaker than the drug use typology for 11- to 12-year olds, for both the total sample and those aged 11–12 in 1976.

For the total NYS sample, both the delinquency typology and the drug use typology show an ordinal progression from nondelinquents (.14) and nonusers (.16) to serious delinquents (.32) and polydrug users (.29) in the probability of future classification as having mental health problems, but both relationships are weak. Among those aged 11–12 in 1976, the ordinal pattern fails to hold, inasmuch as nondelinquents and nonusers are slightly more likely than exploratory delinquents and alcohol users, respectively, to be subsequently classified as having mental health problems. For subsequent mental health problem classification, the crucial distinction among delinquency types appears to be that between serious delinquents and the other three types, with serious delinquents being twice as likely to become problem types on the mental health problem scale. Drug use type is again useless as a predictor for those aged 11–12 in 1976. Mental health problem type, however, is a moderately good predictor of subsequent mental health problem type. Those classified as not having mental health problems in 1976 have a 12% to 13% probability of becoming mental health problem types in 1977–1983, but those classified as having mental health problems in 1976 have a 46% to 51% chance of being subsequently classified as having mental health problems.

For the total NYS sample, then, classification in the most serious category (serious delinquent, polydrug user, mental health problem type) of each typology from 1977 to 1983 is best predicted by the 1976 classification on that same typology. For those aged 11–12 in 1976, the same holds true for delinquency and mental health problems, but because of the very low rates of marijuana and polydrug use among 11- to 12-year olds, the best predictor of polydrug use in 1977–1983 is the delinquency typology rather than the drug use typology. Correlations between typology in 1976 and classification as a serious delinquent, polydrug user, or mental health problem type from 1977 to 1983 are typically about .30 to .35 for the best predictor, except for polydrug use among those aged 11–17 in 1976, for which the correlation is only about half as large (.17), and for which the delinquency typology rather than the drug use typology is the best predictor.

Transitions Between Serious Delinquent and Polydrug User Types

Focusing exclusively on serious delinquency and polydrug use, the transition matrices in Table 7.5 show the annual probability of making the transition among four states: being neither a serious delinquent nor a polydrug user, being a serious delinquent but not a polydrug user, being a polydrug user but not a serious delinquent, and being both a serious delinquent and a polydrug user. Mental health problem type is excluded because the numbers would be too small. For the transition matrices involving those aged 11–12 in 1976, even the cross-classification by serious delinquency and polydrug use produces rows with no cases in 1976–1977 and 1977–1978. Transition matrices are presented for the total NYS sample, for those aged 11–12 in 1976 and for those aged 15–16 in 1976. The use of ages 11–12 and 15–16 in 1976 allows us to look at transitions throughout adolescence, from 11–12 to 12–13 in 1976, through ages 18–19 to 19–20 in 1980. Transitions are presented only for 1976–1977 to 1979–1980, because (as detailed in Chapter 5) we cannot compute annual transition matrices for 1980–1983.

For the general sample, in each period, most begin as neither polydrug users nor serious delinquents, and most people who begin as neither remain neither. Individuals who begin as serious delinquents (only) tend to become neither serious delinquents nor polydrug users, or secondarily, to remain serious delinquents. Transitions to polydrug user, instead of or in addition to serious delinquency, are relatively infrequent. Polydrug users tend primarily to remain polydrug users and, secondarily, to become neither polydrug users nor serious delinquents. Transitions from polydrug users (only) to both polydrug user and serious delinquent are a little more likely than the transition from serious delinquent (only) to both serious delinquent and polydrug user, but still relatively infrequent. Nobody goes directly from being a polydrug user (only) to being a serious delinquent (only). For 1976–1977, those who are both serious delinquents and polydrug users tend to drop both and to become neither serious delinquents nor polydrug users. Remaining both serious delinquents and polydrug users is next most likely, followed by the transition to polydrug user (only). For the other three transition periods, those who begin as both tend to remain both serious delinquents and polydrug users or, secondarily, to become polydrug users (only). Transitions from both serious delinquent and polydrug user to serious delinquent (only) or to neither serious delinquent nor polydrug user vary in probability from one pair of years to another.

For those aged 11–12 in 1976, all except one person were classified as being neither serious delinquents nor polydrug users or as being serious deliquents but not polydrug users. The one exception was classified as both a serious delinquent and a polydrug user, and that individual became

TABLE 7.5. Transitions between serious delinquent and polydrug user types.

	Neither	Serious delinquent	Polydrug user	Both	Neither	Serious delinquent	Polydrug user	Both	Neither	Serious delinquent	Polydrug user	Both
1976–1977												
Neither	.94	.03	.02	.00	.98	.03	.00	.00	.92	.04	.03	.01
Serious	.64	.26	.03	.08	.77	.23	.00	.00	.47	.37	.03	.13
Polydrug	.40	.00	.50	.10	NA[a]	NA	NA	NA	.29	.00	.50	.21
Both	.40	.10	.20	.30	.00	1.00[b]	.00	.00	.27	.09	.27	.36
1977–1978												
Neither	.94	.02	.03	.01	.96	.02	.02	.00	.92	.03	.04	.01
Serious	.56	.36	.04	.04	.33	.61	.06	.00	.72	.28	.00	.00
Polydrug	.38	.00	.56	.06	NA[a]	NA	NA	NA	.40	.00	.52	.08
Both	.14	.19	.33	.33	NA[a]	NA	NA	NA	.00	.23	.39	.39
1978–1979												
Neither	.92	.02	.05	.01	.95	.02	.02	.01	.90	.01	.09	.00
Serious	.54	.22	.03	.02	.40	.30	.00	.30	.71	.14	.10	.05
Polydrug	.25	.00	.63	.11	.00	.00	.63	.38	.31	.00	.59	.09
Both	.00	.00	.42	.58	.00	.00	1.00[c]	.00	.00	.00	.33	.67
1979–1980												
Neither	.94	.01	.05	.00	.94	.03	.03	.01	.94	.00	.05	.01
Serious	.47	.39	.08	.06	.62	.23	.08	.08	.43	.57	.00	.00
Polydrug	.29	.00	.67	.04	.53	.00	.33	.13	.24	.00	.72	.04
Both	.19	.10	.21	.50	.23	.15	.15	.46	.09	.00	.36	.55
Age in 1976:	11–17				11–12				15–16			

[a] No cases in this category at the beginning of the transition period; therefore transition from this category (row) is impossible.
[b] $n = 1$.
[c] $n = 2$.

a serious delinquent only, and not a polydrug user, in 1977. In 1977 (ages 12 and 13), there were only those classified as neither serious delinquents nor polydrug users, and those classified as serious delinquents but not polydrug users. Two (less than 0.5%) of those classified as neither serious delinquents nor polydrug users became classified as both serious delinquents and polydrug users in 1978, and both moved out of serious delinquency and became polydrug users (only) in 1979. Not until 1979 do we see more than ten cases in either or both of the last two categories in Table 7.5. For the two youngest cohorts until ages 14–15, there are too few polydrug users, with or without serious delinquency, to say anything about their patterns of transition. In all four pairs of years, those who are neither serious delinquents nor polydrug users tend to remain so. Transitions from neither serious delinquent nor polydrug user to both polydrug user and serious delinquent are very rare, and transitions to serious delinquent (only) or polydrug user (only) are not much more frequent. Of those individuals initially classified as serious delinquents (only) in all four transition periods, the most likely transition is to neither serious delinquent nor polydrug user, followed by remaining a serious delinquent. In three of the four pairs of years, those who began as serious delinquents (only) were found to be least likely to become polydrug users (only).

For those aged 15–16 in 1976, the most probable transition is again from being neither a serious delinquent nor a polydrug user to that same category in the next year. For each year except 1976, however, the next most likely transition for those who are neither serious delinquents nor polydrug users is becoming a polydrug user (only). Transitions from neither to both, serious delinquent and polydrug user, are rare in all four pairs of years. Of those who begin as serious delinquents (only), the most probable transition in the first three periods (and the second most probable in the last period) is to neither serious delinquent nor polydrug user, and the second most likely outcome (the most likely in 1979–1980) is to remain a serious delinquent (only). Of those who begin as polydrug users only, the majority remain in that category, and the next most likely transition is to become neither serious delinquents nor polydrug users. Nobody goes directly from being a polydrug user (only) to being a serious delinquent (only), but some few go from polydrug user (only) to both. For those who begin any period as both, the most likely outcome is to remain both serious delinquents and polydrug users, followed by a transition to polydrug user (only). There is no consistent pattern of transition from both serious delinquent and polydrug user either to serious delinquent (only) or to neither polydrug user nor serious delinquent.

In any given period, for any given age, most of those who begin as polydrug users (only), or as both polydrug users and serious delinquents, tend to remain polydrug users, and tend not to become or remain serious delinquents. There are a few exceptions to this generality: one individual who went from both to serious delinquent (only) at age 11 or 12 in 1976–1977; 46% of polydrug users (only), who either remained polydrug users (only) or became both polydrug users and serious delinquents in 1978–1979 for those aged 11–12 in 1976; and 67% of those who were both polydrug users and serious delinquents and remained so in 1978–1979 among those who were aged 15–16 in 1976. Overall, however, once one has become a polydrug user, one tends to persist in that category. Across time periods and ages, there is an erratic and usually weak tendency for polydrug users (only) to become serious delinquents in addition to, but never instead of, being polydrug users, and an erratic but stronger probability of becoming neither polydrug users nor serious delinquents. There also appears to be a tendency around ages 14–16 (probability = .23 for those aged 11–12 in 1976 and .27 for those aged 15–16 in 1976) for those who are both serious delinquents and polydrug users to become neither.

Becoming a serious delinquent is not as persistent a status as becoming a polydrug user. For most ages in most time periods, half or more of those who begin as serious delinquents (only) do not end the period as serious delinquents (with or without being polydrug users). Most of those who begin any period as both serious delinquents and polydrug users continue to be polydrug users (except in 1978–1979, for two individuals aged 11–12 in 1976) and, in most but not all periods for each of the age groups considered here, those who begin as both serious delinquents and polydrug users tend to remain serious delinquents as well. There are several exceptions to this latter generalization, most notably in 1976–1977 and 1979–1980 for those aged 15–16 in 1976. Although being a serious delinquent does not seem to enhance appreciably the likelihood of remaining a polydrug user for those who are both serious delinquents and polydrug users, being a polydrug user as well as a serious delinquent does appear to enhance the probability of remaining a serious delinquent. These results suggest that even though drug use may have little impact on the onset of serious delinquency (as evidenced by the temporal priority of Index offenses in Chapter 5), it may contribute to the maintenance or continuation of serious delinquency over time. Serious delinquency, by contrast, may play some role in the onset of polydrug use (or they may both result from a common or similar set of causal variables), but it appears to have little association with the maintenance of polydrug use.

Risk Models for Chronic Delinquency, Drug Use, and Mental Health Problems

Although previous sections have considered various interrelationships between delinquency and ADM problems, the question of whether delinquency, drug use, and mental health problems are additive or interactive in producing future delinquency or drug use has not been formally addressed. This question is concerned with whether certain levels (or types) of delinquency are related to later delinquency or drug use only in the presence of particular levels of drug and/or mental health problems, or whether the effects of these variables on later delinquent behavior or drug use are unrelated.

To examine whether the joint influence of delinquency, drug use, and emotional problems on future delinquency and drug use was additive or interactive, we used the annual delinquency, drug use, and mental health problem types for 1976. The cross-classification of these three typologies, together with measures of future delinquency or drug use were employed in a hierarchical loglinear analysis. As a measure of future delinquency, a future serious career offender status was developed. Classification as serious career offender required two or more consecutive years of involvement in serious delinquency—that is, being placed in the serious offender type for two or more consecutive years from 1977 through 1980. A future chronic drug use status was also developed with chronic drug users defined as persons classified as polydrug users for two or more consecutive years during the 1977–1980 period. Future chronic mental health problem status was likewise defined as having mental health problems for two or more consecutive years from 1977 through 1980. Of those in the sample, 5.6% were classified as chronic serious offenders, 8.6% as chronic polydrug users, and 4.9% as having chronic mental health problems.

In the loglinear analysis of future chronic delinquency,[2] we first discovered that all second- and higher-order interaction terms could be eliminated without significantly (probability ≤ .05) affecting the fit of the model. The first-order interaction between mental health problem type and future chronic delinquency also failed to reach statistical significance ($\chi^2 = 2.44$, df $= 1$, $p = .12$). The interactions between future chronic delinquency and both delinquency type and drug use type are statistically significant, indicating that a simple additive model of future chronic delinquency, with delinquency type and drug use type as predictors, is

---

[2] For discussions of loglinear and logit models, see Aldrich and Nelson (1984), Goodman (1970), Knoke and Burke (1980), and Lindeman, Merenda and Gold (1980). The natural logarithm of the odds ratio (β) is similar to but not the same as a regression coefficient (see Goodman, 1970; Knoke & Burke, 1980). Although some individual category effects in Table 7.1 are not statistically significant, only one variable, drug use type in the explanation of chronic mental health problems, has no statistically significant category effects. This variable is retained in the model on the hierarchical assumption that if a variable is included in a statistically significant interaction effect (in this case, mental health type by drug use type) the variable itself should be retained in the equation (see for example, Lindeman et al., 1980). The natural logarithm of the odds ratio for the polydrug categories is marginally significant ($p = .095$); that is, significant at the .10 level.

appropriate ($\chi^2 = 28.11$, df $= 37$, $p = .85$). Also included in this model are interactions between delinquency type (but not chronic delinquency) and both drug use type and mental health problem type, an indication that the three behavioral typologies are intercorrelated.

For chronic polydrug use, the third-order interaction among chronic polydrug use, delinquency type, drug use type, and mental health problem type could be eliminated without significantly affecting the fit of the model ($\chi^2 = 11.21$, df $= 9$, $p = .26$), as could the second-order interactions with chronic polydrug use, which involved delinquency type and drug use type ($\chi^2 = 11.31$, df $= 9$, $p = .26$) and delinquency type and mental health problem type ($\chi^2 = 7.285$, df $= 3$, $p = .06$), although this latter interaction appears to be marginally significant. We found it necessary, however, to retain the second-order interaction of chronic polydrug use with drug use type and mental health problem type ($\chi^2 = 8.73$, df $= 3$, $p = .03$), as well as the first-order interactions between chronic polydrug use and delinquency type, between delinquency type and drug use type, and between delinquency type and mental health problem type. These interactions, plus those implicit (from the hierarchical model) in the second-order interaction term (chronic polydrug use with drug use type, chronic polydrug use with mental health problem type, mental health problem type with drug use type) provide an adequate fit of the loglinear model ($\chi^2 = 39.19$, df $= 3$, $p = .12$). Except for the absence of any interaction between chronic mental health problems and delinquency type ($\chi^2 = 4.20$, df $= 3$, $p = .24$), the model for chronic mental health problems is similar to that for chronic polydrug use. As does the model for chronic polydrug use, the model for chronic mental health problems involves a second-order interaction among chronic mental health problems, mental health problem type, and drug use type (and implicitly in a hierarchical model, first order interactions of chronic mental health problems with mental health problem type, chronic mental health problems with drug use type, and drug use type with mental health problem type), and first order interactions of delinquency type with both mental health problem type and drug use type. This interactive model provides an adequate fit to the data ($\chi^2 = 36.58$, df $= 33$, $p = .31$).

The results of the hierarchical loglinear analysis were used to specify a multivariate logit model with polytomous independent variables. The results of the logit analysis are presented in Table 7.6. The chi-square statistics, degrees of freedom, and probabilities in parentheses in Table 7.6 are those for the hierarchical loglinear model; the parameters that are not in parentheses are for the logit model. Those effect coefficients that are statistically significant with probability $\leq .05$ are so indicated with an asterisk ($*$).

For chronic serious delinquency the simple additive model with delinquency type and drug use type as independent variables provides a good fit for the data ($\chi^2 = 5.54$, df $= 9$, $p = .78$). Being a serious delinquent or a polydrug user significantly increases the likelihood of subsequently

TABLE 7.6. Logit models of chronic serious delinquency, polydrug use, and mental health problems.[a]

Dependent variable	Likelihood ratio χ^2	Degrees of freedom	Probability	Independent variable	Category[b]	Odds ratio	β (ln of odds ratio)
Chronic serious delinquency	5.54 (28.11)	9 (37)	.785 (.854)	Delinquency type	Nondelinquent	.14	−1.950*
					Exploratory	1.19	.174
					Nonserious	.97	−.030
					Serious	6.09	1.806*
				Drug use type	Nonuser	.97	−.028
					Alcohol	.37	−.990*
					Marijuana	1.24	.212
					Polydrug	2.12	.750*
				Mean effect	(constant)		−2.556*
Chronic polydrug use	25.52 (31.90)	17 (27)	.166 (.236)	Drug use type	Nonuser	.27	−1.309*
					Alcohol	.43	−.848*
					Marijuana	2.44	.890*
					Polydrug	3.55	1.267*
				Mental health type	Nonproblem	1.30	.265*
					Problem	.77	−.265*
				Delinquency type	Nondelinquent	.28	−1.262*
					Exploratory	1.34	.294
					Nonserious	.85	−.161
					Serious	3.09	−1.129*
				Drug use type by mental health type	Nonuser by problem	1.98	.684*
					Alcohol by problem	.82	−.195
					Marijuana by problem	.94	−.062
					Polydrug by problem	.65	−.427

				Delinquency type by mental health type	Nondelinquent by problem	.53	−.628*
Chronic mental health problems	.000 (36.58)	0 (33)	1.000 (.306)		Exploratory by problem	1.28	.250
					Nonserious by problem	.79	−.236
					Serious by problem	1.85	.614*
				Mean effect	(constant)		−1.491*
				Mental health type	Nonuser	.40	−.928*
					Problem	2.53	.928*
				Drug use type	Nonuser	.98	−.021
					Alcohol	1.01	.014
					Marijuana	.56	−.578
					Polydrug	1.79	.585
				Mental health type by drug use type	Problem by nonuser	1.31	.268
					Problem by alcohol	2.29	.827*
					Problem by marijuana	.45	−.798*
					Problem by polydrug	.74	−.297
				Mean effect	(constant)		−2.214*

* Statistically significant ($p \leq .05$).

a Figures in parentheses are for the hierarchical loglinear model from which the logit model was identified.

b In models with interactive terms involving mental health type, the coefficients (β) for the effects of *nonproblem* type, by drug use type or delinquency type are equal to −1 times the coefficient for problem type by drug use or delinquency type; that is, β (nonproblem) $= -\beta$ (problem).

becoming a chronic serious delinquent. Being a nondelinquent or an alcohol user significantly decreases the likelihood of becoming a chronic serious delinquent. None of the other effects is statistically significant, with the exception of the mean effect or constant term. As the magnitude of the effect coefficients indicates, the effects of being a serious delinquent or a nondelinquent are approximately twice as strong as the effects of being an alcohol or polydrug user. It is interesting that being a nonuser has little impact on future chronic serious delinquency. It is possible that an age effect (with younger adolescents more likely to be nonusers) acts to suppress the relationship between being a nonuser and chronic serious delinquency. Alternatively, those who use alcohol (but not drugs, which are illegal for adults) may be more conforming (and thus less likely to engage in chronic delinquency) than those who abstain completely from substance use.

When the model indicated by the hierarchical loglinear analysis was specified for the logit model of chronic polydrug use, the fit to the data was barely adequate ($\chi^2 = 31.18$, df $= 20$, $p = .05$). Reintroduction of interaction between delinquency type and mental health problem type as an independent variable (which was marginally significant in the loglinear analysis as noted above) decreases the χ^2 by 8.66 (df $= 3$, $p < .05$) and provides an adequate fit for the data ($\chi^2 = 25.52$, df $= 17$, $p = .17$). The difference between the significance of the influence of the interaction between delinquency and mental health types for the loglinear and logit models may be explained by the inclusion in the loglinear model of other influences not directly related to chronic poly-drug use.

All of the drug use type categories significantly influence the likelihood of chronic polydrug use in a predictable way—nonuse and alcohol use negatively and marijuana and polydrug use positively. Polydrug users are most likely, and nonusers least likely, to become chronic polydrug users; marijuana users are more, and alcohol users less likely to become chronic polydrug users. However, the effects of being an alcohol or marijuana user are less than those of being a nondelinquent (which decreases the likelihood of becoming a chronic polydrug user nearly as much as does being a nouser) or being a serious delinquent (which increases the likelihood of chronic polydrug use almost as much as does being a polydrug user). Having mental health problems is weakly (but statistically significantly) and *negatively* associated with chronic polydrug use. In addition, for nonusers and for serious delinquents, it *increases* the risk of subsequent chronic polydrug use, but for nondelinquents, having mental health problems decreases the risk of subsequent chronic polydrug use. Overall, more serious delinquency and use of illegal (for adults) drugs increase the likelihood of chronic polydrug use, whereas nondelinquency and abstinence from illegal drugs decrease that likelihood. The relationship between mental health problem type and chronic polydrug use appears to be complex and somewhat inconsistent.

The hierarchical loglinear analysis specified a saturated model for chronic mental health problems, and by definition a saturated model fits the data perfectly. For chronic mental health problems, then, the adequacy of the model, which includes mental health type and drug use type but not delinquency type as predictors, may better be evaluated by the chi-square for the loglinear model (in parentheses in Table 7.6), which indicates an adequate fit to the data. As we might expect, having mental health problems in 1976 increases the risk of chronic mental health problems in 1977–1980. Although drug use type is included in the model, none of the effects of individual categories are statistically significant ($p <$ .05). The interactions between mental health type and drug use type are, however, related to subsequent chronic mental health problems. The combination of having mental health problems and being an alcohol user in 1976 increases the likelihood of chronic mental health problems in 1977–1980, but the influence of having mental health problems and being a marijuana user in 1976 reduces the likelihood of subsequent mental health problems.

In summary, both delinquency and drug use influence the likelihood of subsequent chronic delinquency. The most important influences are those of the extreme categories of the delinquency type. The influence of delinquency, drug use, and mental health problem types on chronic polydrug use is complex. The drug use types influence subsequent chronic polydrug use in a predictable way, and serious delinquency increases the likelihood of subsequent polydrug use. In interaction with drug use types, having mental health problems may increase (for non-users) the likelihood of chronic polydrug use. In interaction with delinquency type, it may increase (for serious delinquents) or decrease (for nondelinquents) the likelihood of chronic polydrug use. Bear in mind that the model for chronic polydrug use has the poorest fit to the data of the three models considered here. Finally, chronic mental health problems are more likely for those with prior mental health problems combined with alcohol use. The combination of mental health problems plus marijuana use significantly reduces the likelihood of subsequent chronic mental health problems. The combined results for chronic polydrug use and chronic mental health problems indicate an overall negative relationship between illegal drug use and mental health problems and, together with the path model in the previous section, they hint that illegal drug use and mental health problems may be alternative responses to similar problems of strain and weak bonding.

Conclusions

As expected, delinquency and drug use were positively correlated. Except for the correlation between two types of drug use (marijuana and polydrug use), however, the correlations were not particularly strong, and reflected only 1% to 12% shared variance. Examination of conditional probabilities, however, indicated that despite low correlations, it is possible to make some strong (90% or more accurate) predictive statements about one type of behavior based on knowledge of another. In particular,

1. If an individual never uses alcohol, that individual will almost never use marijuana (97%–98% accurate) or harder drugs (99%–100% accurate).
2. If an individual never uses marijuana, that individual will almost never use harder drugs (95%–96% accurate).
3. If an individual never commits minor delinquent acts, that individual will almost never commit Index offenses (95%–98%).
4. If an individual never commits a minor delinquent act, that individual will almost never use illegal drugs other than marijuana (92%–93% accurate).

As Table 7.3 indicates, *retrodiction* ("predicting" past events from future events) works even better than prediction. Practically *all* of those who have ever used marijuana or harder drugs have also used alcohol, and nearly all of those who have committed delinquent acts (93%–97% for minor delinquency, 97%–99% for Index offenses) have also used alcohol. The vast majority of those who have ever used marijuana or other illegal drugs, or who have committed Index offenses, have committed minor delinquent acts. These results, plus the temporal analysis of onset (connected with Table 7.4) suggest that

1. Alcohol use is a necessary cause or precursor of illegal drug use (marijuana and polydrug use).
2. Minor offending is a necessary cause or precursor of Index offending. This would be even more the case had we included status offenses in our measure of minor delinquency.
3. Minor offending is a necessary cause or precursor of marijuana and polydrug use. Although this is only 95% to 98% accurate, we would expect these percentages to increase if we included status offenses in our minor offenses measure.

From Tables 7.4 and Chapter 5, it seems clear that, insofar as delinquency and drug use are causally related, it is the onset of delinquency that leads to the onset of drug use, and not vice versa. Beyond the onset of minor delinquency and alcohol use (which, when both occur, involves the onset of minor delinquency *before* alcohol use), the more serious measures of delinquency and drug use appear to be related to one another, but not very strongly. Put another way, the relationships within delinquency and drug use measures are stronger than the relationships between the two types of measures.

In a study of prison inmates, the U.S. Department of Justice (1983) found that prison inmates drank prior to their offenses "no more than would be expected" on any particular day. For YNS respondents the mean frequency per person per year of alcohol use is 7.5 in 1976 (age 11–17), 44.5 in 1980 (ages 15–21), and 58 in 1983 (ages 18–24). Among polydrug users, the most frequent alcohol users, the mean frequencies are 46 in 1976, 123 in 1980, and 118 in 1983. At most, then, alcohol use occurs an average of once every 3 days. If we use this high figure of 33% as a benchmark, it appears that alcohol use immediately prior to the commission of criminal acts does not simply reflect typical alcohol use for those committing the offenses.

For rape in particular, alcohol use immediately prior to the offense is extremely high, two to five times what we would expect from polydrug users or the total sample respectively. Combining the "alcohol" and "both" (alcohol plus drugs) categories from Table 7.3, alcohol use is also higher than expected immediately prior to aggravated assault, lower than expected for robbery, and about as expected for burglary and larceny. For motor vehicle theft, alcohol use is higher than expected in 1979, but lower than expected in 1983, indicating a changing relationship with age.

The mean frequency of marijuana use per person per year is 7 (93 for polydrug users) in 1976, 31 (167 for polydrug users) in 1980, and 33 (128 for polydrug users) in 1983. As with alcohol, 33% provides a reasonable benchmark for comparison with Table 7.3. If polydrug use is added, the increase is small for the general population but may bring the high benchmark up from 33% to 50% for polydrug users. Consequently, it appears that drug use immediately prior to crime is low for rape, aggravated assault, robbery, burglary, and larceny. It is also low for motor vehicle theft in 1979, but high or typical for 1983.

Taken together, these results offer little support for the idea that drug use leads to crime, in either the long term (onset, Chapter 5) or the more immediate time frame (Table 7.3). Alcohol use, by contrast, does appear to be implicated in rape and aggravated assault, both of which are characterized by physical violence, but neither of which is characterized by a utilitarian profit motive. For crimes of profit, alcohol use occurs no more often than we would expect, based on frequency of use within the sample. This result raises the possibility that alcohol is causally related only to nonprofit crimes of violence. Finally, from Table 7.5, it appears that although delinquency is more likely to influence *onset* of drug use than drug use is to influence onset of delinquency, serious drug use (repeated polydrug use) is more likely to influence the *maintenance* of serious delinquency than serious delinquency is to influence the maintenance of polydrug use. Given the nature of the analysis, this conclusion is necessarily tentative.

The temporal order of onset and the developmental pattern of delinquency and drug use are quite clear. Minor delinquency comes first, followed by alcohol use, serious delinquency, and serious drug use. From Table 7.3, it appears that even for the short term, immediately prior to offending, there is increased use of alcohol but not of drugs immediately prior to serious offenses, particularly rape and aggravated assault. Up to this point at least, there is consistency in the temporal pattern. It is only when we begin to explore the maintenance of repeated Index offenses (serious delinquency) or polydrug use that we find some hint that the maintenance of delinquency and drug use may be subject to a reversal of the otherwise apparent temporal or causal flow. If drug use does influence delinquency, it may be by reducing the probability of "dropping out" of delinquent behavior rather than by increasing the probability of initiating delinquent behavior.

8
Summary and Implications

Our purpose in this final chapter is twofold. First, we review the empirical findings presented in the preceding chapters. Second, we discuss the theoretical, methodological, and policy implications of those findings.

We began in Chapter 1 by describing the National Youth Survey (NYS) and discussing the validity of self-report measures of delinquency and drug use. After detailing the construction of the measurement scales used in this book, including the distinction between prevalence rates and general offending rates, typologies for delinquent behavior, drug (including alcohol) use, and mental health problems were presented. As explained in Chapter 1, our coverage of different varieties of delinquent behavior is fairly comprehensive; however, our coverage of drug use is slightly less so, and our coverage of mental health problems is quite limited.

Empirical Findings

THE JOINT OCCURRENCE OF DELINQUENT BEHAVIOR AND ADM PROBLEMS

The general population prevalence rate for youth with multiple delinquent-ADM problems is very small. Only one-half of 1% of adolescents in 1976 exhibited serious levels of all three problems—that is, were serious delinquents, multiple illicit drug users and characterized as having mental health problems; less than 1% were both serious delinquents and polydrug users. Considered separately, the 1976 prevalence rates for serious delinquency and mental health problems were very similar (9%–12%) in the adolescent population, whereas polydrug users comprised only 3.4% of the population in 1976. Five years later, the prevalence rate for polydrug users were more than 12% and the rates for serious delinquents and youth with emotional problems had declined to approximately 5%. More than a third of the youth panel reported nonexperimental use of one or more illicit drugs in 1980, when the panel was aged 15–21. By 1983, serious delinquents constituted less than 3% of the sample, polydrug users had increased to more than 15%, and panel members with mental health problems remained about the same at 6%.

In 1976, when the sample was aged 11–17, 40% of all polydrug users were serious delinquents; however, a relatively small proportion of all serious delinquents were polydrug users (16%). By 1980 half of all serious offenders were also polydrug users, but now only 17% of polydrug users were also serious delinquents. This asymmetry in the relationship between delinquency and drug use is a direct result of the different dynamics of these problems in the general population, and makes it difficult to generalize about the concomitance of these two adolescent problems in either a criminal justice or drug treatment population. The assumption that most serious delinquents are also serious drug users or have problems related to drug use was correct for 1980 and 1983 when the sample's median age was 18 and 21, but it was not true in 1976 when the median age in the sample was 14.

During late adolescence and early adulthood (ages 15–21) there is evidence of a considerable concomitance of ADM problems among the relatively small group of very serious offenders. Nearly 50% were also polydrug users and 82% reported nonexperimental use of at least one illicit drug; 21% were classified as having mental health problems; 56% were experiencing negative social consequences associated with their use of alcohol; 37% were experiencing negative consequences from their illicit drug use; and 14% were classified as having both serious drug and mental health problems. A majority of serious delinquents during late adolescence and early adulthood have more than one problem. There do appear to be multiple problem youth, whether or not there is a multiple problem syndrome.

There is also evidence that the prevalence of multiple problem youth was increasing over time in the youth panel, and this trend also has significance for treatment and policy decisions. Although we did not look specifically at the relationship between joint delinquency–drug problems and the length of serious criminal or drug-using careers, the data are consistent with the hypothesis that multiple problem youth have longer careers, that they are less likely to "mature out" of deviant behavior patterns through normal developmental processes or are less responsive to treatment interventions, or both. There are of course, other possible explanations for our findings. For example, it is possible that those who initiate their careers at a later point in their life span are more likely to be multiple problem youth/young adults. However, this alternative hypothesis seems less likely (but not impossible) given the pattern of initiation rates by age for serious crimes, and it is contrary to the available evidence from crime and delinquency studies on the age of onset and career length (Blumstein et al., 1986).

Demographic Correlates of Delinquency and ADM Behavior

Our analysis of demographic correlates of delinquency and ADM behavior focused on five variables: age, sex, race, parental social class, and urban-rural residence. The data revealed a curvilinear relationship between age and delinquency, with delinquency peaking in mid-adolescence, consistent with past studies. There was a generally positive relationship between age and drug use, with some evidence of a leveling off or reversal in young adulthood, and no significant relationship between mental health problems and age.

Being male is positively associated with prevalence and, to a lesser extent, offending rates for delinquency, and with drug use rates. However, gender was related only weakly or not at all with prevalence for alcohol, marijuana, and polydrug use, including problem use. Being female, by contrast, is associated with having higher rates of depression and mental health service use. Blacks have higher prevalence rates for more serious offenses and mental health problems than whites, but whites have higher prevalence rates for less serious delinquency, alcohol use, marijuana use, polydrug use, and depression. Offending rates and drug use rates do not appear to differ by race; neither do rates of mental health service use.

Prevalence of more serious types of delinquency appears to be higher for the lower class than the middle class, but the relationship between social class and delinquency is otherwise inconsistent or insignificant. Prevalence of substance use is higher among the middle class than the lower class, but this finding reflects the experience of those who have moved beyond adolescence. Among those aged 11–17, there appears to be no difference in substance use by parental social class. For the mental health problem measures, the results are mixed: Depression appears to be unrelated to social class; mental health problems (emotional problems plus social isolation) are higher for the lower class; and mental health service use is higher for the middle class.

Urban residence is associated with higher prevalence and offending rates of delinquency in adolescence, but the relationship between urban residence and delinquency appears to be weaker (albeit in the same direction) at later ages. Alcohol use is not related to urban-rural residence, but marijuana and polydrug use are higher among urban residents than among rural residents. Urban-rural residence does not appear to be significantly related to mental health.

On the whole, as indicated in Chapter 2, demographic variables are weak to moderate predictors of individual-level rates of delinquency, drug use, and mental health. When we examine aggregate age- and period-specific averages for each of the cohorts, however (Chapter 4), age is consistently related to delinquency, drug use, and mental health, and the relationship is usually curvilinear, consistent with the hypothesis of maturational reform. Absolute cohort size (or, alternatively, average parity) is also related to delinquency and ADM problems, more to prevalence than to offending rates, use rates, or mental health problem scale scores. The higher levels of explained variance in the aggregate (cohort) rates is at least in part a result of aggregation, but may also reflect the greater range of ages in this analysis (11–24 years) compared to the single-year analyses in which the range is only 7 years. The age-period-cohort analysis of Chapter 4 opens an important avenue for future research—namely, the construction and testing of models designed to explain the age, period, and cohort effects in terms of variables that are theoretically related to delinquency and ADM problems.

The observation that the age curves for drug use and delinquency are different raises an important question. If both delinquency and drug use are caused by a common etiological configuration, why do these alternative responses to this set of causes follow a different course over the adolescent and early adult years? Although there is little evidence to date for a unique set of causes for one or the other, we cannot, of course, rule out this possibility. It is more likely, however, that factors associated with the maintenance of these behaviors differ. The data presented do suggest a differential maintenance hypothesis. Those forms of delinquent behavior which are characterized by an inverted U-shape age curve or a general declining curve during late adolescence are all offenses with strong sex differentials; that is, they are dominated by males. As the influence of peer groups (especially same-sex peer groups) declines in late adolescence and is replaced by relatively permanent and intimate heterosexual relationships, it is unlikely that the new partners in these relationships will support or tolerate these kinds of offenses. Social supports for these behaviors diminish as the influence of predominantly same-sex adolescent peer groups diminish. Simultaneously the risks and social costs associated with apprehension for these serious forms of crime are also increasing. In contrast, drug use is not strongly related to one's gender, and the possibility for social supports from one's wife or partner and other couples in friendship networks is much greater. Drugs continue to serve a sociability function, and both alcohol and marijuana are widely accepted as normative. The social supports and the low risk/cost associated with drug use serve to extend involvement in these forms of behavior into early adulthood. It is also possible that drug use is a more permanent adaptation and, once started, is more inherently self-rewarding, thereby resulting in varying degrees of physical and psychological dependency. In any case, we believe the explanation for the differences in the dynamics of delinquency and drug use involve differences over time in maintenance factors, in addition to some differences in original initiation factors.

Developmental Patterns

Allowing for problems of left-hand censoring, right-hand censoring, and the gap in the data from 1980 to 1983, it appears that initiation of delinquency, alcohol use, and marijuana use is higher in early adolescence, then tapers off as the sample ages. Initiation of polydrug use and mental health use, both of which are low-prevalence behaviors, shows no clear trend over time. Suspension of delinquency and alcohol use also decline over time, as does suspension of mental health problems, but suspension of polydrug use fluctuates and suspension of marijuana use increases from 1977 to 1983. Alcohol use, marijuana use, and general delinquency are relatively persistent behaviors, once initiated, with an average of more than 4 years of activity after initiation. Index offending, polydrug use, and mental health problems seem to be less persistent, but the reason may be that they are typically initiated later than alcohol use or general delinquency.

With the exception of alcohol use, a substantial proportion (25%–95%) of those who initiate delinquent or ADM problem behavior apparently terminate that behavior (or at least suspend it for some time) prior to the end of adolescence. For Index offenses and mental health problems, the termination rate among ever-active respondents is more than 75%, and for general delinquency and polydrug use it is close to one-half. The demographic correlates of termination are generally the same as those for prevalence of the same behavior.

For the delinquency, drug use, and mental health typologies, the most likely transitions from one year to another are those in which individuals in a given category will either remain in that category or move to an adjacent category. In the latter case, movement to an adjacent category, the more frequent pattern is to move toward less involvement in delinquency or ADM problems rather than more. In general these results suggest the existence of a developmental progression in which less serious involvement in delinquency and drug use is usually prerequisite to more serious involvement. In other words, changes in behavior appear to be gradual, rather than abrupt.

With regard to transitions *between* types of problem behavior, minor delinquency typically occurs first, followed by alcohol use. For those who ever commit Index offenses or have mental health problems, Index offenses and/or mental health problems occur next. When both occur, Index offenses precede mental health problems slightly more often (54%) than mental health problems precede Index offenses (46%). Illegal drug use (marijuana and polydrug use, in that order) typically occur last. With the exception of alcohol use, delinquent behavior tends to precede mental health problems, and both tend to precede illegal drug use in development over the life cycle.

It is our belief that any concern over the temporal sequence of these different problems in an effort to determine *causal* priority is to some extent misdirected. If they have a common etiology, either may precede the other with no causal implications. In addition, one may lead to initiation of a second, but the second may contribute to maintenance or continuation of the first. This conclusion does not negate the fact that there may be a set of typical developmental progressions, but there is no evidence of the inevitability of progressing from one state or stage to another. In fact, the NYS data indicate that the annual transition probabilities are always substantially greater for a regression to a less advanced state than for a progression to a more advanced state of delinquency. Even though it was not always the case for transitions between drug use types, the probability of progression to a more advanced type was always quite low. Further, with respect to temporal ordering, both drug use–delinquency sequences were observed. The NYS data again confirm what other longitudinal studies have found, that the most frequent sequence involves initiation into delinquent behavior followed by initiation into drug use. Nevertheless some youth become involved in both behaviors in the reverse order.

ETIOLOGY

The etiological analysis again confirms the findings from other prospective longitudinal studies that delinquency and drug use are related to a similar set of social psychological and demographic variables. There is a reasonable argument that these two problem forms are different manifestations of a common set of underlying causes. There was, however, some evidence that delinquency and drug use outcomes involved slightly different sets of predictors or different contributions from particular predictors included in the model. In particular, sex is a significant predictor of delinquency but not drug use, and belief is a significant predictor of all three types of drug use (alcohol, marijuana, and polydrug), but not of delinquency. Mental health problems appear to have a very different etiology from that of delinquency or drug use. Even though one behavior increases the probability of the other, the proximate influences are very different. Some indirect influences, however, appear common to all three types of behavior.

As expected, there was an interaction effect between delinquent peer group bonding (DPGB) and conventional bonding. Contrary to expectations, however, this interaction was not the principal etiological path to delinquent behavior, and its effect was negligible for all three types of substance use. (Because DPGB had no influence on mental health problems, the interaction between DPGB and conventional bonding was irrelevant for mental health problems.) The principal influence on both delinquent behavior and substance use is DPGB, and the strength of this relationship relative to other influences is usually modified only slightly by levels of conventional bonding.

PREDICTION ANALYSIS

Correlations among ever-prevalence measures of delinquency and ADM problems are all positive and almost all statistically significant. This indicates that involvement in one type of delinquency or ADM behavior is associated with an increased likelihood of involvement in another. Although we hesitate to infer causality from this pattern, it does appear that some behaviors are usually prerequisite to others: Minor offenses appear to be prerequisite to Index offenses, marijuana use, and polydrug use; and alcohol use appears to be prerequisite to marijuana use and polydrug use.

Although delinquent behavior typically precedes drug use, there is some evidence that drug use subsequently influences delinquent behavior. Alcohol use appears to be implicated in rape and aggravated assault, and drug use may be implicated in motor vehicle theft, based on frequency of use immediately prior to the commission of the offense. Furthermore, although onset of delinquency is more likely to precede onset of drug use than vice versa, serious (polydrug) drug use appears to have more of an influence on the *maintenance* of serius delinquency than serious delinquency has on the maintenance of serious drug use. Finally, in the logistic regression, drug use type is a significant predictor of subsequent chronic serious delinquency, above and beyond the predictive effect of delinquency type. Drug use type (but not delinquency type) is also predictive of chronic mental health problems, as well as chronic polydrug use. For chronic polydrug use, all three types of behavior are predictors. The predictive analysis lends further support to the finding from the etiological analysis that delinquency and mental health problems are less related to one another than either is to drug use.

Implications

METHODOLOGICAL IMPLICATIONS

Menard and Elliott (1988b) have noted that existence of a debate in the literature on crime and delinquency between proponents and critics of longitudinal research. Responding to this debate, they offer empirical evidence that (a) long-term retrospectively collected data do not produce the same results as prospectively collected data with a shorter recall period; (b) period data and cohort data (i.e., cross-sectional vs. longitudinal data) do not lead to the same conclusions about the relationship between age and delinquency; (c) pure cross-sectional and temporally ordered regression models of delinquency and drug use produce results that may be inconsistent with one another; and (d) longitudinal data such as that available from the NYS can be used to make strong tests between hypotheses based on competing theoretical perspectives. We will not go into detail regarding these findings in this book. We do, however, wish to point out the fact that the longitudinal design of the NYS was essential to the examination of trends in the joint occurrence of delinquent and ADM behaviors (Chapter 3); the changes in the demographic correlates of delinquent and ADM behaviors as the NYS sample aged (Chapter 2); the age-period-cohort analysis (Chapter 4); the analysis of temporal and developmental patterns, especially temporal priority and transition patterns (Chapter 5); the proper temporal and causal ordering of the regression model (Chapter 6); and the prediction of chronic serious delinquency, chronic polydrug use, and chronic mental health problems (Chapter 7). In every chapter the ability to make comparisons both across ages and over time has informed and strengthened (in some places by appropriately qualifying) our substantive conclusions.

We have used a fairly broad range of analytical methods, from the simplest comparisons of means and percentages to conditional probabilities and logit models. In several cases different methods were used to analyze the same or similar questions. Although the more sophisticated analytical techniques have helped refine some of the conclusions or assess the strength of relationships more precisely, the general conclusions have usually been little affected by the sophistication of the analysis. For an important exception, however, see the age-period-cohort analysis in Chapter 4. In Chapter 4, the multivariate analysis helped reveal patterns not evident in the bivariate relationships. Powerful methods may be no substitute for good data, but in conjunction with good data they do help us to develop a clearer idea of patterns not readily ascertainable by simpler methods.

Distinctions between prevalence and offending rates appear to be important. In the age-period-cohort analysis of Chapter 4 in particular, it is clear that the influences on prevalence are not necessarily the same as the influences on offending rates. This difference is further documented in Menard and Elliott (1988b). Also, the distinction between onset or initiation and maintenance or continuation of delinquent and ADM problem behavior appears to be a useful one. This distinction is particularly evident when we examine the temporal order of onset of delinquency prior to drug use (Chapters 5 and 7), and contrast it with the apparent effect of drug use on the maintenance of delinquency (Chapter 7).

THEORETICAL IMPLICATIONS

The findings in the present book allow us to draw some conclusions with regard to three theoretical issues. First, what are the respective roles of strain, control, and social learning theory in the explanation of delinquency, drug use, and mental health problems? Second, how well do the Maturational Reform and Easterlin hypotheses explain aggregate age- and period-specific rates of delinquency and ADM problem behavior? Third, what is the evidence in our data for or against the existence of a multiple problem behavior syndrome?

Elliott et al. (1985), using different measures of strain, a different (lagged endogenous) regression model, and no demographic variables, found a common etiological pattern for delinquency and illegal drug use. Actually, their lagged endogenous regression models indicate a common etiology for *change* in delinquency and illegal drug use, in which prior delinquency or drug use and involvement with delinquent peers explain current delinquency or drug use. In part because we do not use lagged endogenous (change) models, and in part because we include demographic as well as theoretical predictor variables, we find some differences in the etiology of delinquency, drug use, and mental health problems.

Despite the differences between the analysis here and in Elliott et al. (1985), however, learning theory (as represented by DPGB) still emerges as the most important direct influence on both delinquency and drug use. Belief, a control theory variable, is important for alcohol and illegal drug use, but not (directly) for delinquency. Both control theory (especially belief) and strain theory (especially school strain) variables have pervasive, indirect influences on delinquency and ADM problem behaviors. For mental health problems, school strain and the family control theory measures (family involvement, family normlessness) have direct effects. Finally, the theoretical variables do not fully explain the relationships between the demographic variables and the dependent variables. One's sex directly influences delinquency, age directly influences alcohol use, and race directly influences mental health problems in Table 6.3. All of the demographic variables have indirect influences on some or all of the dependent variables.

Both the Easterlin hypothesis and the Maturational Reform hypothesis receive considerable support from the analysis in Chapter 4, but their effects are not consistent for every one of the dependent variables. Evidence is *not* strong for the existence of a multiple problem behavior syndrome (Donovan & Jessor, 1985; Jessor & Jessor, 1977). Very few of our respondents were engaged in all three: delinquency, drug use, and mental health problems. Although the three are positively related, there appear to be at least three distinct etiological patterns: one for delinquency (DPGB plus respondent's sex), one for mental health problems (school strain, family involvement, family normlessness, and race), and one for drug use (DPGB, belief, and perhaps one other variable, depending on the particular substance being used). Mental health and delinquency are most distinct from one another, and in the logit model neither was predictive of the other. Although the three types of behavior are clearly correlated and seem to share some indirect influences, it would be a mistake to ignore the differences and construct a single, composite "problem behavior" variable from the three.

Policy Implications

The dynamics of delinquency, drug use, and mental health problems are quite different, and this fact has implications for policy and treatment. Given the different spacing of these problem behaviors over the lifespan, the probability of encountering multiple problem youth in justice, drug treatment, or mental health agency populations is clearly related to age. In early adolescence, youth are most likely to evidence delinquency or mental health problems, and the proportion with multiple problems is likely to be quite low. In most instances, the first contact with an official control or treatment agency will involve the juvenile justice system.

The situation is likely to be quite different during middle to late adolescence for a number of reasons. First, in the adolescent population the proportion of youth involved in serious delinquency who are multiple problem youth is increasing during this part of the lifespan. Second, there is evidence (Elliott and Huizinga, 1984) that delinquent youth with either substance use or mental health problems are at higher risk of arrest, i.e., they are more likely than other delinquent offenders to penetrate the justice system, given a similar level and seriousness of offending. Third, the likelihood of official court sanctions being applied to offenders is clearly related to age, with older offenders more likely to be incarcerated than younger offenders (other things being equal). As a result, the proportion of multiple problem youth among older offenders generally and particularly among those who are incarcerated is likely to be quite high and poses serious problems for our justice system and correctional institutions.

Given these expected high rates of multiple problem youth among older delinquents, it seems obvious that good screening and diagnostic capabilities must be developed and made available to the justice system. Further, given the evidence that drug use and mental health problems may serve to maintain serious delinquent behavior and extend the career into the adult years, any effective rehabilitation program must attend to these other problems.

From a number of perspectives, multiple illicit drug use may be the more serious problem for our society. This form of problem behavior involves a larger proportion of the adolescent population, it is more likely to extend into the adult years, and it appears to represent a more permanent adaptation than delinquent behavior, with higher rates of continuity once youth enter the more serious levels of involvement. It seems clear that involvement in multiple illicit drugs is indicative of a greater commitment to a deviant lifestyle than is either delinquent behavior or mental health problems.

At the same time, there is some evidence in the NYS data that it is *early onset* of illicit drug use that is associated with high risk for other forms of problem behavior. While the absolute numbers of polydrug users increased with age, the proportion with serious delinquency or mental health problems declined quite dramatically with age. It may be that the initiation of illicit drug use after 18 is not linked to either serious criminal behavior or mental health problems, at least in the short run. This does not preclude other negative consequences on adult functioning or even longer-range effects involving crime or mental health problems, but the documentation of these effects requires a longer follow-up than is presently available. In any case, the evidence presented here concerning the stability of polydrug use and its relationship to the continuity of other problem behaviors suggests that drug prevention and treatment must play a central role in our efforts to deal with multiple problem youth.

Many current treatment strategies focus upon building bonds to conventional persons and social institutions and devloping a commitment to conventional values. The findings reported here suggest that eliminating exposure to deviant others and access to deviant opportunity structures is at least as, and perhaps more, important for delinquency and substance abuse treatment. Weak bonds to the conventional social order, in and of themselves were not highly predictive of delinquency and were only weakly predictive of drug use. However, there was some evidence that conventional bonding was a protective factor, i.e., those at high risk of problem behavior by virtue of their involvement in deviant peer groups, were less likely to become involved in delinquency or drug use if they had strong conventional bonds. Still, one implication of these findings is that our treatment and prevention programs must give more attention to the role of the peer group in the onset and maintenance of delinquency and drug use.

In contrast to delinquency and drug use, the most appropriate context for intervention and treatment of the type of mental health problems investigated here is the family, not the peer group. Weak bonding (internal and external) to the family is the best predictor of mental health problems, as measured by the emotional problems/social isolation scale. In addition to strengthening bonds with the family, reduction of school strain (by providing more successful experiences in the school context and greater real and perceived access to higher education) appears to be a potentially successful intervention for reducing these particular forms of adolescent mental health problems. School strain also exerts an indirect influence on delinquency and drug use, so interventions involving the reduction of school strain may affect not only mental health problems, but also (less dramatically) delinquency and drug use.

Given the similarities in etiology and the concomitance of delinquency and ADM problems, a case can be made for the broadening of our intervention treatments to deal with multiple problem youth and redoubling our primary prevention efforts. A high priority should also be given to efforts to prevent the escalation of relatively nonserious forms of these behaviors into more serious forms. A large proportion of youth experiment with both delinquent behavior and drug use, yet relatively few escalate their involvement in these behaviors to serious and dysfunctional levels. Thus the chances of successfully intervening in this deviance developmental process appear to be good if the intervention is early.

With regard to primary prevention, any intervention that is successful in preventing the onset of minor or general delinquency is likely to have a profound preventive impact on serious delinquency and illegal drug use. Further down the developmental path, interventions that reduce polydrug use among serious, polydrug-using delinquents may facilitate the termination of serious delinquent behavior. Our conclusions in this regard are necessarily tentative, but deserve further consideration for program implementation. If we are correct, it may be possible to construct meaningful interventions for some of the most serious multiple problem youth.

Finally, these findings call for a reevaluation of the present structure of treatment and research organizations which tend to focus upon one of these problem behaviors to the exclusion of others. Given the concomitance of a wide range of problem behaviors and the evidence for at least some common factors in their etiology, there is a clear need for interdisciplinary approaches to the study of problem behavior. Further, the findings reported here suggest that there are a number of treatments or interventions which should impact at least two and in some cases all three types of problem behavior. Although the primary arena may vary somewhat by type of problem, interventions aimed at one problem have either a direct or an indirect effect on others. This raises the possibility of treating multiple problems within a single agency or program context, which has the advantage of better coordination of services and the potential for greater effectiveness in dealing with multiple problem cases.

IMPLICATIONS FOR FUTURE RESEARCH

The present study has fairly thoroughly examined the full range of delinquent and criminal behavior for individuals aged 11–24. A reasonably extensive set of subsance-specific drug use behaviors has also been considered. Our data are relatively weak, however, in the area of mental health problems, and a new study, in some ways parallel to the present study, and in which a broader range of mental health problems was considered, could add substantially to our understanding of the epidemiology and social etiology of mental health problems. In particular, such a study could examine more carefully the distribution of different types of mental health problems across sex, race, age, social class, and place of residence; the development of mental health problems over the life cycle, particularly in the adolescent years; and the social correlates of mental health problems, with special attention (suggested in the etiological analysis in Chapter 6) to strain, family normlessness, and family involvement.

Also useful would be an extension of the present analysis of the joint occurrence of delinquent (or criminal) behavior and ADM problems as the NYS sample ages, and an analysis of trends with age in the demographic correlates of delinquent (or criminal) and ADM behavior. With the seventh wave of data collection soon to be available, for respondents aged 21–27, we shall begin this analysis. As a supplement to this longitudinal research effort, a series of self-report studies conducted at regular intervals with nationally representative samples, at least of adolescents but preferably of the population in general, would be useful for monitoring temporal trends in crime, delinquency, and ADM problems. Such a project has already been undertaken for high school seniors with respect to drug use, but the focus of this work needs to be expanded substantially.

Further exploration of the age, period, and cohort size effects documented in Chapter 4 is clearly warranted. First, as data become available for our respondents at later ages, we need to ascertain whether the shift in alcohol and drug use around age 20 represents a leveling off or a reversal of the positive age trend that persisted in adolescence. Second, it would be useful to introduce theoretically relevant explanatory variables into the aggregate analysis to see whether they eliminate (and explain) the direct effects of age, period, and cohort size on delinquency and ADM problem behavior.

Now that we have life cycle data on the temporal order of delinquency, drug use, mental health problems, and variables that theoretically influence those behaviors, the time has come to develop a clearer picture of developmental sequences regarding onset of delinquency and ADM behaviors relative to the onset of DPGB, normlessness, and strain, and the weakening of conventional beliefs and involvement in conventional institutions. In addition to their role in the onset of problem behavior, we need also to examine more carefully the role of theoretically relevant variables in the maintenance and termination of delinquent and ADM problem behaviors. From Chapters 5 and 7, it appears that causal influences, if they exist, may operate in two directions, but may do so at distinctly different times in the developmental sequence or life cycle.

The etiological analysis of Chapter 6 needs to be expanded in order to search more thoroughly for the presence of interactive effects and possible threshold effects. We need to reassess our present approach to causal analysis, to consider adding (not substituting) a search for necessary prerequisites to delinquency and ADM problems, and context-specific sufficient causes of delinquency and ADM problems. Such an analysis would be aided substantially by a better knowledge of life cycle developmental patterns, such as those discussed above, to ascertain more effectively the direction of causal influences at particular ages or particular stages in the developmental cycle.

Clearly, there are other possible avenues for future research. The list presented here is clearly not exhaustive, but it does suggest some areas for further exploration that follow directly from the analysis presented in the preceding chapters. As is so often the case, in answering a few questions we have raised more new ones than we have answered.

References

Abrahamson, M. (1980) *Urban sociology* (2nd ed.). Englewood Cliffs, NJ: Prentice-Hall.

Agresti, A., & Finlay, B. (1986). *Statistical methods for the social sciences* (2nd ed.). San Francisco: Dellen.

Ahlburg, D.A., & Schapiro, M.O. (1984). Socioeconomic ramifications of changing cohort size: An analysis of U.S. postwar suicide rates by age and sex. *Demography, 21,* 97–108.

Akers, R.L. (1964). Socio-economic status and delinquent behavior: A retest. *Journal of Research in Crime and Delinquency, 1,* 28–46.

Akers, R.L., Massey, J., Clarke, W., & Laver, R. (1983). Are self-reports of adolescent deviance valid? Biochemical measures, randomized responses, and the bogus pipeline in smoking behavior. *Social Forces, 672,* 234–251.

Aldrich, J.H., & Nelson, F.D. (1984). *Linear probability, logit, and probit models.* Beverly Hills, CA: Sage.

Allen, D.E., & Sandhu, H.S. (1967). A comparative study of delinquents and non-delinquents: Family affect, religion, and personal income. *Social Forces, 46,* 263–268.

American Psychiatric Association. (1980). *Diagnostic and statistical manual of mental disorders* (3rd ed.). Washington, DC: Author.

Ansel, S., Mandell, W., Matthias, W., Mason, C., & Hocherman, I. (1976). Reliability and validity of self-reported illegal activities and drug use collected from narcotic addicts. *The International Journal of the Addictions, 11,* 325–336.

Arnold, W. 1965. Continuities in research: Scaling delinquent behavior. *Social Problems, 13,* 59–65.

Bachman, J.G. (1987). Changes in deviant behavior during late adolescence and early adulthood. Paper presented at the Meetings of the International Society for the Study of Behavioral Development. July 12–16, Tokyo, Japan.

Bachman, J.G., O'Malley, P., & Johnston, J. (1978). *Youth in transition (Vol. 6). Adolescence to adulthood: Change and stability in the lives of young men.* Ann Arbor: University of Michigan, Institute for Social Research.

Bale, R.N. (1979). The validity and reliability of self-reported data from heroin addicts: Mailed questionnaires compared with face-to-face interviews. *The International Journal of the Addictions, 1467,* 993–1000.

Ball, J.C. (1967). The reliability and validity of interview data obtained from 59 narcotic drug addicts. *American Journal of Sociology, 72,* 650–654.

Basquin, M., & Trystram, D. (1966). Exhibitionism in the adolescent. *Annales Medico-Psychologiques, 2*(4).

Becker, H.S. (1963). *Outsiders: Studies in the sociology of deviance.* New York: Free Press.

Bentler, P.M., & Eichberg, R.H. (1975). A social psychological approach to substance abuse construct validity: Prediction of adolescent drug use from independent data sources. In D.J. LeHieri (Ed.), *Predicting adolescent drug abuse: A review of issues, methods and correlates* (pp. 129–146). Washington, DC: U.S. Government Printing Office.

Biderman, A.D. (1972). Notes on prevalence and incidence, Unpublished monograph. Bureau of Social Science Research, Washington, D.C.

Biles, D. (1971). Birth order and delinquency. *Australian Psychologist, 6,* 189–193.

Blackmore, J. (1974). The relationship between self-reported delinquency and official convictions amongst adolescent boys. *British Journal of Criminology, 14,* 172–176.

Blumstein, A., Cohen, J., Roth, J.A., & Visher C.A. (Eds.). (1986). *Criminal careers and "career criminals"* (Vol. 1). Washington, DC: National Academy Press.

Bohrnstedt, G.W., & Knoke, D. (1982). *Statistics for social data analysis.* Itasca, IL: F.E. Peacock.

Bonito, A.J., Nurco, D.N., & Shaffer, J.W. (1976). The veridicality of addicts' self-reports in social research. *The International Journal of Addictions, 11,* 719–724.

Brennan, T., & Auslander, N. (1979). *Adolescent loneliness: An exploratory study of social and psychological predispositions and theory.* Boulder, CO: Behavioral Research Institute.

Brennan, T., Elliott, D.S., & Knowles, B.A. (1981). *Patterns of multiple drug use* (National Youth Survey Report No. 15). Boulder, CO: Behavioral Research Institute. Boulder, Colorado.

Briar, S., & Piliavin, I. (1965). Delinquency, situational inducements and commitment to conformity. *Social problems, 13,* 35–45.

Cahalan, D. (1970). *Problem Drinkers,* San Francisco: Jossey-Bass.

Chaiken, J., and Chaiken, M. (1982). *Varieties of criminal behavior.* Santa Monica, CA: The Rand Corporation.

Chambliss, W.J., & Nagasawa, R.H. (1969). "On the validity of official statistics: A comparative study of white, black, and Japanese high school boys." *Journal of Research in Crime and Delinquency, 6,* 71–77.

Chilton, R., & Spielberger, A. (197). Is delinquency increasing? Age structure and the crime rate. *Social Forces, 49,* 487–493.

Cicourel, A.V. (1968). *The social organization of juvenile justice.* New York: Wiley.

Clark, J.P., & E.W. Haurek. 1966. "Age and Sex Roles of Adolescents and Their Involvement in Misconduct: A Reappraisal." *Sociology and Social Research* 50:495–508.

Clark, J.P., & Tifft, L.L. (1966). Polygraph and interview validation of self-reported delinquent behavior. *American Sociological Review, 31,* 516–523.

Clark, J.P., & Wenninger, E.P. (1962). Socioeconomic class and area as correlates of illegal behavior among juveniles. *American Sociological Review, 27,* 826–834.

Clinard, M.B., & Meier, R.F. (1979). *Sociology of deviant behavior* (5th ed.). New York: Holt, Rinehart, and Winston.

Cloward, R.A., & Ohlin, L.E. (1960). *Delinquency and opportunity.* New York: Free Press.

Cohen, A.K. (1955). *Delinquent boys: The culture of the gang.* New York: Free Press.

Coleman, J.S., Campbell, E.Q., Hobson, C.J., McPartland, J., Mood, A.M., Weinfeld, F.D. & York, R.L. (1966). *Equality of educational opportunity.* Washington, DC: U.S. Government Printing Office.

Collins, J.J. (1981). *Alcohol use and criminal behavior: An executive summary.* Washington, DC: National Institute of Justice.

Conklin, J.E. (1986). *Criminology* (2nd ed.). New York: Macmillan.

Cox, T.J., & Longwell, B. (1974). Reliability of interview data concerning current heroin use from heroin addicts on methadone. *The International Journal of the Addictions, 9,* 161–165.

Dentler, R.A., & Monroe, L.J. (1961). Social correlates of early adolescent theft. *American Sociological Review, 26,* 733–743.

Dohrenwend, B.P. & Dohrenwend, B.S. (1969). *Social status and psychological disorder: A causal inquiry.* New York: Wiley.

Dohrenwend, B.P. (1975). Sociocultural and social psychological factors in the Genesis of Mental Disorders. *Journal of Health and Social Behavior, 16,* 365–392.

Dohrenwend, B.P., & Dohrenwend, B.S. (1976). Sex differences and psychiatric disorders. *American Journal of Sociology, 81,* 1447–1454.

Donovan, J.E., & Jessor, R. (1985). Structure of problem behavior in adolescence and young adulthood. *Journal of Consulting and Clinical Psychology, 53,* 890–904.

Dunford, F.W., & Elliott, D.S. (1984). Identifying career offenders using self-reported data. *Journal of Research in Crime and Delinquency, 21,* 57–86.

Durkheim, E. (1951). *Suicide.* New York: Free Press.

Easterlin, R.A. (1987). *Birth and fortune* (2nd ed.). Chicago: University of Chicago Press.

Eckerman, W.C., Bates, J.D., Rachal, J.V., & Poole, W.K. (1971). *Drug usage and arrest charges: A study of drug usage and arrest charges among arrestees in six metropolitan areas of the United States.* Bureau of Narcotics and Dangerous Drugs, U.S. Department of Justice. Washington, DC: U.S. Government Printing Office.

Elliott, D.S. (1982). Review essay: *Measuring Delinquency* by M.J. Hindelang, T. Hirschi, and J.G. Weiss, *Criminology, 20,* 527–537.

Elliott, D.S. (1985). The assumption that theories can be combined with increased explanatory power: Theoretical integrations. Pp. 123–150 in R.F. Meier (ed.), *Theoretical Methods in Criminology.* Beverly Hills, CA: Sage.

Elliott, D.S., & Ageton, S.S. (1980). Reconciling race and class differences in self-reported and official estimates of delinquency. *American Sociological Review, 40,* 95–110.

Elliott, D.S., Ageton, S.S., Huizinga, D.H., Knowles, B.A., & Canter, R.J.

(1983). *The prevalence and incidence of delinquent behavior: 1976–1980* (National Youth Survey Report No. 26). Boulder, CO: Behavioral Research Institute.

Elliott, D.S., & Huizinga, D. (1983). Social class and delinquent behavior in a national youth panel: 1976–1980. *Criminology, 21,* 149–177.

Elliott, D.S., & Huizinga, D. (1984). The Relationship Between Delinquent Behavior and ADM Problems. Paper presented at the ADAMHA/OJJDP State-of-the-Art Research Conference on Juvenile Offenders with Serious Drug Alcohol and Mental Health Problems. April 17–18, Rockville, Maryland.

Elliott, D.S., & Huizinga, D. (1988). Improving self-reported measures of delinquency. Paper presented at the NATO Workshop on Self-Reported Measures of Delinquency, Congress Center, The Netherlands, June 26–30.

Elliott, D.S., Huizinga, D., & Ageton, S.S. (1985). *Explaining delinquency and drug use.* Beverly Hills, CA: Sage.

Elliott, D.S., & Voss, H. (1974). *Delinquency and dropout.* Lexington, MA: D. C. Heath.

Ennis, P.H. (1967). Crime, victims, and the police. *Trans-Action, 4,* 36–44.

Epps, E.G. (1967). Socioeconomic status, race, level of aspiration and juvenile delinquency. *Phylon, 28,* 16–27.

Erickson, M.L. & Empey, L.T. (1963). Court records, undetected delinquency and decision making. *Journal of Criminal Law, Criminology, and Police Science, 54,* 456–469.

Erickson, M.L., & Empey, L.T. (1965). Class position, peers, and delinquency. *Sociology and Social Research, 49,* 268–282.

Farris, R.E.L., & Dunham, H.W. (1965). *Mental disorders in urban areas.* Chicago: University of Chicago Press.

Farrington, D.P. (1973). Self-reports of deviant behavior: Predictive and stable? *Journal of Criminal Law and Crimonology, 64,* 99–110.

Farrington, D.P. (1986). Age and crime. In M. Tonry & N. Morris (Eds.), *Crime and justice: An annual review of research* (Vol. 7, pp. 189–250). Chicago: University of Chicago Press.

Feighner, J.P., Robins, E., Guze, S.B., Woodruff, R.A., Winokur, G., & Munoz, R. (1972). Diagnostic criteria for use in psychiatric research. *Archives of General Psychiatry, 26,* 57–63.

Flanagan, T.J., & McGarrell, E.F. (1986). *Sourcebook of criminal justice statistics-1985.* Washington D.C.: U.S. Government Printing Office.

Gandossy, R.P., Williams, J.R., Cohen, J. & Harwood, H.J. (1980). *Drugs and crime.* Washington, DC: U.S. Government Printing Office.

Garofalo, J., & Hindelang, M.J. (1977). *An introduction to the National Crime Survey* (U.S. Department of Justice Analytic Report SD-VAD-4). Washington, DC: U.S. Government Printing Office.

Gibbons, D.C. (1987). *Society, crime, and criminal behavior* (5th ed.). Englewood Cliffs, NJ: Prentice-Hall.

Gibbons, D.C., & Krohn, M.D. (1986). *Delinquent behavior* (4th ed.). Englewood Cliffs, NJ: Prentice Hall.

Gibbs, J. (1966). Conceptions of deviant behavior: The old and the new. *Pacific Sociological Review, 9,* 9–14.

Gibbs, J. (1972). Issues in defining deviant behavior. In R. Scott & J. Douglas (Eds.), *Theoretical perspectives on deviance.* New York: Basic Books.

Gibson, H.B., Morrison, S., & West, D.J. (1970). The confession of known offenses in response to a self-reported delinquency schedule. *British Journal of Crimonology, 10,* 277–280.

Glenn, N. (1976). Cohort analysts' futile quest: Statistical attempts to separate age, period, and cohort effects. *American Sociological Review, 41,* 900–904.

Glenn, N. (1977). *Cohort analysis.* Beverly Hills: Sage.

Glenn, N. (1981). Age, birth cohorts, and drinking: An illustration of the hazards of inferring effects from cohort data. *Journal of Gerontology, 36,* 362–369.

Gold, M. (1966). Undetected delinquent behavior. *Journal of Research in Crime and Delinquency, 3,* 27–46.

Gold, M. (1970). *Delinquent behavior in an American city.* Belmont, CA: Brooks Cole.

Gold, M. (1977). *The validity of self-reports of delinquent behavior.* Unpublished manuscript, Institute for Social Research.

Gold, M., & Reimer, D.J. (1975). Changing patterns of delinquent behavior among Americans 13 to 16 years old: 1967–1972. *Crime and Delinquency Literature, 7,* 483–517.

Goodman, L.A. (1970). The multivariate analysis of qualitative data: interactions among multiple classifications. *Journal of the American Statistical Association, 65,* 226–256.

Gould, L.C. (1968). Who defines delinquency? A comparison of self-reported and officially reported indices of delinquency for three racial groups. *Social Problems, 16,* 325–336.

Graetz, B. (1987). Cohort changes in educational inequality. *Social Science Research, 16,* 329–344.

Graham, M.G. (1987). Controlling drug abuse and crime: A research update. *NIJ Reports,* March/April. Washington, DC: National Institute of Justice.

Greenberg, D.F. (1977). Delinquency and the age structure of society. *Contemporary Crises, 1,* 189–224.

Greenberg, D.F., & Larkin, N.J. (1985). Age-cohort analysis of arrest rates. *Journal of Quantitative Crimonology, 1,* 227–240.

Gropper, B.A. (1985). *Probing the links between drugs and crime.* Washington, DC: National Institute of Justice.

Groves, E.W. (1974). Patterns of college student use and lifestyles. In E. Josephson & E.E. Carrol (Eds). *Drug use: Epidemiology and sociological approaches.* New York: Wiley.

Hackler, J.C., & Lautt, M. (1969). Systematic bias in measuring self-reported delinquency. *Canadian Review of Sciology and Anthropology, 6,* 92–106.

Hammersley, R., & Morrison, V. (1987). Effects of polydrug use on the criminal activities of heroin users. *British Journal of Addiction, 82,* 899–906.

Hardt, R.H., & Peterson-Hardt, S. (1977). On determining the quality of the delinquency self-report method. *Journal of Research in Crime and Delinquency, 14,* 247–261.

Harter, C.L. (1977). The 'good times' cohort of the 1930s. *PRB Report, 3,* 1–4.

Haskell, M., & Yablonsky, L. (1974). *Criminology: Crime and criminality.* Chicago: Rand McNally.

Helzer, J.E., Robins, L.N., Croughan, J.L., & Welner, A. (1981). Renard Diagnostic Interview. *Archives of General Psychiatry, 38,* 393–398.

Hesselbrock, V., Stabenau, J., Hesselbrock, M., Mirkin, P., & Mey, R. (1982). A comparison of two interview schedules. *Archives of General Psychiatry, 39,* 674–677.

Hindelang, M.J. (1978). Race and involvement in common law crimes. *American Sociological Review, 43,* 93–109.

Hindelang, M.J., Hirschi, T., & Weis, J. (1979). Correlates of delinquency: The illusion of discrepancy between self-report and official measures. *American Sociological Review, 44,* 995–1014.

Hindelang, M.J., Hirschi, T., & Weis, J. (1981). *Measuring delinquency.* Beverly Hills: Sage.

Hirschi, T. (1969). *Causes of delinquency.* Berkeley: University of California Press.

Hirschi, T., & Gottfredson, M. (1983). Age and explanation of crime. *American Journal of Sociology, 89,* 552–584.

Hobcroft, J., Menken, J., & Preston, S. (1982). Age, period, and cohort effects in demography: A review. *Population Index, 48,* 4–43.

Hollingshead, A.B., & Redlich, F.C. (1958). *Social class and mental illness.* New York: Wiley, p. 47.

Holzner, A.S., & Ding, L.K. (1973). White Dragon Pearls in Hong Kong: A study of young women drug addicts. *The International Journal of the Addictions, 8*(2).

Hood, R., & Sparks, R. (1970). *Key issues in criminology.* New York: McGraw-Hill.

Horton, P.D. (1973). The mystical experience as a suicide preventive. *American Journal of Psychiatry, 130*(3).

Huba, G.J., & Bentler, P.M. (1984). Causal models of personality, peer culture characteristics drug use and criminal behaviors over a five-year span. Pp. 73–94 in D.W. Goodwin, K.T. VanDuser, and S. A. Mednick (eds) *Longitudinal Research in Alcoholism.* Boston: Kluwer-Nijhof.

Huizinga, D.H., & Eliott, D.S. (1981). *A longitudinal study of delinquency and drug use in a national sample of youth: An assessment of causal order* (National Youth Survey Report No. 16). Boulder, CO: Behavioral Research Institute.

Huizinga, D.H., & Elliott, D.S. (1986). Reassessing the reliability and validity of self-report delinquency measures. *Journal of Quantitative Criminology, 2,* 293–327.

Inciardi, J.A. (Ed.). (1981). *The drugs-crime connection.* Beverly Hills: Sage.

Jensen, G.F., & Rojek, D. (1980). *Delinquency.* Lexington, MA: D.C. Heath.

Jessor, R. (1979). Marihuana: A review of recent psychological research. In R.L. Dupont, A. Goldstein, and J. O'Donnell (Eds.), *Handbook on Drug Abuse* (pp. 337–355). Washington, DC: U.S. Government Printing Office.

Jessor, R., Donovan, J.E., & Widmer, K. (1980). *Adolescent drinking behavior.* Boulder, CO: Institute of Behavioral Science, University of Colorado.

Jessor, R., Graves, T.D., Hanson, R.C., & Jessor, S.L. (1968). *Society, personality and deviant behavior: A study of a tri-ethnic community.* New York: Holt, Rinehart and Winston.

Jessor, R., & Jessor, S.L. (1977). *Problem behavior and psychosocial development: A longitudinal study of youth.* New York: Academic Press.

Johnson, B.D., & Huizinga, D.H. (1983). *The concentration of delinquent offending: The contribution of serious drug involvement to long rate offending.* Paper presented at the 1983 meetings of the American Criminology Association, Denver.

Johnson, B.D., Goldstein, P.J., Preble, E., Schmeidler, J., Lipton, D.S., Spunt, B., and Miller, T. (1985). *Taking Care of Business.* Lexington, MA: Lexington.

Johnston, L.D., Bachman, J.G., & O'Malley, P.M. (1979). *Drugs and the class of '78: Behaviors, attitudes, and recent national trends.* Washington, DC: U.S. Government Printing Office.

Johnston, L.D., O'Malley, P.M., & Eveland, L.K. (1978). Drugs and delinquency: A search for causal connections. In D. B. Kandel (Ed.), *Longitudinal research on drug use,* (pp. 137–156). New York: Wiley.

Johnston, L.D., O'Malley, P.M., & Bachman, J.G. (1984). *Highlights from Drugs and American High School Students 1975–1983.* Washington, DC: U.S. Government Printing Office.

Johnstone, J.W.C. (1978). Social class, social areas, and delinquency. *Sociology and Social Research, 63,* 49–72.

Jones, L.Y. (1980). *Great expectations.* New York: Ballantine.

Kandel, D.B. (1975). States of adolescent involvement in drug use. *Science, 190,* 912–914.

Kandel, D.B. (Ed.). (1978). *Longitudinal research on drug use.* New York: Wiley.

Kandel, D.B. (1980). Drug and drinking behavior among youth. *Annual Review of Sociology, 6,* 235–285.

Kandel, D.B. (1982). Epidemiological and psychosocial perspectives on adolescent drug use. *Journal of the Academy of Child Psychiatry, 21,* 328–347.

Kandel, D.B., & Davies, M. (1928). Epidemiology of depresive mood in adolescents: An empirical study. *Archives of General Psychiatry, 39,* 1205–1212.

Kandel, D.B., & Faust, R. (1975). Sequence and states in patterns of adolescent drug use. *Archives of General Psychiatry, 32,* 923–932.

Kelejian, H.H., & Oates, W.E. (1974). *Introduction to econometrics: Principles and applications.* New York: Harper & Row.

Kessler, R.C., & Greenberg, D.F. (1981). *Linear panel analysis: Models of quantitative change.* New York: Academic Press.

Kessler, R.C., Reuter, J.A., & Greenley, J.R. (1979). Sex differences in the use of psychiatric outpatient facilities. *Social Forces, 58,* 557–571.

Kitsuse, J.I. (1962). Societal reaction to deviant behavior: Problems of theory and method. *Social Problems, 9,* 247–256.

Kitsuse, J.I. (1972). Deviance, deviant behavior and deviants: Some conceptual problems. In W. Filstead (Ed.), *An introduction to deviance: Readings in the process of making deviants.* Chicago: Markham.

Kitsuse, J.I., & Cicourel, A.V. (1963). A note on the uses of official statistics. *Social Problems, 11,* 131–139.

Klein, M.W., Teilman, K.S., Lincoln, S.B., & Labin, S. (1978). *Diversion as operationalization of labelling theory.* Social Science Research Institute, University of Southern California, Los Angeles.

Knoke, D. & Burke, P.J. (1980). Log-linear models. Beverly Hills, CA: Sage.

Konopka, G. (1966). *The adolescent girl in conflict.* Englewood Cliffs, NJ: Prentice-Hall.

Kornhauser, R.R. (1978). *Social sources of delinquency.* Chicago: University of Chicago Press.

Krisberg, B., & Austin, J. (1983). *The impact of juvenile court interventions on delinquent careers: An interim report.* San Francisco: National Council on Crime and Delinquency.

Kulik, J.A., Stein, K.B., & Sarbin, T.R. (1968). Dimensions and patterns of adolescent antisocial behavior. *Journal of Consulting and Clinical Psychology, 32,* 375–382.

Lander, B. (1954). *Towards an understanding of juvenile delinquency.* New York: Columbia University Press.

Lees, J.P., & Newson, L.J. (1954). Family or sibship position and some aspects of juvenile delinquency. *British Journal of Delinquency, 5,* 46–65.

Lemert, E.M. (1951). *Social pathology.* New York: McGraw-Hill.

Lemert, E.M. (1972). Social problems and the sociology of deviance. In E.M. Lemert (Ed.), *Human deviance social problems and social control* (pp. 3–25). Englewood Cliffs, NJ: Prentice-Hall.

Lemert, E.M. (1974). Beyond Mead: The societal reaction to deviance. *Social Problems, 21,* 457–468.

Liker, J.K., Augustyniak, S., & Duncan, G.J. (1985). Panel data and models of change: A comparison of first difference and conventional two-wave models. *Social Science Research, 14,* 80–101.

Lindeman, R.H., Merenda, P.F., & Gold, R.Z. (1980). *Introduction to bivariate and multivariate analysis.* Glenview, IL: Scott-Foresman.

Little, C.B. (1983). *Understanding deviance and control: Theory, research and social policy.* Itasca, IL: F.E. Peacock.

Loftus, E.F., and Marberger, W. (1983). Since the eruption of Mt. St. Helens has anyone beaten you up? Improving the accuracy of retrospective reports with landmark events. *Memory and Cognition, 116*(2), 114–120.

Markus, G.B. (1978). *Analyzing panel data.* Beverly Hills, CA: Sage.

Marquis, K.H., & Abner, P.A. (1981). *Quality of prisoner reports: Arrest and conviction response errors.* Santa Monica, CA: The Rand Corporation, R-2637-DOJ.

Mason, K.O., Mason, W.M., Winsborough, H.H., & Poole, W.K. (1973). Some methodological issues in cohort analysis of archival data. *American Sociological Review, 38,* 242–258.

Mason, W.M., Mason, K.O., & Winsborough, H.H., (1976). Reply to Glenn. *American Sociological Review, 41,* 904–905.

Matza, D. (1964). *Delinquency and drift.* New York: Wiley.

Maxim, P.S. (1985). Cohort size and juvenile delinquency: A test of the Easterlin Hypothesis. *Social Forces, 63,* 661–681.

McDonald, L. (1969). *Social class and delinquency.* Hamden, CT: Archon.

Megargee, E.I. (1972). *The California Psychological Inventory Handbook.* San Francisco: Jossey-Bass.

Menard, S. (1981). The test score decline: An analysis of available data. In B.E. Mercer & S.C. Hey (Eds.), *People in Schools* (pp. 183–209). Cambridge, MA: Schenkman.

Menard, S. (1987). Short-term trends in crime and delinquency: A comparison of UCR, NCS, and self-report data. *Justice Quarterly, 4,* 455–474.

Menard, S., & Elliott, D.S. (1988a). *Age, period, and cohort effects on self-reported delinquent behavior* (National Youth Survey Report No. 40). Boulder, CO: Institute of Behavioral Science.

Menard, S. & Elliott, D.S. (1988b). *Longitudinal and cross-sectional data collection and analysis in the sociological study of crime and delinquency* (National Youth Survey Report No. 42). Boulder, CO: Institute of Behavioral Science.

Menard, S., & Huizinga, D. (1988). *Age, period, and cohort effects on self-reported drug use.* (National Youth Survey Report No. 41). Boulder, CO: Institute of Behavioral Science.

Menard, S., & Morse, B.J. (1984). A structuralist critique of the IQ-delinquency hypothesis: Theory and evidence. *American Journal of Sociology, 89,* 1347–1378.

Menard, S., & Morse, B.J. (1986). IQ and delinquency: A response to Harry and Minor. *American Journal of Sciology, 91,* 962–968.

Merton, R.K. (1938). Social structure and anomie. *American Sociological Review, 3,* 672–682.

Merton, R.K. (1968). *Social theory and social structure* (enlarged ed.). New York: Free Press.

Murphy, J.M., Sobol, A.M., Neff, R.K., Olivier, D.C. & Leighton, A.H. (1984). Stability of prevalence. *Archives of General Psychiatry, 41,* 990–997.

Nettler, G. (1974). *Explaining crime.* New York: McGraw-Hill.

Nurco, D.N., Shaffer, J.N., Ball, J.C., & Kinlock, T.W. (1984). Trends in the commission of crime among narcotic addicts over successive periods of addiction and nonaddiction. *American Journal of Drug and Alcohol Abuse, 10,* 481–489.

Nye, F.I., & Short, J.F., Jr. (1957). Scaling delinquent behaviors. *American Sociological Review, 22,* 326–331.

Nye, F.I., Short, J.F., Jr., & Olson, V. (1958). Socioeconomic status and delinquent behavior. *American Journal of Sociology, 63,* 381–389.

O'Brien, R.M. (1985). *Crime and victimization data.* Beverly Hills: Sage.

Osgood, D.W., Johnston, L.O., O'Malley, P.M., and Bachman, J.G. (1988). The generality of deviance. *American Sociological Review, 53,* 81–93.

Parker, H., & Newcombe, R. (1987). Heroin use and acquisitive crime in an English community. *British Journal of Sociology, 38,* 331–350.

Parry, H.J., Balter, M.B., & Cisin, I.H. (1971). Primary levels of underreporting psychotropic drug use. *Public Opinion Quarterly, 34,* 582–592.

Penning, M., & Barnes, G.E. (1982). Adolescent marijuana use: A review. *The International Journal of the Addictions, 17,* 749–791.

Petersilia, J. (1978). The validity of criminality data derived from personal interviews. In C. Welford (Ed.), *Quantitative studies in criminology.* Beverly Hills: Sage.

Petersilia, J., Greenwood, P.W., & Lavin, M. (1978). *Criminal careers of habitual felons.* Santa Monica, CA: The Rand Corporation.

Petzel, T.P., Johnson, J.E., & McKillip, J. (1973). Response bias in drug surveys. *Journal of Consulting and Clinical Psychology, 40,* 437–439.

Pfuhl, E.H., Jr. (1970). Mass media and reported delinquent behavior: A negative case. In M.E. Wolfgang, L. Savitz, & N. Johnston (Eds.)., *The Sociology of Crime and Delinquency* (2nd ed., pp. 509–523). New York: Wiley.

Pine, G. (1965). Social class, social mobility, and delinquent behavior. *The Personnel and Guidance Journal, 43,* 770–774.

Pittel, S.M., Calef, V., Gryler, R.B., Hilles, L., Hofer, R., & Kempner, P. (1971).

Developmental factors in adolescent drug use: A study of psychedelic drug users. *Journal of the American Academy of Child Psychiatry, 10*(4), 640–660.

Pope, C.E., & McNeely, R.L. (1981). Introduction. In R.L. McNeely & L.E. Pope (Eds.), *Race, Crime and Criminal Justice* (pp. 9–27). Beverly Hills: Sage.

Porterfield, A.L. (1943). Delinquency and its outcome in court and college. *American Journal of Sociology, 49,* 199–208.

Porterfield, A. (1946). *Youth in trouble.* Fort Worth: Leo Potishman Foundation.

Pullum, T.W. (1977). Parameterizing age, period, and cohort effects: An application to U.S. delinquency rates, 1964–1973. In K. F. Schuessler (Ed.), *Sociological methodology 1978* (pp. 116–140). San Francisco: Jossey-Bass.

Rahav, G. (1980). Birth order and delinquency. *British Journal of Criminology, 20,* 385–395.

Regier, D.A., Myers, J.K., Kramer, M., Robins, L.N., Blazer, D.G., Hough, R.L., Eaton, W.W., & Locke, B.Z. (1984). The NIMH Epidemiological Catchment Area (ECA) program: Historical context, major objectives, and study population characteristics. *Archives of General Psychiatry, 41,* 934–941.

Reiss, A.J., Jr. (1975). Inappropriate theories and inadequate methods as policy plagues: Self-reported delinquency and the law. N.J. Demerath III (Eds.). In *Social policy and sociology* (pp. 211–222). New York: Academic Press.

Reiss, A.J., Jr., & Rhodes, A.L. (1961). The distribution of juvenile delinquency in the social class structure. *American Sociological Review, 26,* 720–732.

Robins, L.N. (1975). History of Drug Use. In J. Elinson & D. Nurco (Eds.), *Operational definitions in socio-behavioral drug use research* (NIDA Research Monograph Series).

Robins, L.N., Helzer, J.E., Croughan, J., Williams, J.B.W., & Spitzer, R.L. (1981a). *NIMH Diagnostic Interview Schedule: Version III.* Washington, DC: U.S. Department of Health and Human Services.

Robins, L.N., Helzer, J.E., Croughan, J., Williams, J.B.W., & Spitzer, R.L. (1981b). The NIMH Diagnostic Interview Schedule: Its history, characteristics, and validity. *Archives of General Psychiatry, 38,* 381–389.

Robins, L.N., Helzer, J.E., Ratcliff, K., & Seyfried, W. (1982). Validity of the Diagnostic Interview Schedule, Version II, DSM-III Diagnoses. *Psychological Medicine 12,* 855–870.

Robins, L.N., Helzer, J.E., Weissman, M.M., Orvaschol, H., Gruenberg, E., Burke, J.D. & Regier, D.A. (1984). Lifetime prevalence rates of specific psychiatric disorders in three sites. *Archives of General Psychiatry, 41,* 949–958.

Rosenberg, C.M. (1969). Young alcoholics. *British Journal of Psychiatry, 115,* 519.

Rosenhan, D.L. (1973). On being sane in insane places. *Science, 1979,* 250–258.

Russell, D.H. (1973). Emotional aspects of shoplifting. *Psychiatric Annals, 3*(5).

Sarri, R. (1983). Gender issues in juvenile justice. *Crime and Delinquency, 29,* 381–397.

Schuerman, L. & Kobrin, S. (1986). Community careers and crime. Pp. 67–100 in A. J. Reiss & M. Tonry (Eds.), *Communities and Crime,* Chicago: University of Chicago Press.

Schur, E.M. (1969). Reactions to deviance: A critical assessment. *American Journal of Criminology, 75,* 309–322.

Sellin, T., & Wolfgang, M.E. (1964). *The measurement of delinquency.* New York: Wiley.

Shapiro, S., Skinner, E.A., Kessler, L.G., Von Korff, M., German, P.S., Tischler, G.L., Leaf, P.J., Benham, L., Cottler, L., & Regier, D.A. (1984). Utilization of health and mental health services. *Archives of General Psychiatry, 41,* 971–982.

Shaw, C.R., & McKay, H.D. (1942). *Juvenile delinquency in urban areas.* Chicago: University of Chicago Press.

Short, J.F., Jr., & Nye, F.I. (1957). Reported behavior as a criterion of deviant behavior. *Social Problems, 5,* 207–213.

Short, J.F., Jr., & Nye, F.I. (1958). Extent of unrecorded juvenile delinquency: Tentative conclusions. *Journal of Criminal Law and Criminology, 49,* 296–302.

Single, E., Kandel, D., & Johnson, B.D. (1975). The reliability and validity of drug use responses in a large-scale longitudinal study. *Journal of Drug Issues, 5,* 426–443.

Skogan, W. (1976). The victims of crime: Some national survey results. In A. L. Guenther (Ed.), in *Criminal Behavior and Social Systems* (2nd ed. pp. 131–148). Chicago: Rand McNally.

Slocum, W.L., & Stone, C.L. (1963). Family culture patterns and delinquent-type behavior. *Marriage and Family Living, 25,* 202–208.

Smith, M.D. (1986). The era of increased violence in the United States: Age, period, or cohort effect? *Sociological Quarterly, 27,* 239–251.

Sparks, R.F. (1981). Survey of victimization: an optimistic assessment. Pp. 1–60 in Tonry, M. and Morris, N. (Eds.) *Crime and Justice: An Annual Review, Vol. 3.* Chicago: University of Chicago Press.

Spitzer, R.L., Endicott, J., & Robins, E. (1978). Research diagnostic criteria. *Archives of General Psychiatry, 35,* 773–782.

Srole, L., & Langner, T.S. (1979). Socioeconomic status groups: Their mental health composition. In S.K. Weinberg (Ed.), *The sociology of mental disorders* (pp. 33–47). Chicago: Aldine.

Srole, L., Langner, T.S., Michael, S.T., Opler, M.K., & Rennie, T.A.C. (1962). *Mental health in the metropolis: The Midtown Manhattan Study.* New York: McGraw-Hill.

Steffensmeier, D., & Harer, M.D. (1987). Is the crime rate really falling? An 'aging' U.S. population and its impact on the nation's crime rate 1980–84. *Journal of Research in Crime and Delinquency, 24,* 23–48.

Steffensmeier, D., Streifel, C., & Harer, M.D. (1987). Relative cohort size and youth crime in the United States, 1953–1984. *American Sociological Review, 52,* 702–710.

Sudman, S., & Bradburn, N.M. (1983). *Asking questions.* San Francisco: Jossey-Bass.

Szasz, T.S. (1974). *The myth of mental illness* (revised ed.). New York: Harper & Row.

Tanner, I.J. (1973). *Loneliness: The fear of love.* New York: Harper & Row.

Tittle, C.R. (1977). Sanction fear and the maintenance of social order. *Social Forces, 55,* 579–596.

Tittle, C.R., Villemez, W.J., & Smith, D.A. (1978). The myth of social class and criminology: An empirical assessment of the empirical evidence. *American Sociological Review, 43,* 643–656.

Tracy, P.E. (1978). An analysis of the incidence and seriousness of self-reported delinquency and crime. Ph.D. Dissertation, University of Pennsylvania. Ann Arbor. University Microfilms International.

U.S. Bureau of the Census (1975). *Historical statistics of the United States, colonial times to 1970.* Washington, DC: U.S. Government Printing Office.

U.S. Department of Justice. (1983). *Report to the nation on crime and justice: The data.* Rockville, MD: National Criminal Justice Reference Service.

Vold, G.B., & Bernard, T.J. (1986). *Theoretical criminology* (3rd ed.). New York: Oxford.

Voss, H.L. (1966). Socioeconomic status and reported delinquent behavior. *Social problems, 13,* 314–324.

Weisberg, S. (1980). *Applied linear regression.* New York: Wiley.

Weiss, R.S. (1973). *Loneliness: The experience of emotional and social isolation.* Cambridge, MA: MIT Press.

West, D.J. (1973). *Who becomes delinquent?* London: Heinemann.

Williams, J.R., & Gold, M. (1972). From delinquent behavior to official delinquency. *Social problems, 20,* 209–229.

Zabin, L.S., Hardy, J.B., Smith, E.A., & Hirsch, M.B. (1986). Substance use and its relation to sexual activity among inner-city adolescents. *Journal of Adolescent Health Care, 7,* 320–331.

Zajonc, R.B. (1976). Family configuration and intelligence. *Science, 192,* 227–236.

Zajonc, R.B., & Markus, G.B. (1975). Birth order and intellectual development. *Psychological Review, 82,* 74–88.

Appendix A
Frequency of Alcohol Use

In the National Youth Survey (NYS), frequency of alcohol use was measured in two different ways. The first was a single item asking how often in the past year the respondent had used alcohol. This single-item approach was used in waves 1, 4, 5, and 6, and in the National Institute of Mental Health (NIMH) subsample for waves 2 and 3. The second approach was to sum three items: frequency of use of beer, wine, and hard liquor. This three-item approach was used in waves 4 and 5, and in the office of Juvenile Justice and Delinquency Prevention (OJJDP) subsample for waves 2 and 3. It would be desirable to have a single measure of frequency of alcohol use for all waves and all subsamples. In an attempt to derive such a measure, bivariate regression was performed on waves 4 and 5, with frequency of alcohol use (single item) as dependent variable and frequency of beer, wine, and hard liquor use (summed three-item scale) as the independent variable. For both wave 4 and wave 5, the equation obtained from the regression analysis was

$$\text{Frequency of alcohol use} = 0.6 \times (\text{frequency of beer plus wine plus hard liquor use}) + 5 \tag{1}$$

The variance explained in frequency of alcohol use (squared correlation coefficient) was .61 for wave 4 and .63 for wave 5. Examination of the scatterplot revealed three obvious outliers, all with alcohol use greater than two times per day, and two of the three with low frequencies of beer, wine, and hard liquor use. Elimination of the three outliers from the analysis resulted in the equation

$$\text{Frequency of alcohol use} = 0.6 \times (\text{frequency of beer plus wine plus hard liquor use}) + 6 \tag{2}$$

and explained variances of .65 and .71 for waves 4 and 5, respectively. Given the consistency of the results, no further refinements of the analysis were attempted.

Different combinations of beer, wine, and hard liquor use were also used as predictors of (single-item) alcohol use. As a single-item indicator, wine use was the worst and beer use the best predictor, although beer use was neither quite as strong a predictor nor quite as consistent over time (the slope was .7 for wave 4 and .8 for wave 5). Of the two-item predictors, beer plus wine use was the best, with 1% to 2% less explained variance (squared correlations of .60–.69, depending on wave and whether outliers were included in the analysis). The equation

$$\text{Frequency of alcohol use} = .7 \times \text{(frequency of}$$
$$\text{beer plus wine)} + 7 \qquad (3)$$

was consistent for both waves, regardless of the inclusion or exclusion of outliers.

The results of the bivariate regression analysis are moderately encouraging. The explained variance, though less than might be desired, is substantial. More important, the parameter estimates for the equation for alcohol use frequency (computed from beer, wine, and hard liquor use frequency) are consistent for both waves 4 and 5, suggesting that they may be generalized to waves 2 and 3 as well. It is clear, however, that the three-item and one-item indicators cannot be used interchangeably without some transformation because both the slope and the intercept indicate that one (untransformed) would be a biased indicator of the other. Equation 1, however, provides a linear unbiased estimate of alcohol use frequency, based on beer plus wine plus hard liquor use.

Since the sum of beer, wine, and hard liquor use frequencies is greater than the single-item indicator of alcohol use frequency (this is to be expected, since one may use more than one type of alcoholic beverage on a single occasion), and since it seems reasonable that a nonuser according to one measure should be a nonuser according to the other, one modification was made in actually computing the alcohol use frequency scores from beer, wine, and hard liquor use scores for waves 2 and 3. For those with a total beer, wine, and hard liquor use frequency less than or equal to once per month (12 times per year), no transformation of the data was performed. This adjustment allows the alcohol use frequency to vary from 0 to 999, instead of forcing it to have a minimum of 5 (the intercept in Equation 1), and maintains alcohol use frequency at a level less than or equal to beer plus wine plus hard liquor use. For frequencies over 12 (more than once per month), the transformation is applied. In effect, we are correcting for what would be distortions at the lower end of the scale, resulting in a very slight departure from linearity but allowing the inclusion of values of 0 through 4, which would be excluded if the transformation were applied to the data at the lower end of the frequency continuum. The correction results in a very slight improvement in explained variance.

Appendix B
Mental Health Measures

The definition of crime is relatively straightforward and objective. Although laws vary across jurisdictions, what is defined as crime within a particular jurisdiction is fairly clearly specified. Every state in the United States has a legal definition of crime, and these definitions agree on the crucial points that the crime must be an act or omission performed with criminal intent or criminal negligence in violation of criminal law, in which act there is joint operation of act or omission and intent or negligence, and for which act punishment is provided by law (Haskell & Yablonsky, 1974, pp 4–8). Other forms of unethical, immoral, or rule-violating behavior are not criminal, but may instead be deviant. The law provides a relatively objective standard for deciding what constitutes crime.

The definition of juvenile delinquency is slightly more problematic, but still relatively objective compared to other behavioral science concepts. Acts performed by minors that would be crimes if committed by adults are considered delinquent in the juvenile court statutes of all states in the United States, but all jurisdictions except the federal have defined other acts as also being delinquent (Sellin & Wolfgang, 1964, pp. 71–72). These acts, including runaway, truancy, incorrigibility, and use of alcohol or tobacco before attaining the legal age to do so, vary from one jurisdiction to another and, in some jurisdictions, may be vaguely defined. The result is that we may be certain that when we are dealing with acts that would be crimes if committed by an adult, we are definitely dealing with delinquent acts; but other acts, depending on statutes specific to a given jurisdiction, may or may not be delinquent.

In contrast to crime and delinquency (and to physical illness), "mental health" and "mental illness" lack clear, relatively objective definitions. With the exception of organic disorders, in which the behavior in question may be traced to some brain injury or other physiological disorder, mental illness is commonly defined in terms of normality or abnormality of behavior, which may vary not only across societies but also within societies, from one social context to another (Clinard & Meier, 1979, pp.

464–470). Both the definition and the diagnosis of mental disorders other than organic disorders are highly problematic. At one extreme, Szasz (1974) suggests that the term "mental illness" is inappropriate, and what we term mental illness is not in fact an illness, but instead a set of problems in dealing with life situations.

Clinard and Meier (1979, pp. 457–458) cite evidence for the lack of reliability and validity of psychiatric diagnoses, even for such severe mental disorders as schizophrenia. Rosenhan (1973) found that psychiatric professionals were unable to detect people who had been misleadingly diagnosed as schizophrenic. It is also important to observe that, like crime and juvenile delinquency, mental illness is not a single type of behavior. There are 17 major categories of mental disorder (of which one is organic disorder) listed by the American Psychiatric Association (1980), and these can be further refined into specific disorders. Unlike crime and delinquency, however, there appears to be a lack of consensus, at least in diagnosis, about which mental disorder is indicated by a particular type of behavior.

Even in a clinical diagnostic setting, then, the absence of clear, objective standards of mental health and problems of unreliability of diagnosis would hinder our efforts to measure mental illness. The problem is compounded in the present study by our use of interview data collected by interviewers who were not psychiatric or psychological professionals, and by our reliance on self-reports of how respondents think that others perceive them (the respondents), rather than objective measures of how others, in fact, perceive our respondents. It is also important to realize that we did not attempt to measure all mental disorders or mental health problems, but limited ourselves primarily to two, feelings of isolation and feelings of being regarded by family members and friends as having emotional problems. These correspond most closely to the categories "affective disorders" or "personality disorders" in the American Psychiatric Association's classification scheme, but they are not formal psychiatric diagnoses.

Isolation, Emotional Problems, and Mental Health Service Use

Table B.1 presents a list of the mental health measures used in this validation, along with the abbreviations used in subsequent tables. In the first five waves of the data collection, only the measures of emotional problems and isolation or loneliness were collected. In wave 6, two new measures of mental health were introduced, replacing isolation and emotional problems. One was a clinical depression scale, used in the clinical diagnosis of depression. The second was a series of questions asking respondents how often in the past they had sought help for emotional problems from friends, clergy, medical and mental health

TABLE B.1. Variables used in Tables B.2 to B.4.

Abbreviation	Variable
NSYMP8	Number of symptoms of depression reported by respondent.
SYMP8	Whether symptoms of depression were reported by respondent (yes/no).
NOWDPP8	Whether respondent is currently depressed (yes/no).
EVDEP8	Whether respondent has ever felt depressed (yes/no).
MHUSE8	Frequency with which respondent has sought help for emotional or mental health problems from a psychologist or psychiatrist, physician, mental health clinic, hospital emergency room, or outpatient facility of a hospital or mental health clinic (number of times).
MHUSP8	Whether respondent has ever sought help for emotional or mental health problems from a psychologist or psychiatrist, physician, mental health clinic, hospital emergency room, or outpatient facility of a hospital or mental health clinic (yes/no).
MHALL8	Frequency with which respondent has sought help for emotional or mental health problems from anyone, including professionals, friends, clergy, social service agencies, spiritualists, herbalists, etc. (number of times).
MHALP8	Whether respondent has sought help for emotional or mental health problems from anyone (see MHALL8 above) (yes/no).
LABCFAM5	Emotional problems labeling by family, fifth wave (numeric score).
LABCFAM8	Emotional problems labeling by family, sixth wave, year 8 (numeric score).
LABCPFA8	Serious emotional problems labeling by family (no for score 12 or under, yes for score over 12).
EMOT5	Emotional problems labeling by family and friends (numeric score).
EMOTP5	Serious emotional problems labeling by family and friends (no for score 24 or under, yes for score over 24).
ISO5	Isolation from friends and family (numeric score).
ISOP5	Serious isolation from friends and family (no for score 26 or under, yes for score over 26).
NSPSH8	Did not seek professional help but should have (no/yes).

professionals, and others. The latter set of measures is perhaps as close as we can get to an objective measure of self-perceived mental health problems. From this set of measures, two measures of mental health service use were constructed. The first was an omnibus measure, constructed by combining all of the separate items (friends, professionals, others). The second was more specific, and was constructed by adding the frequencies with which respondents had sought help from psychiatrists or psychologists, physicians, or mental health centers for emotional or psychological problems.

Validation consisted of comparing mental health service use with each of three measures of mental health, emotional, or psychological problems: isolation, measured as feelings of isolation from friends and family; emotional problems, measured as perceptions of being labeled as "sick" or "messed up" or having emotional problems by friends and family; and depression, as measured by the clinical depression scale. Additionally, the emotional problems (family) scale was considered separately because information on this variable, but not the other measures of isolation or emotional problems, was available for the sixth wave of data collection. In addition to frequencies and absolute scores, categorical scores were constucted for all four sets of indicators. For isolation and emotional problems, scores were constructed by separating those who reported themselves as being severely isolated or who saw themselves as being perceived as having serious problems from those who did not. For depression and mental health service use, ever-prevalence scores were used. For depression, those who reported themselves as having ever been depressed were separated from those who did not; those who reported themselves as being currently depressed were separated from those who did not; and those who had self-reported symptoms of depression were separated from those who did not. For mental health service use, those who had ever sought help for emotional problems (from anyone for one measure, from professionals for the other) were separated from those who had not. One additional measure, whether the respondent had ever thought he or she needed professional help but failed to seek it, was also included in the analysis.

The results of the correlation analysis are presented in Table B.2. It is readily apparent that correlations among different measures of depression are high (from .683 to .868), those among different measures of mental health service use are moderate (.299 to .871), and other correlations are relatively small. Almost all of the correlations are statistically significant at the .05 level (most are significant at the .001 level). Correlations of depression with mental health service use range between .120 and .375; those for emotional problems from .056 to .136; and those for isolation from −.028 to .088. Emotional problems by the family has correlations with mental health service use ranging from .052 to .246. It is important to note that the measures for isolation and emotional problems were collected three years before those for mental health use, but those for depression and for emotional problems by family (presented in the table as LABCFAM8 and LABCPFA8, continuous and dichotomous scores, respectively) were collected at the same time as those for mental health service use. It does appear that the time lag may have some impact on the relationship between mental health problems and mental health service use, possibly as a result of "telescoping" effects (seeing oneself as depressed in the past if one sees oneself as depressed now, or reporting "ever" use of mental health services based primarily on current use).

The correlations among the four types of measures are low. This is to be expected, for two reasons. First, not everyone with a mental health problem makes use of mental health services. Second, and more important, not everyone who makes use of mental health services has the same problem; many people use mental health services who do not fall into any of our three categories (depressed, isolated, emotional problems). A more appropriate test of the validity of our mental health measures would be to

TABLE B.2. Zero-order correlations among mental health measures.

	NSYMP8	SYMP8	NOWDPP8	EVDEP8	MHUSE8	MHUSP8	MHALL8	MHALP8
NSYMP8	1.000	.803	.788	.683	.170	.375	.181	.333
SYMP8		1.000	.868	.850	.130	.298	.143	.330
NOWDPP8			1.000	.447	.157	.339	.169	.321
EVDEP8				1.000	.108	.255	.120	.308
MHUSE8					1.000	.544	.871	.234
MHUSP8						1.000	.516	.431
MHALL8							1.000	.299
MHALP8								1.000

	LABCFAM5	LABCFAM8	LABCPFA8	EMOT5	EMOTP5	ISO5	ISOP5	NSPSH8
NSYMP8	.140	.301	.241	.132	.134	.059	.120	.336
SYMP8	.134	.263	.199	.130	.124	.052	.074	.248
NOWDPP8	.107	.179	.151	.101	.078	-.007	.086	.293
EVDEP8	.127	.272	.198	.127	.132	.046	.057	.223
MHUSE8	.106	.119	.101	.080	.079	.058	.068	.073
MHUSP8	.135	.246	.243	.108	.136	.039	.088	.230
MHALL8	.134	.117	.093	.099	.088	.053	.056	.081
MHALP8	.052	.137	.136	.050	.056	-.028	.036	.226
LABCFAM5	1.000	.505	.228	.980	.392	.829	.194	.140
LABCFAM8		1.000	.485	.505	.227	.425	.109	.224
LABCPFA8			1.000	.210	.317	.109	.134	.225
EMOT5				1.000	.371	.849	.175	.127
EMOTP5					1.000	.189	.222	.138
ISO5						1.000	.282	.056
ISOP5							1.000	.058

see what percentage of those who describe themselves as being depressed (or isolated or having emotional problems) use mental health services, and what percentage of those who do not so describe themselves use mental health services. This measure will still be confounded by the fact that many who use mental health services do so for problems we have not measured in the present study, but if those who report having a mental health problem are more likely to use mental health services, particularly professional services, our confidence in the validity of our indicators is increased.

Tables B.3 and B.4 present the results of comparing those who report being (a) depressed, (b) labeled as having serious emotional problems, and (c) seriously isolated, with those who do not, on use of mental health services. Again, emotional problems by family, measured at the same time as mental health service use, is included as an alternative to emotional problems by family and friends, measured 3 years before

TABLE B.3. Depression and mental health service use.

		EVDEP8		NOWDPP8		SYMP8	
		No	Yes	No	Yes	No	Yes
MHUSP8	No	920	373	980	14	1014	279
row %		71.2	28.8	96.6	1.4	78.4	21.6
column %		92.7	74.3	88.8	43.8	92.7	69.8
	Yes	72	129	124	18	80	121
row %		35.8	64.2	87.3	12.7	39.8	60.2
column %		7.3	25.7	11.2	56.3	7.3	30.3
		$\chi^2 = 95.75^*$		$\chi^2 = 127.35^*$		$\chi^2 = 130.39^*$	
		Pearson's $r = .255^*$		Pearson's $r = .339^*$		Pearson's $r = .298^*$	
		Use ratio = 3.5		Use ratio = 5.0		Use ratio = 4.2	

		EVDEP8		NOWDPP8		SYMP8	
		No	Yes	No	Yes	No	Yes
MHALP8	No	647	165	659	5	703	109
row %		79.7	20.3	99.2	0.8	86.6	13.4
column %		65.3	32.9	59.7	15.6	64.3	27.3
	Yes	344	337	444	27	390	291
row %		50.5	49.5	94.3	5.7	57.3	42.7
column %		34.7	67.1	40.3	84.4	35.7	72.8
		$\chi^2 = 139.86^*$		$\chi^2 = 23.15^*$		$\chi^2 = 160.71^*$	
		Pearson's $r = .307^*$		Pearson's $r = .148^*$		Pearson's $r = .330^*$	
		Use ratio = 1.9		Use ratio = 2.1		Use ratio = 2.0	

* $p \leq .001$

TABLE B.4. Isolation, emotional problems and mental health service use.

		ISOP5		EMOTP5		LABCPFA8	
		No	Yes	No	Yes	No	Yes
MHUSP8	No	1194	22	1179	36	1244	48
row %		98.2	1.8	97.0	3.0	96.4	3.6
column %		87.2	66.7	87.7	63.2	88.6	53.4
	Yes	175	11	165	21	160	41
row %		94.1	5.9	88.7	11.3	79.6	20.4
column %		12.8	33.3	12.3	36.8	11.4	46.6
		$\chi^2 = 10.11^*$		$\chi^2 = 25.57^*$		$\chi^2 = 85.18^*$	
		Pearson's $r = .092^*$		Pearson's $r = .143^*$		Pearson's $r = .243^*$	
		Use ratio $= 2.6$		Use ratio $= 3.0$		Use ratio $= 4.1$	

		ISOP5		EMOTP5		LABCPFA8	
		No	Yes	No	Yes	No	Yes
MHALP8	No	754	14	744	23	787	24
row %		98.2	1.8	97.0	3.0	97.0	3.0
column %		55.1	42.4	55.4	40.4	56.1	27.3
	Yes	615	19	600	34	616	64
row %		97.0	3.0	94.6	5.4	90.6	9.4
column %		44.9	57.6	44.6	59.6	43.9	72.7
		$\chi^2 = 1.60$		$\chi^2 = 4.38^{**}$		$\chi^2 = 26.56^*$	
		Pearson's $r = .039$		Pearson's $r = .060^{**}$		Pearson's $r = .136^*$	
		Use ratio $= 1.3$		Use ratio $= 1.3$		Use ratio $= 1.7$	

* $p \le .001$.
** $p \le .05$.

mental health service use. For all of the mental health problem measures, the proportion using mental health services is higher for those with the mental health problem than for those without it. The relationship is affected by the time lag, since emotional problems by family at time 8 is much more strongly related to professional mental health service use at time 8 than emotional problems by both family and friends at an earlier date, and more closely related to professional mental health service use than serious emotional problems by family at time 5. Emotional problems by family at time 5 is more closely related than emotional problems by family at time 8 to isolation at time 5 (and, perforce, to emotional problems, which is a combination of emotional problems by family and friends). It is also significant that the use ratios are higher for the use of professional mental health services than for the omnibus measure. This finding suggests that we are indeed tapping the domain of concern to mental health professionals, and not just a more general measure of need for emotional support.

Conclusion

Problems in the definition and diagnosis of mental illness abound even in clinical, diagnostic settings. Not only may there be difficulty in distinguishing one mental disorder from another, but mistaken or misleading diagnoses of some individuals may go unnoticed by mental health professionals. Additionally, when one examines only selected types of mental illness, the correlation between mental illness and mental health service use is likely to be small. Despite these problems, we believe that we have derived two acceptable indicators of specific mental health problems: social isolation and emotional problem behavior. Both of these are positively correlated with mental health service use, although the correlations are weak. More important, employing mental health service use as a relatively objective criterion of mental health problems, both measures of mental health problems have predictive validity in that individuals who have either problem are more likely than individuals who do not have that problem to seek assistance, particularly professional assistance, for mental health problems.

We cannot say whether assistance was sought for the specific problems we have measured or, instead, for other problems. Out data indicate, however, that the different mental health problems are not strongly related to one another. Separate analysis (not presented in detail here) indicates that the ratio of those with emotional problems who are also isolated, to those with emotional problems who are not also isolated, varies between 1.1 : 1 and 14.4 : 1. The ratio of those who feel isolated and who also had emotional problems varies between 1.1 : 1 and 11.4 : 1. The ratio of those who are isolated and also depressed to those who are isolated but not depressed is 1.2 : 1 to 2.1 : 1. The ratio of those who were depressed and isolated to those who were depressed but not isolated was 1.2 : 1 to 1.6 : 1. The ratio of those who had emotional problems and depressed to those who had emotional problems and not depressed ranged from 2.7 : 1 to 3.7 : 1 (3.8 : 1 to 4.8 : 1 for emotional problems by family). The ratio of those who were depressed with emotional problems to those were depressed and did not have emotional problems was a fairly consistent 2.0 : 1 to 2.4 : 1 (2.3 : 1 to 3.3 : 1 for emotional problems by family). Overall, the correlations and ratios indicate not only some limited association and overlap among the mental health measures, but a considerable degree of independence as well.

Given these results, we have chosen to proceed with our analysis of selected mental health problems, to see whether these problems are related to delinquent behavior and drug use. Our conclusions must be qualified by noting the limitation of our measures, especially with regard to the full universe of mental health problems.

Appendix C
Prevalence and Offending Use Rates for Multiple Problem Types[1]

[1] The general offending rates presented in Appendix C are rates per person, not per 100 persons as used in the earlier tables. The "percent of total" refers to the percent of the total number of offenses committed in the sample that are committed by individuals in each particular type or subtype. Note that the felony theft scale includes a non-Index offense (bought stolen goods), so nonoffenders, who cannot have an Index offense by definition, may nevertheless have a felony theft offense.

TABLE C.1.

1976	N No MH problem 1483	N MH problem 204	Felony assault						Felony thefts					
			No mental health problem			Mental health problem			No mental health problem			Mental health problem		
			Preva-lence	Offend-ing rate	Percent of total	Preva-lence	Offend-ing rate	Percent of total	Preva-lence	Offend-ing rate	Percent of total	Preva-lence	Offend-ing rate	Percent of total
Nondelinquent														
Nonuser	782	74	0.0	.00	0	0.0	.00	0	0.1	.01	0	0.0	.00	0
Alcohol user	97	11	0.0	.00	0	0.0	.00	0	1.0	.01	0	9.1	.18	0
Marijuana user	33	5	0.0	.00	0	0.0	.00	0	3.0	.06	0	20.0	.20	0
Polydrug user	8	3	0.0	.00	0	0.0	.00	0	0.0	.00	0	33.3	.33	NA
Exploratory delinquent														
Nonuser	167	27	25.7	.26	5	48.1	.48	2	10.8	.14	2	11.1	.11	0
Alcohol user	61	8	13.1	.13	1	0.0	.00	0	19.7	.26	1	0.0	.00	0
Marijuana user	31	4	29.0	.29	1	0.0	.00	0	25.8	.39	1	0.0	.00	0
Polydrug user	8	0	12.5	.13	0	NA	NA	NA	37.5	.50	0	NA	NA	NA
Nonserious delinquent														
Nonuser	103	9	40.8	.67	8	66.7	1.11	1	19.4	.40	4	33.3	.89	1
Alcohol user	45	7	20.0	.29	2	28.6	.43	0	35.6	3.80	15	28.6	1.43	1
Marijuana user	33	12	39.4	.61	2	25.0	.50	1	45.5	1.45	4	41.7	1.00	1
Polydrug user	11	4	45.5	.64	1	25.0	.25	0	54.5	1.55	1	75.0	4.25	1
Serious Delinquent														
Nonuser	43	19	86.0	5.77	29	84.2	2.95	7	48.8	1.53	6	42.1	1.58	3
Alcohol user	27	6	88.9	3.78	12	66.7	2.67	2	48.1	1.74	4	66.7	1.50	1
Marijuana user	19	7	94.7	6.47	14	85.7	2.14	2	57.9	3.58	6	100.0	8.57	5
Polydrug user	15	8	100.0	4.67	8	100.0	3.25	3	86.7	28.67	38	62.5	4.25	3

1976	N No MH problem 1483	N MH problem 204	Robbery — No mental health problem Prevalence	Offending rate	Percent of total	Robbery — Mental health problem Prevalence	Offending rate	Percent of total	Index offenses — No mental health problem Prevalence	Offending rate	Percent of total	Index offenses — Mental health problem Prevalence	Offending rate	Percent of total
Nondelinquent														
Nonuser	782	74	0.0	.00	0	0.0	.00	0	0.0	.00	0	0.0	.00	0
Alcohol user	97	11	0.0	.00	0	0.0	.00	0	0.0	.00	0	0.0	.00	0
Marijuana user	33	5	0.0	.00	0	0.0	.00	0	0.0	.00	0	0.0	.00	0
Polydrug user	8	3	0.0	.00	0	0.0	.00	NA	0.0	.00	0	0.0	.00	NA
Exploratory delinquent														
Nonuser	167	27	3.0	.03	1	7.4	.07	0	31.1	.31	3	63.0	.63	1
Alcohol user	61	8	3.3	.03	0	25.0	.25	0	23.0	.23	1	25.0	.25	0
Marijuana user	31	4	3.2	.03	0	0.0	.00	0	35.5	.35	1	0.0	.00	0
Polydrug user	8	0	0.0	.00	0	NA	NA	NA	25.0	.25	0	NA	NA	NA
Nonserious delinquent														
Nonuser	103	9	9.7	.14	3	0.0	.00	0	47.6	.82	5	77.8	1.22	1
Alcohol user	45	7	0.0	.00	0	14.3	.29	0	26.7	.40	1	57.1	1.00	0
Marijuana user	33	12	0.0	.00	0	0.0	.00	0	48.5	.79	2	58.3	.92	1
Polydrug user	11	4	18.2	.27	1	0.0	.00	0	72.7	1.27	1	25.0	.25	0
Serious Delinquent														
Nonuser	43	19	48.8	2.72	24	57.9	1.74	7	100.0	9.07	23	100.0	5.84	7
Alcohol user	27	6	25.9	6.19	34	50.0	4.83	6	100.0	10.96	17	100.0	8.67	3
Marijuana user	19	7	26.3	1.95	8	42.9	1.14	2	100.0	9.89	11	100.0	9.00	4
Polydrug user	15	8	46.7	2.33	7	50.0	4.13	7	100.0	17.73	16	100.0	7.88	4

TABLE C.1. *Continued*

1976	N No MH problem 1483	N MH problem 204	Minor assaults						Minor thefts					
			No mental health problem			Mental health problem			No mental health problem			Mental health problem		
			Preva-lence	Offend-ing rate	Percent of total	Preva-lence	Offend-ing rate	Percent of total	Preva-lence	Offend-ing rate	Percent of total	Preva-lence	Offend-ing rate	Percent of total
Nondelinquent														
Nonuser	782	74	27.7	.43	3	27.0	.42	0	4.5	.06	2	2.7	.04	0
Alcohol user	97	11	27.8	.45	0	54.5	.64	0	15.5	.19	1	0.0	.00	0
Marijuana user	33	5	24.2	.36	0	0.0	.00	0	21.2	.30	0	0.0	.00	0
Polydrug user	8	3	25.0	.38	0	0.0	.00	0	0.0	.00	0	0.0	.00	0
Exploratory delinquent														
Nonuser	167	27	86.2	3.00	4	74.1	2.33	0	24.0	.41	2	11.1	.33	2
Alcohol user	61	8	73.8	2.07	1	100.0	3.50	0	37.7	.75	2	37.5	.50	2
Marijuana user	31	4	64.5	1.58	0	25.0	.25	0	45.2	1.16	1	25.0	.75	1
Polydrug user	8	0	75.0	1.38	0	NA	NA	NA	50.0	1.25	0	NA	NA	NA
Nonserious delinquent														
Nonuser	103	9	89.3	16.11	13	77.8	9.78	1	35.0	2.03	7	22.2	1.89	1
Alcohol user	45	7	73.3	11.0	4	71.4	175.43	10	53.3	5.91	9	28.6	2.29	1
Marijuana user	33	12	87.9	13.73	4	91.7	13.08	1	81.8	6.52	8	75.0	2.33	1
Polydrug user	11	4	100.0	6.64	1	50.0	3.00	0	54.5	4.82	2	50.0	4.75	1
Serious Delinquent														
Nonuser	43	19	90.7	65.67	22	94.7	43.68	6	55.8	2.65	4	52.6	38.84	26
Alcohol user	27	6	96.3	45.33	10	83.3	2.00	0	66.7	10.70	10	66.7	2.50	1
Marijuana user	19	7	94.7	53.21	8	100.0	12.57	1	42.1	2.26	2	100.0	16.57	4
Polydrug user	15	8	100.0	91.73	11	75.0	7.38	0	86.7	28.00	15	50.0	2.38	1

1976	N No MH problem 1483	N MH problem 204	Illegal services — No mental health problem Preva-lence	Offend-ing rate	Percent of total	Mental health problem Preva-lence	Offend-ing rate	Percent of total	Public disorder — No mental health problem Preva-lence	Offend-ing rate	Percent of total	Mental health problem Preva-lence	Offend-ing rate	Percent of total
Nondelinquent														
Nonuser	782	74	0.4	.00	0	0.0	.00	0	14.2	.81	6	17.6	.30	0
Alcohol user	97	11	0.0	.00	0	0.0	.00	0	52.6	2.06	2	54.5	1.18	0
Marijuana user	33	5	6.1	.09	0	0.0	.00	0	63.6	2.03	1	80.0	33.40	1
Polydrug user	8	3	25.0	.38	0	0.0	.00	0	50.0	2.63	0	66.7	3.67	0
Exploratory delinquent														
Nonuser	167	27	0.6	.01	0	3.7	.04	0	56.6	2.07	3	48.1	1.41	0
Alcohol user	61	8	1.6	.02	0	0.0	.00	0	86.9	4.80	3	75.0	2.00	0
Marijuana user	31	4	32.3	1.00	2	50.0	1.75	0	90.3	8.87	2	100.0	5.50	0
Polydrug user	8	0	12.5	.25	0	NA	NA	NA	75.0	5.63	0	NA	NA	NA
Nonserious delinquent														
Nonuser	103	9	0.0	.00	0	0.0	.00	0	69.9	7.82	7	33.3	8.33	1
Alcohol user	45	7	2.2	.04	0	0.0	.00	0	86.7	14.04	6	57.1	9.71	1
Marijuana user	33	12	33.3	1.52	3	41.7	1.67	1	93.8	24.16	7	100.0	60.00	6
Polydrug user	11	4	72.7	5.45	3	100.0	37.75	8	100.0	19.36	2	75.0	107.75	4
Serious Delinquent														
Nonuser	43	19	7.0	.14	0	11.1	.22	0	72.1	23.40	9	63.2	7.00	1
Alcohol user	27	6	3.8	.35	0	0.0	.00	0	85.2	15.67	4	66.7	15.67	1
Marijuana user	19	7	31.6	33.37	33	57.1	1.71	1	84.2	60.74	10	100.0	22.29	1
Polydrug user	15	8	86.7	22.47	18	87.5	73.13	30	100.0	132.80	18	87.5	36.88	3

TABLE C.1. *Continued*

1976	N No MH problem 1483	N MH problem 204	Vandalism						General delinquency					
			No mental health problem			Mental health problem			No mental health problem			Mental health problem		
			Prevalence	Offending rate	Percent of total	Prevalence	Offending rate	Percent of total	Prevalence	Offending rate	Percent of total	Prevalence	Offending rate	Percent of total
Nondelinquent														
Nonuser	782	74	19.3	.51	9	36.5	1.08	2	36.6	.64	2	40.5	.73	0
Alcohol user	97	11	20.6	.58	1	27.3	.64	0	67.0	1.16	0	81.8	1.27	0
Marijuana user	33	5	18.2	.61	0	0.0	.00	0	66.7	1.24	0	40.0	.80	0
Polydrug user	8	3	12.5	.50	0	33.3	.33	0	62.5	1.38	0	33.3	.33	0
Exploratory delinquent														
Nonuser	167	27	43.1	1.38	5	44.4	1.52	1	100.0	5.18	3	100.0	4.48	0
Alcohol user	61	8	45.9	1.36	2	62.5	2.00	0	100.0	5.82	1	100.0	5.88	0
Marijuana user	31	4	71.0	1.87	1	50.0	.75	0	100.0	7.10	1	100.0	6.00	0
Polydrug user	8	0	50.0	2.75	0	NA	NA	NA	100.0	6.25	0	NA	NA	NA
Nonserious delinquent														
Nonuser	103	9	58.3	3.24	5	33.3	3.33	1	100.0	25.64	10	100.0	21.67	1
Alcohol user	45	7	60.0	3.29	3	28.6	.71	0	100.0	31.91	5	100.0	189.00	5
Marijuana user	33	12	69.7	5.00	4	75.0	2.50	1	100.0	34.64	4	100.0	58.08	3
Polydrug user	11	4	81.8	5.73	1	50.0	.75	0	100.0	28.00	1	100.0	54.25	1
Serious Delinquent														
Nonuser	43	19	81.4	17.91	17	73.7	3.47	1	100.0	100.35	16	100.0	107.56	7
Alcohol user	27	6	70.4	16.07	9	50.0	3.00	0	100.0	99.08	9	100.0	15.17	0
Marijuana user	19	7	68.4	68.63	28	100.0	6.29	1	100.0	173.00	12	100.0	54.71	1
Polydrug user	15	8	93.3	20.27	7	62.5	2.50	0	100.0	233.53	13	100.0	97.63	3

1976	N No MH problem 1483	N MH problem 204	Alcohol use						Marijuana use					
			No mental health problem			Mental health problem			No mental health problem			Mental health problem		
			Prevalence	Offending rate	Percent of total	Prevalence	Offending rate	Percent of total	Prevalence	Offending rate	Percent of total	Prevalence	Offending rate	Percent of total
Nondelinquent														
Nonuser	782	74	23.3	.47	3	18.9	.38	0	2.3	.05	0	1.4	.03	0
Alcohol user	97	11	100.0	16.55	13	100.0	21.82	2	14.4	.29	0	27.3	.55	0
Marijuana user	33	5	87.9	12.30	3	100.0	20.00	1	100.0	26.94	7	100.0	16.80	1
Polydrug user	8	3	100.0	23.63	2	66.7	22.00	1	75.0	51.00	3	66.7	78.33	2
Exploratory delinquent														
Nonuser	167	27	37.7	.75	1	22.2	.44	0	6.6	.13	0	3.7	.07	0
Alcohol user	61	8	100.0	12.89	6	100.0	11.00	1	23.0	.46	0	12.5	.25	0
Marijuana user	31	4	90.3	25.61	6	100.0	31.50	1	100.0	52.65	14	100.0	38.00	1
Polydrug user	8	0	100.0	20.38	1	NA	NA	NA	100.0	92.38	6	NA	NA	NA
Nonserious delinquent														
Nonuser	103	9	34.0	.68	1	22.2	.44	0	5.8	.12	0	0.0	.00	0
Alcohol user	45	7	100.0	26.49	9	100.0	9.14	1	31.1	.62	0	28.6	.57	0
Marijuana user	33	12	100.0	33.48	9	100.0	24.75	2	100.0	48.45	13	100.0	65.25	6
Polydrug user	11	4	100.0	44.91	4	100.0	49.00	2	90.9	63.55	6	100.0	168.75	6
Serious Delinquent														
Nonuser	43	19	39.5	.79	0	42.1	.84	0	7.0	.14	0	5.3	.11	0
Alcohol user	27	6	100.0	26.89	6	100.0	80.50	4	14.8	.67	0	33.3	.67	0
Marijuana user	19	7	100.0	48.32	7	100.0	48.14	3	100.0	45.89	7	100.0	65.43	4
Polydrug user	15	8	93.3	71.60	9	100.0	56.25	4	93.3	118.33	15	87.5	106.75	7

TABLE C.1. Continued

| | | | Polydrug use | | | | | |
| | | | No mental health problem | | | Mental health problem | | |
1976	N No MH problem 1483	N MH problem 204	Prevalence	Offending rate	Percent of total	Prevalence	Offending rate	Percent of total
Nondelinquent								
Nonuser	782	74	0.3	.01	0	0.0	.00	0
Alcohol user	97	11	1.0	.02	0	0.0	.00	0
Marijuana user	33	5	12.1	.24	0	0.0	.00	0
Polydrug user	8	3	100.0	40.13	17	100.0	116.33	19
Exploratory delinquent								
Nonuser	167	27	0.6	.01	0	0.0	.00	0
Alcohol user	61	8	0.0	.00	0	12.5	.25	0
Marijuana user	31	4	19.4	.39	1	50.0	1.00	0
Polydrug user	8	0	100.0	7.50	3	NA	NA	NA
Nonserious delinquent								
Nonuser	103	9	1.9	.04	0	0.0	.00	0
Alcohol user	45	7	4.4	.09	0	0.0	.00	0
Marijuana user	33	12	18.2	.36	1	8.3	.17	0
Polydrug user	11	4	100.0	36.82	22	100.0	23.25	5
Serious delinquent								
Nonuser	43	19	0.0	.00	0	0.0	.00	0
Alcohol user	27	6	3.7	.07	0	0.0	.00	0
Marijuana user	19	7	10.5	.21	0	42.9	.86	0
Polydrug user	15	8	100.0	16.20	13	100.0	41.63	18

1976	N No MH problem 1483	N MH problem 204	Mental health problems			
			No mental health problem		Mental health problem	
			Prevalence	Mean scale Score	Prevalence	Mean scale Score
Nondelinquent						
Nonuser	782	74	0.0	36.62	100.0	51.61
Alcohol user	97	11	0.0	36.93	100.0	54.00
Marijuana user	33	5	0.0	36.67	100.0	57.60
Polydrug user	8	3	0.0	41.88	100.0	57.00
Exploratory delinquent						
Nonuser	167	27	0.0	38.35	100.0	54.79
Alcohol user	61	8	0.0	37.56	100.0	54.25
Marijuana user	31	4	0.0	38.48	100.0	55.00
Polydrug user	8	0	0.0	39.13	NA	NA
Nonserious delinquent						
Nonuser	103	9	0.0	39.86	100.0	54.33
Alcohol user	45	7	0.0	38.16	100.0	50.57
Marijuana user	33	12	0.0	39.76	100.0	54.17
Polydrug user	11	4	0.0	41.82	100.0	50.50
Serious delinquent						
Nonuser	43	19	0.0	40.94	100.0	53.91
Alcohol user	27	6	0.0	41.78	100.0	55.50
Marijuana user	19	7	0.0	39.00	100.0	49.71
Polydrug user	15	8	0.0	44.53	100.0	54.33

TABLE C.2.

1980	N No MH problem 1406	N MH problem 83	Felony assault						Felony thefts					
			No mental health problem			Mental health problem			No mental health problem			Mental health problem		
			Preva-lence	Offend-ing rate	Percent of total	Preva-lence	Offend-ing rate	Percent of total	Preva-lence	Offend-ing rate	Percent of total	Preva-lence	Offend-ing rate	Percent of total
Nondelinquent														
Nonuser	411	21	0.0	.00	0	0.0	.00	0	0.7	.01	0	0.0	.00	0
Alcohol user	382	16	0.0	.00	0	0.0	.00	0	0.5	.01	0	0.0	.00	0
Marijuana user	176	7	0.0	.00	0	0.0	.00	0	2.8	.03	1	0.0	.00	0
Polydrug user	48	4	0.0	.00	0	0.0	.00	0	4.2	.04	0	0.0	.00	0
Exploratory delinquent														
Nonuser	23	3	39.1	.39	2	33.3	.33	0	8.7	.09	0	33.3	.33	0
Alcohol user	56	7	14.3	.14	2	42.9	.43	1	16.1	.29	2	0.0	.00	0
Marijuana user	67	4	19.4	.19	3	0.0	.00	0	19.4	.30	3	50.0	.50	0
Polydrug user	33	3	3.0	.03	0	0.0	.00	0	15.2	.21	1	0.0	.00	0
Nonserious delinquent														
Nonuser	16	0	25.0	.50	2	NA	NA	NA	18.8	.25	1	NA	NA	NA
Alcohol user	36	0	25.0	.42	4	NA	NA	NA	19.4	.28	2	NA	NA	NA
Marijuana user	44	1	34.1	.45	5	0.0	.00	0	22.7	.61	4	100.0	1.00	0
Polydrug user	62	3	22.6	.35	5	66.7	.67	0	27.4	.53	5	33.3	.33	0
Serious Delinquent														
Nonuser	8	1	62.5	2.38	4	100.0	3.00	1	25.0	.88	1	0.0	.00	0
Alcohol user	5	1	100.0	7.60	9	0.0	.00	0	60.0	1.60	1	100.0	7.00	1
Marijuana user	16	3	81.3	4.25	16	66.7	6.33	4	62.5	4.13	10	66.7	5.67	3
Polydrug user	23	9	82.6	4.52	24	88.9	8.33	18	82.6	10.61	37	77.8	18.56	26

1980	N No MH problem 1406	N MH problem 83	Robbery — No mental health problem			Robbery — Mental health problem			Index offenses — No mental health problem			Index offenses — Mental health problem		
			Prevalence	Offending rate	Percent of total	Prevalence	Offending rate	Percent of total	Prevalence	Offending rate	Percent of total	Prevalence	Offending rate	Percent of total
Nondelinquent														
Nonuser	411	21	0.0	.00	0	0.0	.00	0	0.0	.00	0	0.0	.00	0
Alcohol user	382	16	0.0	.00	0	0.0	.00	0	0.0	.00	0	0.0	.00	0
Marijuana user	176	7	0.0	.00	0	0.0	.00	0	0.0	.00	0	0.0	.00	0
Polydrug user	48	4	0.0	.00	0	0.0	.00	0	0.0	.00	0	0.0	.00	0
Exploratory delinquent														
Nonuser	23	3	4.3	.04	1	0.0	.00	0	47.8	.48	1	33.3	.33	1
Alcohol user	56	7	0.0	.00	0	0.0	.00	9	21.4	.21	1	42.9	.43	1
Marijuana user	67	4	0.0	.00	0	25.0	.25	1	29.9	.30	2	25.0	.25	2
Polydrug user	33	3	0.0	.00	0	0.0	.00	0	12.1	.12	0	0.0	.00	0
Nonserious delinquent														
Nonuser	16	0	12.5	.25	3	NA	NA	NA	37.5	.75	1	NA	NA	NA
Alcohol user	36	0	2.8	.05	1	NA	NA	NA	33.3	.56	2	NA	NA	NA
Marijuana user	44	1	9.1	.16	5	0.0	.00	0	52.3	.80	4	100.0	1.00	0
Polydrug user	62	3	1.6	.03	1	0.0	.00	0	33.9	.53	4	66.7	1.00	0
Serious Delinquent														
Nonuser	8	1	12.5	6.25	32	0.0	.00	0	100.0	9.50	8	100.0	3.00	0
Alcohol user	5	1	20.0	1.00	3	0.0	.00	0	100.0	9.60	5	100.0	3.00	0
Marijuana user	16	3	18.8	.31	3	33.3	4.00	8	100.0	7.81	14	100.0	14.00	5
Polydrug user	23	9	30.4	1.87	28	44.4	2.56	15	100.0	11.35	29	100.0	21.78	22

TABLE C.2. *Continued*

			Minor assaults						Minor thefts					
			No mental health problem			Mental health problem			No mental health problem			Mental health problem		
1980	N No MH problem	N MH problem	Preva-lence	Offend-ing rate	Percent of total	Preva-lence	Offend-ing rate	Percent of total	Preva-lence	Offend-ing rate	Percent of total	Preva-lence	Offend-ing rate	Percent of total
	1406	83												
Nondelinquent														
Nonuser	411	21	11.7	.17	4	4.8	.14	0	2.4	.03	1	4.8	.10	0
Alcohol user	382	16	7.9	.12	3	0.0	.00	0	3.9	.05	1	0.0	.00	0
Marijuana user	176	7	6.8	.12	1	14.3	.29	0	5.7	.09	1	0.0	.00	0
Polydrug user	48	4	6.3	.10	0	0.0	.00	0	10.4	.17	0	0.0	.00	0
Exploratory delinquent														
Nonuser	23	3	69.6	2.00	3	100.0	2.00	0	17.4	.26	0	33.3	.67	0
Alcohol user	56	7	58.9	1.55	5	71.4	2.00	1	33.9	.91	3	28.6	.29	3
Marijuana user	67	4	31.3	.67	3	75.0	1.50	0	38.8	1.07	4	100.0	3.50	4
Polydrug user	33	3	24.2	.48	1	33.3	3.00	1	27.3	.91	2	0.0	.00	2
Nonserious delinquent														
Nonuser	16	0	50.0	2.00	2	NA	NA	NA	6.3	.31	0	NA	NA	NA
Alcohol user	36	0	61.1	2.94	6	NA	NA	NA	38.9	1.28	3	NA	NA	NA
Marijuana user	44	1	56.8	3.68	9	0.0	.00	1	52.3	9.55	26	0.0	.00	0
Polydrug user	62	3	30.6	1.55	5	0.0	.00	0	45.2	3.32	13	0.0	.00	0
Serious Delinquent														
Nonuser	8	1	87.5	12.88	6	0.0	.00	0	50.0	1.50	1	100.0	1.00	0
Alcohol user	5	1	100.0	5.60	2	100.0	1.00	0	60.0	1.80	1	100.0	16.00	1
Marijuana user	16	3	68.8	3.44	3	33.3	9.33	2	62.5	6.81	7	33.3	4.00	1
Polydrug user	23	9	69.6	5.57	7	88.9	74.56	38	73.9	13.70	19	100.0	26.89	15

1980	N No MH problem 1406	N MH problem 83	Illegal services — No mental health problem Prevalence	Offending rate	Percent of total	Illegal services — Mental health problem Prevalence	Offending rate	Percent of total	Public disorder — No mental health problem Prevalence	Offending rate	Percent of total	Public disorder — Mental health problem Prevalence	Offending rate	Percent of total
Nondelinquent														
Nonuser	411	21	0.2	.01	0	0.0	.00	0	11.2	.33	1	23.8	.95	0
Alcohol user	382	16	0.0	.00	0	0.0	.00	0	40.6	2.30	6	62.5	3.00	0
Marijuana user	176	7	6.3	.12	0	0.0	.00	0	54.0	4.01	5	57.1	4.00	0
Polydrug user	48	4	8.3	.21	0	0.0	.00	0	79.2	9.71	3	100.0	41.50	1
Exploratory delinquent														
Nonuser	23	3	4.3	.09	0	0.0	.00	0	56.5	1.30	0	100.0	1.33	0
Alcohol user	56	7	5.4	.09	0	0.0	.00	0	83.6	7.40	3	85.7	15.86	1
Marijuana user	67	4	31.3	.78	1	25.0	.50	0	94.0	17.19	7	75.0	12.75	0
Polydrug user	33	3	54.5	2.55	1	66.7	2.33	0	84.8	16.03	3	100.0	175.67	3
Nonserious delinquent														
Nonuser	16	0	6.3	.63	0	NA	NA	NA	37.5	3.70	0	NA	NA	NA
Alcohol user	36	0	2.8	.28	0	NA	NA	NA	80.6	20.75	5	NA	NA	NA
Marijuana user	44	1	38.6	5.64	4	0.0	.00	0	86.4	37.34	11	100.0	1.00	0
Polydrug user	62	3	64.5	22.48	21	66.7	138.33	6	95.2	58.18	23	100.0	36.67	1
Serious Delinquent														
Nonuser	8	1	0.0	.00	0	0.0	.00	0	37.5	27.50	1	0.0	.00	0
Alcohol user	5	1	20.0	.40	0	0.0	.00	0	100.0	39.00	1	0.0	.00	0
Marijuana user	16	3	50.0	3.94	1	66.7	1.33	0	87.5	21.50	2	100.0	7.67	0
Polydrug user	23	9	87.0	58.57	20	77.8	337.00	45	87.0	70.13	10	100.0	176.22	10

Table C.2. Continued

1980	N No MH problem 1406	N MH problem 83	Vandalism						General delinquency					
			No mental health problem			Mental health problem			No mental health problem			Mental health problem		
			Prevalence	Offending rate	Percent of total	Prevalence	Offending rate	Percent of total	Prevalence	Offending rate	Percent of total	Prevalence	Offending rate	Percent of total
Nondelinquent														
Nonuser	411	21	6.1	.16	7	0.0	.00	0	19.5	.31	1	14.3	.33	0
Alcohol user	382	16	6.5	.19	8	6.3	.13	0	26.2	.46	1	25.0	.31	0
Marijuana user	176	7	6.3	.14	3	14.3	.57	0	39.8	.76	1	71.4	1.14	0
Polydrug user	48	4	4.2	.65	3	0.0	.00	0	45.8	.98	0	50.0	1.25	0
Exploratory delinquent														
Nonuser	23	3	43.5	.87	2	33.3	3.33	1	100.0	4.26	0	100.0	6.67	0
Alcohol user	56	7	25.0	.54	3	42.9	1.43	1	100.0	5.52	1	100.0	4.86	0
Marijuana user	67	4	31.3	.87	6	75.0	2.25	1	100.0	5.79	2	100.0	7.25	0
Polydrug user	33	3	24.2	.67	2	66.7	1.33	0	100.0	6.42	1	100.0	8.00	0
Nonserious delinquent														
Nonuser	16	0	31.3	.81	1	NA	NA	NA	100.0	46.44	3	NA	NA	NA
Alcohol user	36	0	41.7	1.97	8	NA	NA	NA	100.0	29.61	5	NA	NA	NA
Marijuana user	44	1	27.3	1.50	7	0.0	.00	0	100.0	47.61	10	100.0	367.00	2
Polydrug user	62	3	37.1	.95	6	0.0	.00	0	100.0	71.73	21	100.0	156.00	2
Serious Delinquent														
Nonuser	8	1	75.0	5.75	5	0.0	.00	0	100.0	54.25	2	100.0	4.00	0
Alcohol user	5	1	80.0	3.80	2	0.0	.00	0	100.0	115.40	3	100.0	24.00	0
Marijuana user	16	3	81.3	7.75	13	66.7	8.00	3	100.0	49.81	4	100.0	158.67	2
Polydrug user	23	9	60.9	2.57	6	100.0	13.13	11	100.0	121.48	13	100.0	592.67	25

1980	N No MH problem 1406	N MH problem 83	Alcohol use — No mental health problem Prevalence	Offending rate	Percent of total	Alcohol use — Mental health problem Prevalence	Offending rate	Percent of total	Marijuana use — No mental health problem Prevalence	Offending rate	Percent of total	Marijuana use — Mental health problem Prevalence	Offending rate	Percent of total
Nondelinquent														
Nonuser	411	21	40.1	.78	0	28.6	.57	0	5.6	.08	0	9.5	.14	0
Alcohol user	382	16	100.0	32.71	19	100.0	25.69	1	23.0	.45	0	18.8	.31	0
Marijuana user	176	7	97.7	59.60	16	85.7	97.43	1	100.0	32.34	12	100.0	74.57	1
Polydrug user	48	4	100.0	90.44	7	100.0	55.75	0	95.8	104.60	11	100.0	18.00	0
Exploratory delinquent														
Nonuser	23	3	65.2	1.35	0	100.0	2.33	0	13.0	.17	0	0.0	.00	0
Alcohol user	56	7	100.00	63.36	5	100.0	22.57	0	26.8	.55	0	42.9	2.43	0
Marijuana user	67	4	100.0	70.24	7	100.0	17.50	0	100.0	48.30	7	100.0	189.00	2
Polydrug user	33	3	93.9	124.00	6	100.0	119.34	1	100.0	153.55	11	100.0	203.33	1
Nonserious delinquent														
Nonuser	16	0	81.3	1.56	0	NA	NA	NA	18.8	.19	0	NA	NA	NA
Alcohol user	36	0	100.0	70.17	4	NA	NA	NA	16.7	.56	0	NA	NA	NA
Marijuana user	44	1	95.5	109.66	7	100.0	30.00	0	100.0	74.86	7	100.0	6.00	0
Polydrug user	62	3	100.0	140.52	13	100.0	100.67	0	96.8	182.34	24	100.0	488.00	3
Serious Delinquent														
Nonuser	8	1	50.0	1.25	0	100.0	2.00	0	25.0	.50	0	0.0	.00	0
Alcohol user	5	1	100.0	110.00	1	100.0	30.00	0	80.0	1.60	0	0.0	.00	0
Marijuana user	16	3	100.0	101.67	0	100.0	105.25	4	100.0	78.33	1			
Polydrug user	23	9	100.0	161.17	6	100.0	132.33	2	100.0	210.48	10	100.0	289.89	6

TABLE C.2. Continued

1980	N No MH problem 1406	N MH problem 83	Polydrug use						Problem substance use			
			No mental health problem			Mental health problem			No mental health problem		Mental health problem	
			Preva-lence	Offend-ing rate	Percent of total	Preva-lence	Offend-ing rate	Percent of total	Preva-lence	Offend-ing rate	Preva-lence	Scale score
Nondelinquent												
Nonuser	411	21	0.0	.00	0	0.0	.00	0	0.2	2.38	0.0	1.95
Alcohol user	382	16	1.6	.03	0		.06	0	3.1	6.67	0.0	6.50
Marijuana user	176	7	14.8	.23	0	0.0	.00	0	6.3	10.91	0.0	9.86
Polydrug user	48	4	100.0	23.92	14	100.0	9.00	0	12.5	11.69	25.0	13.25
Exploratory delinquent												
Nonuser	23	3	0.0	.00	0	0.0	.00	0	0.0	4.22	0.0	5.33
Alcohol user	56	7	3.6	.05	0	0.0	.00	0	17.9	8.16	42.9	10.86
Marijuana user	67	4	11.9	.18	0	25.0	.50	0	17.9	12.27	0.0	12.75
Polydrug user	33	3	100.0	25.58	10	100.0	26.00	1	33.3	14.88	100.0	25.67
Nonserious delinquent												
Nonuser	16	0	0.0	.00	0	NA	NA	NA	0.0	5.25	NA	NA
Alcohol user	36	0	2.8	.06	0	NA	NA	NA	25.0	7.97	NA	NA
Marijuana user	44	1	25.0	.41	0	0.0	.00	0	22.7	12.57	0.0	11.0
Polydrug user	62	3	100.0	41.87	32	100.0	152.33	6	38.7	14.92	100.0	18.00
Serious Delinquent												
Nonuser	8	1	0.0	.00	0	0.0	.00	0	0.0	2.86	0.0	5.00
Alcohol user	5	1	0.0	.00	0	0.0	.00	0	60.0	13.2	0.0	7.00
Marijuana user	16	3	25.0	.38	0	33.3	.33	0	56.3	17.63	66.7	13.67
Polydrug user	23	9	100.0	61.91	17	100.0	165.00	18	65.2	17.13	100.0	22.11

1980	N No MH problem 1406	N MH problem 83	Mental health problems			
			No mental health problem		Mental health problem	
			Prevalence	Mean scale score	Prevalence	Mean scale score
Nondelinquent						
Nonuser	411	21	0.0	33.15	100.0	52.86
Alcohol user	382	16	0.0	33.42	100.0	53.06
Marijuana user	176	7	0.0	34.93	100.0	52.86
Polydrug user	48	4	0.0	35.30	100.0	54.00
Exploratory delinquent						
Nonuser	23	3	0.0	35.00	100.0	52.67
Alcohol user	56	7	0.0	33.86	100.0	49.00
Marijuana user	67	4	0.0	36.43	100.0	50.00
Polydrug user	33	3	0.0	39.85	100.0	47.00
Nonserious delinquent						
Nonuser	16	0	0.0	33.56	NA	NA
Alcohol user	36	0	0.0	35.92	NA	NA
Marijuana user	44	1	0.0	36.41	100.0	52.00
Polydrug user	62	3	0.0	36.71	100.0	57.00
Serious delinquent						
Nonuser	8	1	0.0	37.63	100.0	46.00
Alcohol user	5	1	0.0	38.00	100.0	50.00
Marijuana user	16	3	0.0	41.38	100.0	53.00
Polydrug user	23	9	0.0	40.57	100.0	53.67

TABLE C.3.

1983	N No MH problem 1400	N MH problem 86	Felony assault						Felony thefts					
			No mental health problem			Mental health problem			No mental health problem			Mental health problem		
			Prevalence	Offending rate	Percent of total	Prevalence	Offending rate	Percent of total	Prevalence	Offending rate	Percent of total	Prevalence	Offending rate	Percent of total
Nondelinquent														
Nonuser	267	13	0.0	.00	0	0.0	.00	0	0.0	.00	0	0.0	.00	0
Alcohol user	573	18	0.0	.00	0	0.0	.00	0	0.5	.01	1	0.0	.00	0
Marijuana user	176	7	0.0	.00	0	0.0	.00	0	4.5	.06	1	0.0	.00	0
Polydrug user	81	4	0.0	.00	0	0.0	.00	0	3.0	.11	1	0.0	.00	0
Exploratory delinquent														
Nonuser	8	1	25.0	.25	1	100.0	1.00	0	25.0	.38	0	0.0	.00	0
Alcohol user	60	6	25.0	.25	7	50.0	.50	1	21.7	.32	3	16.7	.17	0
Marijuana user	34	3	26.5	.26	4	66.7	.67	1	8.8	.12	1	33.3	1.67	1
Polydrug user	44	7	9.1	.09	2	0.0	.00	0	5.9	.48	3	42.9	1.00	1
Nonserious delinquent														
Nonuser	7	0	0.0	.00	0	NA	NA	NA	57.1	.86	1	NA	NA	NA
Alcohol user	35	3	28.6	.54	8	33.3	.67	1	17.1	.91	5	33.3	.33	0
Marijuana user	28	7	25.0	.39	5	42.9	.43	1	25.0	.46	2	28.6	.57	1
Polydrug user	58	7	15.5	.21	5	57.1	1.00	3	10.4	1.19	10	28.6	.43	0
Serious Delinquent														
Nonuser	0	0	NA	NA	NA	NA	NA	NA	NA	NA	NA	NA	NA	NA
Alcohol user	3	0	100.0	3.00	4	NA	NA	NA	0.0	.00	0	NA	NA	NA
Marijuana user	7	2	100.0	2.57	8	100.0	3.00	3	57.1	5.57	6	50.0	.50	0
Polydrug user	19	8	68.4	4.21	36	100.0	2.75	10	7.4	17.79	51	87.5	10.00	12

	N No MH problem 1400	N MH problem 86	Robbery No mental health problem Prevalence	Offending rate	Percent of total	Robbery Mental health problem Prevalence	Offending rate	Percent of total	Index offenses No mental health problem Prevalence	Offending rate	Percent of total	Index offenses Mental health problem Prevalence	Offending rate	Percent of total
Nondelinquent														
Nonuser	267	13	0.0	.00	0	0.0	.00	0	0.0	.00	0	0.0	.00	0
Alcohol user	573	18	0.0	.00	0	0.0	.00	0	0.0	.00	0	0.0	.00	0
Marijuana user	176	7	0.0	.00	0	0.0	.00	0	0.0	.00	0	0.0	.00	0
Polydrug user	81	4	0.0	.00	0	0.0	.00	0	0.0	.00	0	0.0	.00	0
Exploratory delinquent														
Nonuser	8	1	12.5	.13	20	0.0	.00	0	37.5	.38	1	100.0	1.00	0
Alcohol user	60	6	1.7	.17	20	0.0	.00	0	36.7	.37	4	66.7	.67	1
Marijuana user	34	3	0.0	.00	0	0.0	.00	0	26.5	.26	2	66.7	.67	0
Polydrug user	44	7	0.0	.00	0	0.0	.00	0	18.2	.18	2	14.3	.14	0
Nonserious delinquent														
Nonuser	7	0	14.3	.14	20	NA	NA	NA	28.6	.57	1	NA	NA	NA
Alcohol user	35	3	0.0	.00	0	0.0	.00	0	31.4	.60	4	66.7	1.00	1
Marijuana user	28	7	0.0	.00	0	0.0	.00	0	35.7	.57	3	42.9	.57	1
Polydrug user	58	7	1.7	.03	40	0.0	.00	0	24.1	.34	4	57.1	1.00	1
Serious Delinquent														
Nonuser	0	0	NA	NA	NA	NA	NA	NA	NA	NA	NA	NA	NA	NA
Alcohol user	3	0	0.0	.00	0	NA	NA	NA	100.0	3.00	2	NA	NA	NA
Marijuana user	7	2	0.0	.00	0	0.0	.00	0	100.0	7.14	10	100.0	3.50	1
Polydrug user	44	7	0.0	.00	0	0.0	.00	0	100.0	12.74	47	100.0	9.75	15

TABLE C.3. Continued

1983	N No MH problem 1400	N MH problem 86	Minor assaults						Minor thefts					
			No mental health problem			Mental health problem			No mental health problem			Mental health problem		
			Preva-lence	Offend-ing rate	Percent of total	Preva-lence	Offend-ing rate	Percent of total	Preva-lence	Offend-ing rate	Percent of total	Preva-lence	Offend-ing rate	Percent of total
Nondelinquent														
Nonuser	267	13	1.9	.02	2	15.4	.15	1	1.9	.03	1	7.7	.15	0
Alcohol user	573	18	4.0	.07	12	0.0	.00	0	4.0	.05	3	11.1	.11	0
Marijuana user	176	7	1.1	.02	1	0.0	.00	0	6.3	.10	2	0.0	.00	0
Polydrug user	81	4	2.5	.02	1	0.0	.00	0	7.4	.11	1	0.0	.00	0
Exploratory delinquent														
Nonuser	8	1	25.0	.63	2	0.0	.00	0	27.5	.88	1	0.0	.00	0
Alcohol user	60	6	16.7	.42	8	16.7	.50	1	20.0	.68	4	16.7	.83	0
Marijuana user	34	3	11.8	.35	4	0.0	.00	0	29.4	.91	3	0.0	.00	0
Polydrug user	44	7	29.5	.43	6	0.0	.00	0	27.3	.98	4	42.9	1.00	1
Nonserious delinquent														
Nonuser	7	0	0.0	.00	0	NA	NA	NA	42.9	1.43	1	NA	NA	NA
Alcohol user	35	3	17.1	.94	10	66.7	2.00	2	17.1	1.71	5	66.7	1.67	0
Marijuana user	28	7	17.9	.57	5	14.3	.14	0	32.1	1.43	4	42.9	1.00	1
Polydrug user	58	7	13.8	.43	8	57.1	2.57	6	43.1	6.17	32	28.6	.57	0
Serious Delinquent														
Nonuser	0	0	NA	NA	NA	NA	NA	NA	NA	NA	NA	NA	NA	NA
Alcohol user	3	0	33.3	7.00	7	NA	NA	NA	33.3	20.0	5	NA	NA	NA
Marijuana user	7	2	28.6	1.86	4	0.0	.00	0	57.1	4.57	3	50.0	1.00	0
Polydrug user	19	8	31.6	3.68	22	37.5	.50	1	42.1	10.84	19	87.5	15.00	11

| | | | Illegal services | | | | | | Public disorder | | | | | |
| | | | No mental health problem | | | Mental health problem | | | No mental health problem | | | Mental health problem | | |
1983	N No MH problem 1400	N MH problem 86	Prevalence	Offending rate	Percent of total	Prevalence	Offending rate	Percent of total	Prevalence	Offending rate	Percent of total	Prevalence	Offending rate	Percent of total
Nondelinquent														
Nonuser	267	13	0.0	.00	0	0.0	.00	0	9.4	.23	1	7.7	.15	0
Alcohol user	573	18	0.2	.00	0	0.0	.00	0	38.6	2.54	13	55.6	2.61	0
Marijuana user	176	7	1.7	.03	0	0.0	.00	0	54.5	3.35	5	42.9	22.57	1
Polydrug user	81	4	3.7	.06	0	0.0	.00	0	67.9	8.21	6	75.0	76.50	3
Exploratory delinquent														
Nonuser	8	1	0.0	.00	0	0.0	.00	0	50.0	2.00	0	100.0	3.00	0
Alcohol user	60	6	1.7	.07	0	0.0	.00	0	81.7	7.02	4	83.3	4.67	0
Marijuana user	34	3	32.4	1.09	1	0.0	.00	0	82.4	10.79	3	33.3	3.33	0
Polydrug user	44	7	40.9	1.61	1	28.6	2.00	0	93.2	15.64	6	85.7	12.57	1
Nonserious delinquent														
Nonuser	7	0	28.6	43.14	6	NA	NA	NA	71.4	5.00	0	NA	NA	NA
Alcohol user	35	3	0.0	.00	0	0.0	.00	0	80.0	25.40	8	100.0	33.33	1
Marijuana user	28	7	60.7	7.00	4	42.9	5.28	1	85.7	21.25	5	85.7	29.71	2
Polydrug user	58	7	56.9	24.07	26	85.7	76.14	10	91.4	47.21	25	85.7	13.29	1
Serious Delinquent														
Nonuser	0	0	NA	NA	NA	NA	NA	NA	NA	NA	NA	NA	NA	NA
Alcohol user	3	0	0.0	.00	0	NA	NA	NA	100.0	26.33	1	NA	NA	NA
Marijuana user	7	2	42.9	4.86	1	50.0	4.50	0	100.0	12.43	1	50.0	6.50	0
Polydrug user	19	8	57.9	140.21	49	87.5	14.13	2	84.2	51.74	9	100.0	48.88	4

TABLE C.3. *Continued*

1983	N No MH problem 1400	N MH problem 86	Vandalism						General delinquency					
			No mental health problem			Mental health problem			No mental health problem			Mental health problem		
			Preva- lence	Offend- ing rate	Percent of total	Preva- lence	Offend- ing rate	Percent of total	Preva- lence	Offend- ing rate	Percent of total	Preva- lence	Offend- ing rate	Percent of total
Nondelinquent														
Nonuser	267	13	0.7	.03	2	0.0	.00	0	11.2	.18	0	30.8	.46	0
Alcohol user	573	18	2.1	.04	6	0.0	.00	0	22.0	.39	1	22.2	.33	0
Marijuana user	176	7	2.3	.02	1	28.6	.29	1	31.3	.56	1	14.3	.29	0
Polydrug user	81	4	2.5	.03	1	0.0	.00	0	40.7	.74	0	25.0	.50	0
Exploratory delinquent														
Nonuser	8	1	12.5	.13	0	0.0	.00	0	100.0	5.25	0	100.0	1.00	0
Alcohol user	60	6	15.0	.35	6	16.7	.33	1	100.0	5.52	2	100.0	3.33	0
Marijuana user	34	3	14.7	.24	2	0.0	.00	0	100.0	5.68	1	100.0	4.33	0
Polydrug user	44	7	13.6	.41	5	0.0	.00	0	100.0	6.77	2	100.0	5.57	0
Nonserious delinquent														
Nonuser	7	0	28.6	.57	1	NA	NA	NA	100.0	83.00	3	NA	NA	NA
Alcohol user	35	3	11.4	.26	2	0.0	.00	0	100.0	73.03	14	100.0	32.67	1
Marijuana user	28	7	17.9	.39	3	14.3	.43	1	100.0	52.25	8	100.0	73.57	3
Polydrug user	58	7	31.0	.84	13	42.9	1.00	2	100.0	69.00	22	100.0	188.29	7
Serious Delinquent														
Nonuser	0	0	NA	NA	NA	NA	NA	NA	NA	NA	NA	NA	NA	NA
Alcohol user	3	0	33.3	20.00	16	NA	NA	NA	100.0	35.00	1	NA	NA	NA
Marijuana user	7	2	57.1	4.86	9	0.0	.00	0	100.0	36.71	1	100.0	15.00	0
Polydrug user	19	8	57.9	4.26	22	50.0	2.38	5	100.0	256.53	27	100.0	77.88	3

	N No MH problem 1400	N MH problem 86	No mental health problem			Mental health problem		
1983			Prevalence	Offending rate	Percent of total	Prevalence	Offending rate	Percent of total
Nondelinquent								
Nonuser	267	13	41.9	.82	0	46.2	.92	0
Alcohol user	573	18	100.0	51.57	34	100.0	65.50	1
Marijuana user	176	7	97.7	63.59	13	100.0	57.71	5
Polydrug user	81	4	98.8	83.63	8	100.0	102.50	0
Exploratory delinquent								
Nonuser	8	1	75.0	1.25	0	100.0	3.00	0
Alcohol user	60	6	100.0	64.07	4	100.0	108.17	1
Marijuana user	34	3	97.1	103.12	4	100.0	18.67	0
Polydrug user	44	7	97.7	113.93	6	100.0	137.71	1
Nonserious delinquent								
Nonuser	7	0	42.9	.86	0	NA	NA	NA
Alcohol user	35	3	100.0	89.34	4	100.0	83.33	0
Marijuana user	28	7	100.0	105.18	3	100.0	108.29	1
Polydrug user	58	7	98.3	135.47	9	100.0	117.71	1
Serious delinquent								
Nonuser	0	0	NA	NA	NA	NA	NA	NA
Alcohol user	3	0	100.0	189.67	1	NA	NA	NA
Marijuana user	7	2	100.0	75.71	1	50.0	2.50	0
Polydrug user	19	8	100.0	214.89	5	100.0	129.88	1

TABLE C.3. Continued

1983	N No MH problem 1400	N MH problem 86	Marijuana use						Polydrug use					
			No mental health problem			Mental health problem			No mental health problem			Mental health problem		
			Preva-lence	Offend-ing rate	Percent of total	Preva-lence	Offend-ing rate	Percent of total	Preva-lence	Offend-ing rate	Percent of total	Preva-lence	Offend-ing rate	Percent of total
Nondelinquent														
Nonuser	267	13	5.2	.09	0	7.7	.08	0	1.1	.02	0	0.0	.00	0
Alcohol user	573	18	20.2	.36	0	33.3	.67	0	3.8	.06	0	5.6	.06	0
Marijuana user	176	7	100.0	66.89	24	100.0	87.57	1	19.3	.36	1	14.3	.43	0
Polydrug user	81	4	86.4	73.68	12	100.0	266.75	2	100.0	25.88	17	100.0	228.50	7
Exploratory delinquent														
Nonuser	8	1	12.5	.25	0	100.0	1.00	0	0.0	.00	0	0.0	.00	0
Alcohol user	60	6	35.0	.70	0	50.0	1.67	0	8.3	.18	0	16.7	.33	0
Marijuana user	34	3	100.0	44.29	3	100.0	125.67	1	14.7	.29	0	0.0	.00	0
Polydrug user	44	7	88.6	72.02	6	100.0	163.57	2	100.0	37.50	13	100.0	48.86	3
Nonserious delinquent														
Nonuser	7	0	0.0	.00	0	NA	NA	NA	0.0	.00	0	NA	NA	NA
Alcohol user	35	3	22.9	.49	0	0.0	.00	0	5.7	.06	0	0.0	.00	0
Marijuana user	28	7	100.0	106.96	6	100.0	108.14	2	35.7	.61	0	14.3	.29	0
Polydrug user	58	7	94.8	195.50	23	100.0	205.71	3	100.0	45.28	21	100.0	85.14	5
Serious Delinquent														
Nonuser	0	0	NA	NA	NA	NA	NA	NA	NA	NA	NA	NA	NA	NA
Alcohol user	3	0	66.7	1.33	0	NA	NA	NA	0.0	.00	0	NA	NA	NA
Marijuana user	7	2	100.0	113.14	2	100.0	5.00	0	28.6	.57	0	50.0	1.00	0
Polydrug user	19	8	89.5	233.21	9	100.0	149.50	2	100.0	187.95	29	100.0	46.63	3

1983	N No MH problem 1400	N MH problem 86	Problem substance use			
			No mental health problem		Mental health problem	
			Prevalence	Mean scale score	Prevalence	Mean scale score
Nondelinquent						
Nonuser	267	13	0.0	2.49	0.0	2.69
Alcohol user	573	18	1.9	6.79	0.0	7.90
Marijuana user	176	7	8.0	12.19	0.0	11.32
Polydrug user	81	4	12.3	16.33	25.0	19.69
Exploratory delinquent						
Nonuser	8	1	12.5	5.16	0.0	13.75
Alcohol user	60	6	8.3	8.53	40.0	14.40
Marijuana user	34	3	14.7	12.92	0.0	11.25
Polydrug user	44	7	13.6	17.48	28.6	20.04
Nonserious delinquent						
Nonuser	7	0	0.0	2.68	NA	NA
Alcohol user	35	3	11.4	7.86	0.0	7.00
Marijuana user	28	7	17.9	14.87	42.9	16.39
Polydrug user	58	7	37.9	19.38	57.1	26.79
Serious delinquent						
Nonuser	0	0	NA	NA	NA	NA
Alcohol user	3	0	33.3	11.50	NA	NA
Marijuana user	7	2	42.9	17.46	50.0	17.50
Polydrug user	19	8	42.1	25.09	50.0	26.59

TABLE C.3. *Continued*

1983	N No MH problem 1400	N MH problem 86	Mental health problems (Sick labeling—family)				Depression					
			No mental health problem		Mental health problem		No mental health problem			Mental health problem		
			Prevalence	Mean scale score	Prevalence	Mean scale score	Prevalence	Mean symptoms	Percent of total	Prevalence	Mean symptoms	Percent of total
Nondelinquent												
Nonuser	267	13	0.0	7.38	100.0	14.77	19.1	.46	12	61.5	1.46	2
Alcohol user	573	18	0.0	7.40	100.0	14.41	23.4	.59	32	66.7	2.78	5
Marijuana user	176	7	0.0	7.76	100.0	14.57	23.3	.58	10	71.4	2.57	2
Polydrug user	81	4	0.0	8.14	100.0	13.50	37.0	1.14	9	50.0	2.50	1
Exploratory delinquent												
Nonuser	8	1	0.0	7.88	100.0	15.00	12.5	.38	0	100.0	4.00	0
Alcohol user	60	6	0.0	7.45	100.0	14.50	26.7	.77	4	66.7	2.17	1
Marijuana user	34	3	0.0	8.12	100.0	14.33	26.5	.76	2	66.7	2.00	1
Polydrug user	44	7	0.0	8.50	100.0	14.57	38.6	.91	4	71.4	2.00	1
Nonserious delinquent												
Nonuser	7	0	0.0	7.86	NA	NA	14.3	.29	0	NA	NA	NA
Alcohol user	35	3	0.0	7.78	100.0	14.33	26.8	.77	3	0.0	.00	0
Marijuana user	28	7	0.0	8.54	100.0	15.71	28.6	.71	2	42.9	1.57	1
Polydrug user	58	7	0.0	8.31	100.0	14.43	32.8	.76	4	57.1	2.86	2
Serious Delinquent												
Nonuser	0	0	NA	NA	NA	NA	NA	NA	NA	NA	NA	NA
Alcohol user	3	0	0.0	7.67	NA	NA	0.0	.00	0	NA	NA	NA
Marijuana user	7	2	0.0	8.43	100.0	16.50	0.0	.00	0	100.0	2.50	0
Polydrug user	19	8	0.0	10.96	100.0	14.38	36.8	1.21	2	50.0	1.63	1

1983	N No MH problem 1400	N MH problem 86	Mental health service use (annual)						DUI drugs/alcohol					
			No mental health problem			Mental health problem			No mental health problem			Mental health problem		
			Prevalence	Rate	Percent of total	Prevalence	Rate	Percent of total	Prevalence	Offending rate	Percent of total	Prevalence	Offending rate	Percent of total
Nondelinquent														
Nonuser	267	13	7.1	.35	8	7.7	.45	0	2.2	.67	0	0.0	.00	0
Alcohol user	573	18	4.4	.66	31	38.9	3.40	4	39.5	2.95	5	16.7	.17	0
Marijuana user	176	7	8.0	.68	10	57.1	24.17	12	59.0	25.79	18	50.0	17.17	0
Polydrug user	81	4	9.9	1.82	11	25.0	5.00	2	96.0	47.44	11	66.7	10.00	0
Exploratory delinquent														
Nonuser	8	1	12.5	.25	0	100.0	2.00	0	0.0	.00	0	NA	NA	NA
Alcohol user	60	6	5.0	.27	1	16.7	.67	0	50.0	3.58	1	50.0	7.50	0
Marijuana user	34	3	2.9	.03	0	0.0	.00	0	64.3	12.43	2	0.0	.00	0
Polydrug user	44	7	4.5	.81	3	14.3	2.50	1	71.6	46.64	6	100.0	50.00	1
Nonserious delinquent														
Nonuser	7	0	14.3	3.86	2	NA	NA	NA	16.7	.33	0	NA	NA	NA
Alcohol user	35	3	5.7	.20	1	0.0	.00	0	50.0	11.37	2	66.7	9.33	0
Marijuana user	28	7	10.7	.48	1	42.9	2.40	1	88.9	47.72	4	42.9	24.71	1
Polydrug user	58	7	12.1	.55	2	57.1	14.00	7	91.3	150.41	33	83.3	32.17	1
Serious Delinquent														
Nonuser	0	0	NA	NA	NA	NA	NA	NA	NA	NA	NA	NA	NA	NA
Alcohol user	3	0	0.0	.00	0	NA	NA	NA	0.0	.00	0	NA	NA	NA
Marijuana user	7	2	0.0	.00	0	0.0	.00	0	50.0	4.50	0	0.0	.00	0
Polydrug user	19	8	15.8	.71	1	12.5	.14	0	82.4	150.76	12	87.5	62.63	2

Appendix D
Annual Transition Matrices for Problem Behavior Types

TABLE D.1. Annual transition matrices for self-reported delinquency types. 1976–1983.

1976–1977	(1)	(2)	(3)	(4)	1977–1978	(1)	(2)	(3)	(4)
(1) Nonoffender	.81	.12	.06	.01	(1)	.82	.11	.06	.02
(2) Exploratory	.46	.31	.15	.08	(2)	.51	.26	.16	.07
(3) Nonserious	.29	.27	.33	.11	(3)	.38	.31	.23	.09
(4) Serious	.22	.18	.25	.35	(4)	.33	.12	.28	.27

1978–1979	(1)	(2)	(3)	(4)	1979–1980	(1)	(2)	(3)	(4)
(1)Nonoffender	.84	.10	.04	.02	(1)	.88	.07	.04	.00
(2) Exploratory	.45	.34	.16	.05	(2)	.47	.31	.17	.05
(3) Nonserious	.33	.26	.33	.09	(3)	.30	.24	.39	.08
(4) Serious	.14	.12	.32	.43	(4)	.14	.14	.19	.53

1980–1983	(1)	(2)	(3)	(4)	1976–1983	(1)	(2)	(3)	(4)
(1) Nonoffender	.86	.09	.06	.00	(1)	.83	.08	.07	.01
(2) Exploratory	.69	.14	.14	.03	(2)	.72	.12	.11	.05
(3) Nonserious	.49	.20	.26	.05	(3)	.67	.19	.12	.02
(4) Serious	.33	.19	.19	.28	(4)	.54	.16	.21	.10

TABLE D.2. Annual transition matrices for drug user types. 1976–1983.

1976–1977	(1)	(2)	(3)	(4)	1977–1978	(1)	(2)	(3)	(4)
(1) Nonuser	.70	.23	.06	.01	(1)	.75	.17	.07	.02
(2) Alcohol	.12	.59	.25	.04	(2)	.15	.60	.22	.03
(3) Marijuana	.13	.11	.56	.20	(3)	.05	.17	.63	.14
(4) Polydrug	.07	.11	.26	.56	(4)	.05	.05	.27	.63

1978–1979	(1)	(2)	(3)	(4)	1979–1980	(1)	(2)	(3)	(4)
(1) Nonuser	.75	.16	.06	.02	(1)	.67	.24	.08	.01
(2) Alcohol	.21	.58	.17	.03	(2)	.10	.72	.15	.03
(3) Marijuana	.09	.14	.55	.22	(3)	.04	.19	.60	.17
(4) Polydrug	.02	.03	.15	.80	(4)	.02	.07	.19	.72

1980–1983	(1)	(2)	(3)	(4)	1976–1983	(1)	(2)	(3)	(4)
(1) Nonuser	.47	.43	.08	.03	(1)	.24	.49	.16	.12
(2) Alcohol	.11	.71	.12	.07	(2)	.11	.53	.21	.16
(3) Marijuana	.07	.34	.33	.27	(3)	.06	.29	.22	.44
(4) Polydrug	.03	.15	.31	.51	(4)	.07	.30	.33	.30

TABLE D.3. Annual transition matrices for mental health problem types, 1976–1983.

1976–1977	(1)	(2)	1977–1978	(1)	(2)
(1) Nonproblem	.96	.04	(1)	.96	.04
(2) Problem	.62	.38	(2)	.63	.37

1978–1979	(1)	(2)	1979–1980	(1)	(2)
(1) Nonproblem	.96	.04	(1)	.97	.03
(2) Problem	.60	.40	(2)	.60	.40

1980–1983	(1)	(2)	1976–1983	(1)	(2)
(1) Nonproblem	.96	.04	(1)	.95	.05
(2) Problem	.64	.36	(2)	.84	.16

Author Index

Subject Index